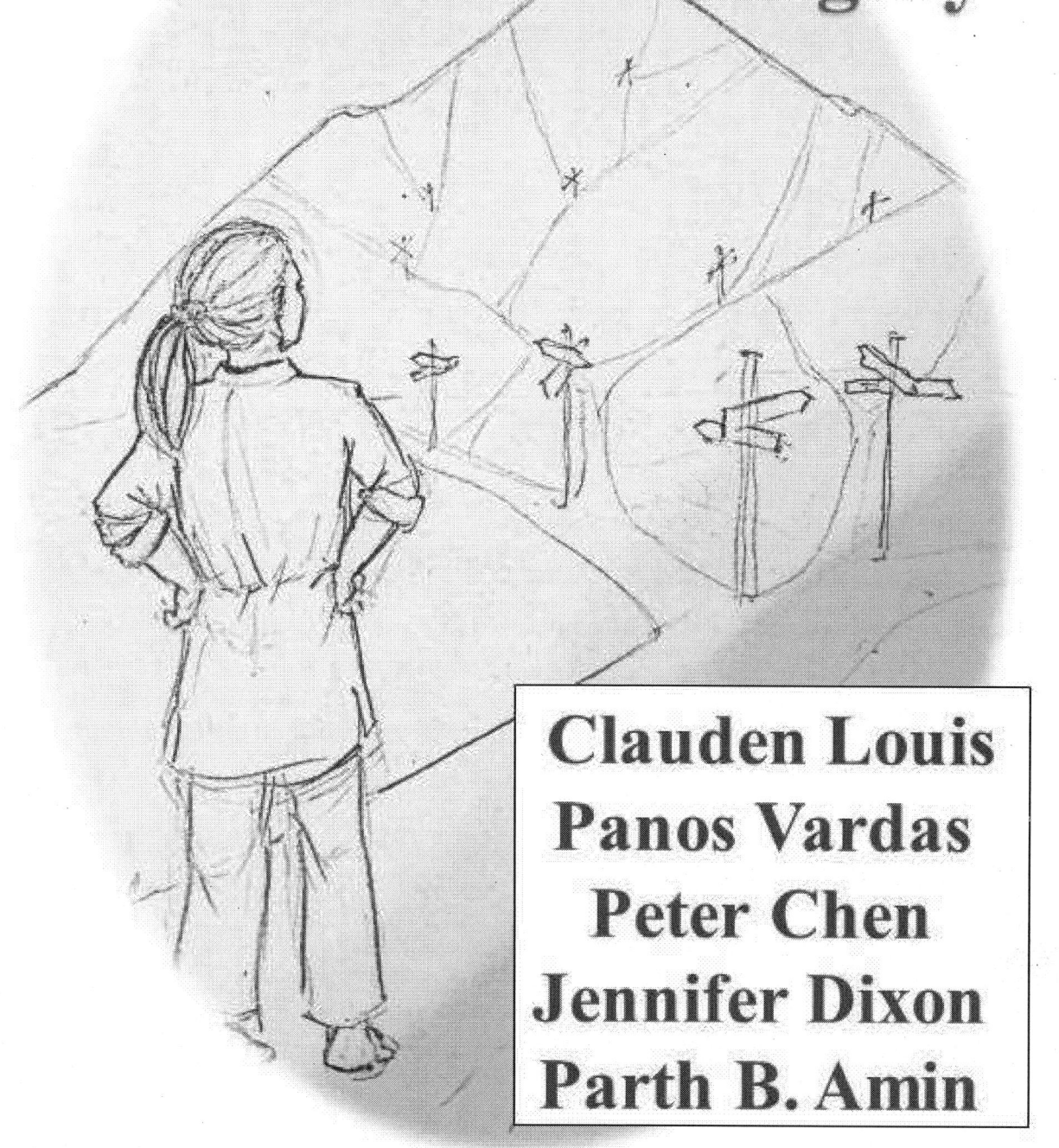

TSRA Decision Algorithms in Cardiothoracic Surgery

Clauden Louis
Panos Vardas
Peter Chen
Jennifer Dixon
Parth B. Amin

TSRA Decision Algorithms in Cardiothoracic Surgery

Clauden Louis MD, MS Projects Chair TSRA 2019 – 2020

Integrated Cardiothoracic Resident, University of Rochester; Rochester, NY

Editor

Panos Vardas MD, Vice President TSRA 2017 – 2018

Assistant Professor Cardiothoracic Surgery, University of Alabama; Birmingham, AL

Cardiac section editor

Peter Chen MD, President TSRA 2018 – 2019

Congenital Cardiac Surgery Fellow, University of Pennsylvania; Philadelphia, PA

Congenital section editor

Jennifer Dixon MD, TSRA 2018 – 2019

Attending Thoracic Surgeon, St. Charles Healthcare; Bend, OR

Thoracic section editor

Parth Amin MD, TRSA 2013-2015

Clinical Assistant Professor Cardiothoracic and Vascular Surgery Western Michigan University

Bronson Methodist Hospital

Kalamazoo, MI

Senior Editor

Thoracic Surgery Residents Association

www.tsranet.org

Copyright © 2019 by the Thoracic Surgery Residents Association

Clauden Louis, Panos Vardas, Peter Chen, Jennifer Dixon, Parth B. Amin

TSRA / TSDA

633 N. Saint Clair Street

Suite 2320

Chicago, IL 60611

www.tsranet.org

All rights reserved. This book is protected by copyright. No part of this book may be reproduced in any form or by any means, electronic or mechanical, including photocopying or the use of any information storage and retrieval system without written permission from the copyright owners.

Disclaimer

TSRA resources are provided as a basic guideline for the study of cardiothoracic surgery and should be used in conjunction with a variety of other educational references and resources. TSRA resources should not be construed as definitive study guides for either the TSDA In-Training Exam or the ABTS Part I (Written) and Part II (Oral) Certification Exams. TSRA makes no claims regarding the study guide's value in preparing for, or its contribution toward performance on, either the TSDA In-Training Exam or the ABTS Certification Exams. TSRA resources are educational tools only and any medical decisions should be made only after discussions with appropriate healthcare providers.

Foreword

The Thoracic Surgery Directors Association (TSDA) and the Thoracic Surgery Residents Association (TSRA) have a clear and sustained commitment to education. The previous textbooks created under the auspices of these two organizations are among the most dense, most affordable, and most practical manuscripts we have come across. It is our hope to provide this addition to the growing TSDA/TSRA library under the same tradition.

Although medicine and surgery is ever changing, many of the basic principles remain the same: *Primum non nocere*. Cardiothoracic surgery surgeons are in a unique role in that what we do to cure, by its very nature a form of harm. It is our burden to stratify risks, convey them to patients, all the while realizing the limitations that exist in what can possibly be done.

We have limitations in that guidelines are often based on "expert" opinion, many randomized trials are small and from single institutions and institutional biases vary across the country. Nevertheless, there are basic frameworks that are shared. Our goal with this nearly four-year project was to come up with a compendium of about 100 algorithms from common problems that could be used by those taking care of cardiothoracic patients.

We would like to thank the numerous TSRA contributors along with the corresponding national faculty for their efforts in creating this reference.

Clauden Louis
Panos Vardas
Peter Chen
Jennifer Dixon
Parth B. Amin

Acknowledgements

We would like to thank the Thoracic Surgery Directors Association (TSDA) for their support with this project and all other initiatives. We would particularly like to thank the TSRA committee members and the multiple contributors that made the creation of this book possible.

We would also like to thank both Vakhtang Tchantchaleishvili MD and Justin Watson MD for their contributions and involvement with the manuscript.

"Special thanks to the yED Graph Editor software by yWorks "the diagramming company" for its high-quality diagrams: https://www.yworks.com/yed"

Artwork by Fabio Sagebin MD

To my wife Silvia, my son Jalen and unborn daughter for their patience and support. To Jean and Verana for their uplift.
To my mentors, for their guidance and vision, to countless others who have served as motivators unbeknownst
Clauden Louis.

To my wife Christiana and my son Nicolas, for their infinite kindness, love and support
To my mentors, for their trust and wisdom
Panos N. Vardas

To my family. teachers and patients
Peter Chen

Many thanks to my loving family, Tryge, Aurora, and Jude, I am so lucky to be on this crazy journey with you all
To the many mentors that have inspired and taught me along the way
Thank you for allowing me to grow into the surgeon I have become
Jenn Dixon

To my teachers and my patients
Parth Amin

To all cardiothoracic surgery residents, present and future.

Contributors

Cardiopulmonary Bypass Troubleshooting
Caleb Matthews, Panos N. Vardas

Difficulty Weaning from Cardiopulmonary Bypass
Ashok Venkataraman, Anthony Perez-Tamayo

Elective evaluation for CABG
Parth Amin

ST Elevation Myocardial Infarction (STEMI)
William S. Ragalie, Clauden Louis, Peyman Banharash

Cardiogenic Shock Post STEMI
Clauden Louis, Jessica G.Y Luc, Sunil Prasad

Intraoperative management of ascending atheroma in CABG
Jared P. Beller, Leora T. Yarboro

Management of combined Coronary Artery Bypass Grafting and Carotid Endarterectomy
Sandeep Sainathan, Luigi Lagazzi

Intraoperative Decision Making for OPCAB
Michael O. Kayatta, Omar M. Lattouf

Moderate and Severe Aortic Stenosis
Gregory Pattakos, Joseph Coselli

Transcatheter Aortic Valve Replacement
Michael Kayatta, Vinod Thourani

Aortic Insufficiency
Yogesh Patel, Philip Hess

Management of Small Aortic Root
Carlo Maria Rosati, Christopher Lau

Non-cardiac Surgery and Aortic Valve Endocarditis
Parth Amin, Ryan Plichta

Indications for Surgical Intervention in Tricuspid Disease at Time of Left-Sided Disease
Rahul R. Handa,, Spencer J. Melby

Mitral regurgitation – Valve reconstruction options
Sudhan Nagarajan, Percy Boateng

Mitral regurgitation - Indications for Surgery
Sudhan Nagarajan, Percy Boateng

Mitral Stenosis
Clauden Louis, Sunil Prasad

Management of Type A Aortic Dissection
Awais Ashfaq, Howard Song

Management of Type B Aortic Dissection
Laura Seese, Christopher Sciortino

Ascending Aortic Aneurysm
Tedi Vlahu, Jeffrey Schwartz

Aortic Root Aneurysms
Kevin Graham, Joel Corvera

Descending Thoracic Aortic Aneurysms
Carlo Maria Rosati, Leonard Girardi

Extracorporeal Membrane Oxygenation
Saikus CE, Piercecchi CW, Blum JM

Left Ventricular Assist Device
Marvin Atkins, Pavin Atluri

Right Ventricular Assist Device
Awais Ashfaq, Fred Tibayan

Pump Thrombosis
J Hunter Mehaffey, Leora Yarboro

Orthotopic Heart Transplantation
Brittany A. Zwischenberger, Carmelo A. Milano

Hypertrophic Cardiomyopathy
Yuriy Dudiy, Howard Song

Cardiac Tumors
Michael Kasten and Mark Turrentine

Sternal Wound Infection
Stevan Pupovac, Frank Manetta

Penetrating Chest Trauma
Tedi Vlahu, Jason Frazier

Blunt Thoracic Trauma
Reilly D. Hobbs, Kiran H. Lagisetty

Endocarditis
Daniel J Weber, Tobias Deuse

Pericardial Disease
Makato Mori, Arnar Geirsson

Tracheal Trauma
Fatima Wilder, Sarah Minasyan

Tracheal Tumors
Fatima Wilder and Sarah Minasyan

Tracheal Stenosis
Fatima Wilder, Sarah Minasyan

Pulmonary Nodules
Stephanie G. Worrell, Andrew C. Chang

Pleural Effusion
Catherine Bixby, Kirk McMurtry

Bronchopulmonary Carcinoid
Caitlin Harrington, Brandon Tieu

Small Cell Carcinoma
Julie Stortz, Vincent Daniel

Surgical Management of Early Stage Non-Small Cell Lung Cancer
Michael A. Archer, Eric S. Lambright

Locally Advanced Lung Cancer
Barry Gibney, Michael Jaklitsch

Stage IV Lung Cancer
Daniel E. Mansour, Robert E. Merritt

Physiologic Assessment for Thoracic Surgery
Meghan Halub, Christopher Komanapalli

Superior Sulcus Tumors
Sudhan Nagarajan, Andrew Kaufman

Mediastinal Staging for Non-Small Cell Lung Cancer
Smarika Shrestha, Michael Flored Reed

Pulmonary Metastatectomy
Sudhan Nagarajan, Andrew Kaufman

Postoperative Surveillance for Lung Cancer
Syed Razi, Nestor Villamizar

Pulmonary Tuberculosis
Parth Amin

Interstitial Lung Disease
Clauden Louis, Christian Peyre

Lung Volume Reduction Surgery
Clauden Louis, Christian Peyre

Evaluation and Approach to Lung Transplant
Pauline Go, John Keech

Empyema
Catherine Bixby, Kirk McMurtry

Spontaneous Pneumothorax
Jennifer Burg, Paul Schipper

Post-pneumonectomy Bronchopleural Fistula
Justin Watson, Brandon Tieu

Chylothorax
Smarika Shrestha, Michael F. Reed

Pleural Mesothelioma
Panos Vardas, Jennifer Dixon, Parth Amin

Caustic Injury
Barry Gibney, Daniel Wiener

Esophageal Perforation
Stevan Pupovac, Paul C. Lee

Acquired Trachea-esophageal Fistula
Justin Watson, Paul Schipper

Management of Leiomyoma
Awais Ashfaq, Paul Schipper

Surgical Approach to Esophageal Cancer
Shane P. Smith, Brian Louie

Choosing Esophageal Conduit
Monisha Sudarshan, Sahar Saddoughi, Dennis Wigle

Determining resectability of Esophageal Adenocarcinoma
Michal J. Lada, Carolyn E. Jones

Post Esophagectomy Anastomotic Leak
Mark Mankins, Thomas Birdas

Gastroesophageal Reflux Disease
Robert Lyons, Jane Yanagawa

Primary Esophageal Motility Disorders
Michal J. Lada, Carolyn E. Jones

Management of Barrett's Esophagus
Michal J. Lada, Carolyn E. Jones

Hiatal Hernia
Jennifer Dixon, Parth Amin

Spontaneous Pneumomediastinum
Velu Balasubramanian, Kalpaj Parekh

Diaphragmatic Injury
Shane P. Smith, Alexander S. Farivar

Anterior Mediastinal Mass
Carlo Rosati, Kenneth Kesler

Thoracic Outlet Syndrome
Shane P. Smith, Kaj H. Johansen

Chest Wall Tumors
Panos Vardas, Jennifer Dixon

Patent Ductus Arteriosus
Awais Ashfaq, Ashok Muralidaran

Atrial Septal Defect (ASD)
Sandeep Sainathan, Carl Backer

Evaluation of Aortopulmonary window
Edo Bedzra, Lester Permut

Cor Triatriatum
Corinne Tan, Carlos Mery

Ventricular Septal Defect (VSD)
David Blitzer, John Brown

Coarctation of the Aorta
Corinne Tan, Carlos M. Mery

Tetralogy of Fallot with Pulmonary Stenosis
Kyle Riggs, Vincent Parnell

Transposition of the Great Arteries
Mahim Malik, Lester Permut

Pulmonary Atresia, Ventricular Septal Defect Major Aortopulmonary Collaterals (PA VSD MAPCAs)
Christopher Greenleaf, Ali Dodge-Khatami

Pulmonary Atresia with Intact Ventricular Septum
Christopher Greenleaf, Ali Dodge-Khatami

Neonatal Ebstein's Anomaly
W. Hampton Gray, S. Ram Kumar

Left Ventricular Outflow Tract Obstruction
Awais Ashfaq, Ashok Muralidaran

Coronary Anomalies
Corinne Tan, Carlos M. Mery

Hypoplastic Left Heart Syndrome
Peter Chen, John E. Mayer

Vascular ring and Pulmonary Artery Sling
Sudhan Nagarajan, Khanh Nguyen

Pediatric heart Failure/Heart Transplant
Joshua Rosenblum/Kirk Kanter

Interrupted Aortic Arch with VSD
Joshua Rosenblum, Kirk Kanter

Functional Single Ventricle Palliation
Bartholomew V. Simon, Michael F. Swartz, George M. Alfieris

Truncus Arteriosus
Christopher Greenleaf, Ali Dodge-Khatami

Evaluation of Complete Atrioventricular Canal Defect
Edo Bedzra, Lester Permut

Double Outlet Right Ventricle
Christopher Greenleaf, Ali Dodge-Kamati

Congenital Pulmonary Veins Anomalies
Bartholomew V. Simon, Michael F. Swartz, George M. Alfieris

Congenital Mitral Stenosis
Kyle Riggs, David LS Morales

Abbreviations

ABC, Airway, Breathing, Circulation;
Abx, antibiotics;
ACEi, angiotensin converting enzyme inhibitor;
ACT, activated clotting time;
ADA, Adenosine deaminase,
Admin, administration;
Adv, advance;
AF, atrial fibrillation;
AFP, alpha fetoprotein;
AHA/ACC, American Heart Association/American College of Cardiology
AI, Aortic Insufficiency
AICD, automated implantable cardioverter-defibrillator;
AJCC, American Joint Committee on Cancer;
ALAD, Anomalous left anterior descending artery;
ALCAPA, anomalous L coronary from
ALCA-R, Anomalous left coronary from the right sinus;
ALCx, Anomalous left circumflex artery;
Alt, alternative;
AMM, anterior mediastinal mass;
ANA, Anti-nucleic acid
Ao, Aorta;
AP, Aortopulmonary; ECG, electrocardiogram;
AR, aortic regurgitation;
ARCA-L, Anomalous right coronary from the left sinus
ARDS, Acute respiratory distress syndrome;
ARE, aortic root enlargement;
Art, arterial;
AS, Aortic stenosis;
ASA, Aspirin;
Asc, ascending;
ASD, atrial septal defect
ASO, arterial switch operation;
ATIII, antithrombin III;
AV, Aortic Valve or Atrioventricular
AVA, Aortic valve area;
AVCD, Atrioventricular canal defect;
Avg, average;
AVR, Aortic Valve Replacement;
BAL, bronchoalveolar lavage;
BAV, balloon aortic valvuloplasty;

BE, Barrett's Esophagus
bHCG, beta human chorionic gonadotropin;
BIMA, bilateral internal mammary arteries;
BiV, biventricular
BIVAD, Biventricular assist device;
BMI, Body Mass Index
BMS, Bare Metal Stent.
BP, blood pressure
BT, Blalock Taussig;
Bx, biopsy;
CABG, Coronary Artery Bypass Grafting;
CAD, coronary artery disease;
CAP, Coronary Anomalies Program.
CCB, Calcium Channel Blocker;
CEA, Carotid Endarterectomy
CF, continuous flow
CFA, Common femoral artery;
CFD, Clampless facilitating device
CF-LVAD, continuous-flow left ventricular assist device;
CHF, Congestive heart failure,
CHX/RTX, chemotherapy/radiotherapy,
CI, cardiac index;
Circ, circuit;
CKD, Chronic Kidney Disease;
CNB, core needle biopsy;
CNS, Central nervous system;
CO, cardiac output;
COPD, chronic obstructive pulmonary disorder;
CP, cardioplegia;
CPB, cardiopulmonary bypass;
CPET, cardiopulmonary exercise testing;
Cr Cl, Creatinine clearance;
CRT, cardiac resynchronization therapy;
CS, coronary sinus;
CSF, cerebrospinal fluid;
CT, Computed Tomography; Cardiothoracic; Chest Tube
CTA, Computed tomographic angiogram;
CTD, connective tissue disease;
CVA, cerebrovascular accident;
CVG, Composite Valve Graft;
CVP, Central venous pressure;
CW, Continuous Wave,

Cx, Circumflex coronary artery;
CXR, Chest X ray;
DCI, distal contractile integral;
DES, distal esophageal spasm; Drug eluting stent
Dexa, dexamethasone;
DHCA, deep hypothermic circulatory arrest;
Diff, differential;
Dist, distance;
DKS, Damus-Kaye-Stansel;
DL, distal latency;
DLCO, Diffusion capacity of lung for carbon monoxide;
DM, diabetes mellitus;
DO2, oxygen delivery;
DOE, Dyspnea on exertion
DORV, Double-outlet right ventricle;
DTA, descending thoracic aorta;
EAC, esophageal adenocarcinoma;
EBRT, External Beam Radiation Therapy
EBUS, Endobronchial ultrasound;
ECG, electrocardiogram;
ECHO, Echocardiogram;
ECMO, Extra Corporeal Membrane Oxygenation;
EF, Ejection Fraction;
EGD, Esophagogastroduodenoscopy;
EKG, electrocardiogram;
EKG, Electrocardiogram;
EMR, endoscopic mucosal resection;
EOA, effective orifice area;
EpiAo, epiaortic;
ERO, Effective regurgitant orifice
ESRD, End Stage Renal Disease;
Est, establish;
EUS, endoscopic ultrasound; PET-CT, positron emission tomography-computed tomography;
F, French;
FAST, Focused Assessment with Sonography in Trauma;
Fem, femoral;
FEV1, forced expiratory volume in 1 second;
FNA, Fine needle aspiration;
FNAB, fine needle aspiration biopsy;
Fnx, function;
GCT, germ cell tumor;

GERD, gastroesophageal reflux disease;
GFR, Glomerular filtration rate;
GOS, Great Ormond Street;
Grd, grade;
GSV, greater saphenous vein;
H&P, history and physical;
HCM, hypertrophic cardiomyopathy,
Hct, Hematocrit,
hep, heparin;
Hep2, hepatic;
HF, heart failure
HGD, high-grade dysplasia;
hr, hour;
HRCT, high-resolution computed tomography;
Ht, heart;
HTN, hypertension;
Hx, history;
IAA, interrupted aortic arch;
IABP, Intra-aortic Balloon Pump.
ICD, implantable cardioverter defibrillator;
ICH, Intracranial hemorrhage;
ICU, Intensive Care Unit;
IEOA, indexed effective orifice area;
ILD, Interstitial Lung Disease
IMA, internal mammary artery;
inc, increase;
iNO, nitric oxide;
INR, International Normalized Ratio;
INTERMACS, Interagency Registry for Mechanically Assisted Circulatory Support;
IPF, Idiopathic Pulmonary Fibrosis;
IRA, infarct-related artery;
IRP, integrated relaxation pressure; EGJ, esophagogastric junction;
IV abx, intravenous antibiotics;
IV, intravenous;
IVC, inferior vena cava;
IVFs, intravenous fluids
IVIG, intravenous immunoglobulin;
K+, potassium;
LA, Left atrium;
LAD, Left Anterior Descending artery;
LAM, lymphangioleiomyomatosis;
LBBB, left bundle branch block;

LC, left coronary;
LDH, Lactate Dehydrogenase;
LGD, low-grade dysplasia;
LIMA left internal mammary artery;
LPA, Left pulmonary artery;
LSA, Left subclavian artery;
LSVC, left superior vena cava;
LV, left ventricle;
LVAD, Left ventricular assist device;
LVEDD, Left ventricular end-diastolic dimension;
LVEF, Left Ventricular Ejection Fraction;
LVESD, Left ventricular end-systolic dimension;
LVOT, left ventricular outflow tract;
LVOTO, left ventricular outflow tract obstruction;
M, Describes metastasis;
MAP, mean arterial pressure;
mBTT, modified Blalock-Thomas-Taussig;
MCT, medium chain triglycerides;
MG, myasthenia gravis;
MI, myocardial infarction;
MLND, Mediastinal lymph node dissection
Mod, moderate
MOF, multiorgan failure;
MPA, Main pulmonary artery;
MR, Magnetic Resonance;
MRA, magnetic resonance angiogram;
MRI, Magnetic resonance imaging;
MS, mitral stenosis;
MV, mitral valve;
MVA, mitral valve area;
MVR, mitral valve surgery (repair or replacement);
N, Lymph Nodes involved;
N2,N3 – mediastinal nodal disease;
NC, noncoronary;
NDBE, non-dysplastic Barrett's Esophagus;
NO, nitric oxide;
Non ST Elevation Myocardial Infarction;
NPO, nothing by mouth;
NSAIDs, Nonsteroidal Anti-inflammatory drugs
NSCLC, non-small cell lung cancer;
NSR, normal sinus rhythm;
NSTEMI, Non-ST segment myocardial infarction;

NYHA, New York Heart Association
OHT, Orthotopic Heart Transplant
OM, obtuse marginal artery;
OMT, Optimal medical therapy;
ONCAB, on-pump coronary artery bypass grafting;
OR, Operating Room;
PA, pulmonary atresia; Pulmonary artery
PAB, pulmonary artery band;
PADP, Pulmonary artery diastolic pressure;
PAH, pulmonary arterial hypertension
PAP, pulmonary artery pressure
PAPVR, partial anomalous pulmonary venous return;
PASP, pulmonary artery systolic pressure;
PBF, pulmonary blood flow;
PCI, Percutaneous Coronary Intervention.
PCWP, pulmonary capillary wedge pressure;
PDA, patent ductus arteriosus;
PDT, photodynamic therapy;
PE, Pulmonary embolism; Pulmonary edema
PEDS, Pediatrics
PEP, panesophageal pressurization;
PET, Positron emission tomography;
PF, pleural fluid,
pfHgb, plasma free hemoglobin
PFO, patent foramen ovale;
PFT, pulmonary function testing;
PGE, prostaglandin E1;
PHTN, pulmonary hypertension
pHTN, Pulmonary Hypertension,
Pks, packs;
PLE, protein losing enteropathy;
PMBC, percutaneous mitral balloon commissurotomy.
POEM, peroral endoscopic myotomy
Porc Ao, porcelain aorta;
PPI, proton-pump inhibitor;
PPM, patient-prosthesis mismatch;
PPO, Percent Predicted Postoperative Lung Function
ppoDLCO, predicted post-operative diffusion limiting capacity of carbon monoxide;
ppoFEV1, predicted post-operative forced expiratory volume,
preop, preoperative;
Prox, proximal;
PTX, Pneumothorax;

PV, pulmonary valve;
PVR, Peripheral Vascular Resistance;
QOL, quality of life;
Qp, pulmonary flow;
Qs, systemic flow;
R0 – negative microscopic margins
R1 – positive microscopic margins,
R2 – positive macroscopic margins
RA, Rheumatoid arthritis; Right atrium
RAP, Right atrial pressure;
RC, right coronary;
RCP, regional/cerebral perfusion;
Res, reservoir;
REV, Reparation a l'etage ventriculaire.
RF, Regurgitant fraction;
RFA, radiofrequency ablation;
RIJ, Right internal jugular;
RSA – Right subclavian artery;
RT, radiation therapy; LN, lymph node;
RV, Right Ventricle; Residual volume
RVAD, Right ventricular assist device;
RVDCC, RV dependent coronary circulation;
RVH, right ventricular hypertrophy;
RVol, Regurgitant volume;
RVOT, right ventricular outflow tract;
RVOTO, right ventricular outflow tract obstruction;
RV-PA, right ventricle-pulmonary artery;
RX, medication;
SAM, systolic anterior motion.
SAVR, surgical aortic valve replacement;
SBP, Systolic Blood pressure
SBRT, stereotactic body radiation therapy
SCD, sudden cardiac death;
SCLC, small cell lung cancer;
SCT, Stair Climbing Test
SLE, systemic lupus erythematosus;
SPM, Spontaneous Pneumomediastinum;
SSV, small saphenous vein
Std, standard;
STEMI, ST Elevation Myocardial Infarction.
STM, serum tumor markers;
STS PROM, Society of Thoracic Surgeons predicted risk of mortality;

SVC, superior vena cava;
SvO2, mixed venous saturation of oxygen;
SVR, systemic vascular resistance;
SWT, Shuttle Walk Test
sys, systemic;
T, Tumor Size;
T1, first thoracic;
TA, Transannular; Tricuspid Annulus
TAH, Total artificial heart.
TAPSE, Tricuspid annular plane systolic excursion;
TAPVC, total anomalous pulmonary venous connection;
TAVR, transcatheter aortic valve replacement;
TCA, tricyclic antidepressant;
TEE, Transesophageal Echocardiography;
TEVAR, thoracic endovascular aortic repair
TF, transfemoral
TG, triglycerides;
TGA, transposition of great arteries;
ThRCRI, Thoracic Revised Cardiac Risk Index
TIA, Transient Ischemic Attacks;
TLC, total lung capacity.
TOF, Tetralogy of Fallot;
TPA, Tissue Plasminogen Activator.
TPG, trans-pulmonary gradient
TPN, total parenteral nutrition;
TR, Tricuspid Regurgitation;
TTE, Transthoracic Echocardiogram
TV, tricuspid valve;
TVR, Tricuspid Valve Repair
Tx, therapy
U/S, ultrasound,
UIP, Usual Interstitial Pneumonia,
UNOS, United Network for Organ Sharing
US, ultrasound;
VA ECMO, Veno-arterial extracorporeal membrane oxygenation;
VA, Veno-arterial;
Vac, vacuum-assisted;
VATS, video assisted thoracoscopic surgery
V-A-V, Veno-arterial-venous;
VE-CO2, minute ventilation-to-carbon dioxide output;
VEDP, Ventricular end diastolic pressure
Vel, Velocity

Ven, venous;
Vent, ventilation;
VIP- etoposide, ifosfamide, cisplatinum
VO2 max, maximum oxygen uptake;
Vol, volume;
VR, venous return;
VSD, ventricular septal defect
VT/VF, Ventricular tachycardia, ventricular fibrillation;
VV, Veno-venous;
w, with;
WU, Wood units;
Δ, change

Table of Contents
Introduction……………...………………………………..……………..………..2
- Authors 2
- Disclaimer 4
- Foreword 5
- Acknowledgements 6
- Contributors 9
- Abbreviations 17

Adult Cardiac Surgery…………..…..…………………………..……..…..…..…..31
1. Cardiopulmonary Bypass
    A. Troubleshooting CBP problems 31
    B. Approach to difficulty weaning off bypass 35
2. Coronary Disease
    A. Preoperative CABG evaluation 39
    B. Management of STEMI 40
    C. Cardiogenic shock 5 days post STEMI 44
    D. Intraoperative management of ascending atheroma in CABG 47
    E. Management of combined carotid/CABG 50
    F. Intraoperative decision-making for OPCAB 51
3. Aortic Valve
    A. Aortic stenosis 54
    B. TAVR 57
    C. Aortic regurgitation 59
    D. Small aortic root 60
    E. Non-cardiac surgery and aortic valve endocarditis 63
4. Mitral/Tricuspid
    A. TR in setting of other valvular disease 66
    B. Mitral regurgitation - Surgery
        1. Reconstruction 68
        2. Indications 71
    C. Mitral stenosis 72
5. Aorta
    A. Type A dissection 75
    B. Type B dissection 76
    C. Ascending aortic aneurysm 79
    D. Aortic root aneurysms 82
    E. Descending thoracic aorta aneurysms 85
6. Heart failure
    A. Extracorporeal Membrane Oxygenation 88

B. Left Ventricular Assist Device 92
  C. Right Ventricular Assist Device 93
  D. Pump thrombosis 94
  E. Orthotopic Heart Transplantation 95
Miscellaneous
  A. Hypertrophic Cardiomyopathy 98
  B. Cardiac tumors 100
  C. Approach to sternal wound infections 102
  D. Penetrating chest trauma 104
  E. Blunt chest trauma 108
  F. Endocarditis 109
  G. Pericardial disease 113

General Thoracic Surgery..…………...………...110
1. Trachea
    A. Tracheal trauma 114
    B. Tracheal tumors 115
    C. Tracheal stenosis 116
2. Lungs
    A. Pulmonary nodules 118
    B. Approach to pleural effusion 120
    C. Pulmonary carcinoid 121
    D. Small cell lung cancer 122
    E. Surgical Management of Early Stage Non-Small Cell Lung Cancer 123
    F. Locally Advanced Lung Cancer 124
    G. Stage IV non-small cell 125
    H. Approach to physiologic readiness for thoracic surgery 129
    I. Superior sulcus tumors 130
    J. Mediastinal Staging for Non-Small Cell Lung Cancer 131
    K. Pulmonary Metastatectomy 133
    L. Postoperative Surveillance for lung cancer 134
    M. Pulmonary Tuberculosis 135
    N. Interstitial lung disease 136
    O. Lung Volume Reduction Surgery 137
    P. Evaluation and approach to lung transplant 138
    Q. Empyema 141
    R. Spontaneous pneumothorax 142
    S. Post-pneumonectomy Bronchopleural Fistula 143
    T. Chylothorax 144
    U. Pleural Mesothelioma 145
3. Esophagus
    A. Esophageal caustic injury 146
    B. Esophageal perforation 147
    C. Acquired Trachea-esophageal Fistula 148
    D. Management of leiomyoma 149
    E. Surgical Approach to Esophageal Cancer 150
    F. Choosing esophageal conduits 151
    G. Determining resectability of esophageal cancer 152
    H. Post Esophagectomy Anastomotic Leak 153
    I. Gastroesophageal Reflux Disease 154
    J. Primary Esophageal Motility Disorders 155
    K. Management of Barrett's Esophagus 156
    L. Management of Paraesophageal Hernia 157
4. Mediastinum

  A. Spontaneous Pneumomediastinum 158
  B. Diaphragmatic injury 159
  C. Thymoma/MG/mediastinal mass 160
5. Other
  A. Thoracic outlet syndrome 162
  B. Chest wall tumors 163

Congenital Heart Surgery..164
1. Patent Ductus Arteriosus (PDA) 164
2. Atrial Septal Defect (ASD) 165
3. Aortopulmonary window (APW) 166
4. Cor triatriatum 167
5. Ventricular Septal Defect (VSD) 168
6. Coarctation of the Aorta 169
7. Tetralogy of Fallot with Pulmonary Stenosis (TOF/PS) 170
8. Transposition of Great Arteries (TGA) 171
9. Pulmonary Atresia with Ventricular Septal Defect with Multiple Aorto-pulmonary Collaterals (PA/VSD/MAPCAs) 172
10. Pulmonary Atresia with Intact Ventricular Septum (PA/IVS) 173
11. Ebstein's Anomaly 174
12. Left Ventricular Outflow Tract (LVOT) obstruction 175
13. Coronary anomalies 176
14. Hypoplastic Left Heart Syndrome (HLHS) 178
15. Vascular rings/PA slings 180
16. Pediatric Heart Failure/Transplant 181
17. Interrupted Aortic Arch with VSD (IAA/VSD) 183
18. Single Ventricle Pathway/Fontan 184
19. Truncus Arteriosus 187
20. Complete Atrioventricular (AV) Canal 189
21. Double Outlet Right Ventricle (DORV) 190
22. Congenital Pulmonary Vein Anomalies 195
23. Congenital Mitral Stenosis (MS) 196
References..197

Cardiopulmonary Bypass Troubleshooting
Caleb Matthews, Panos N. Vardas

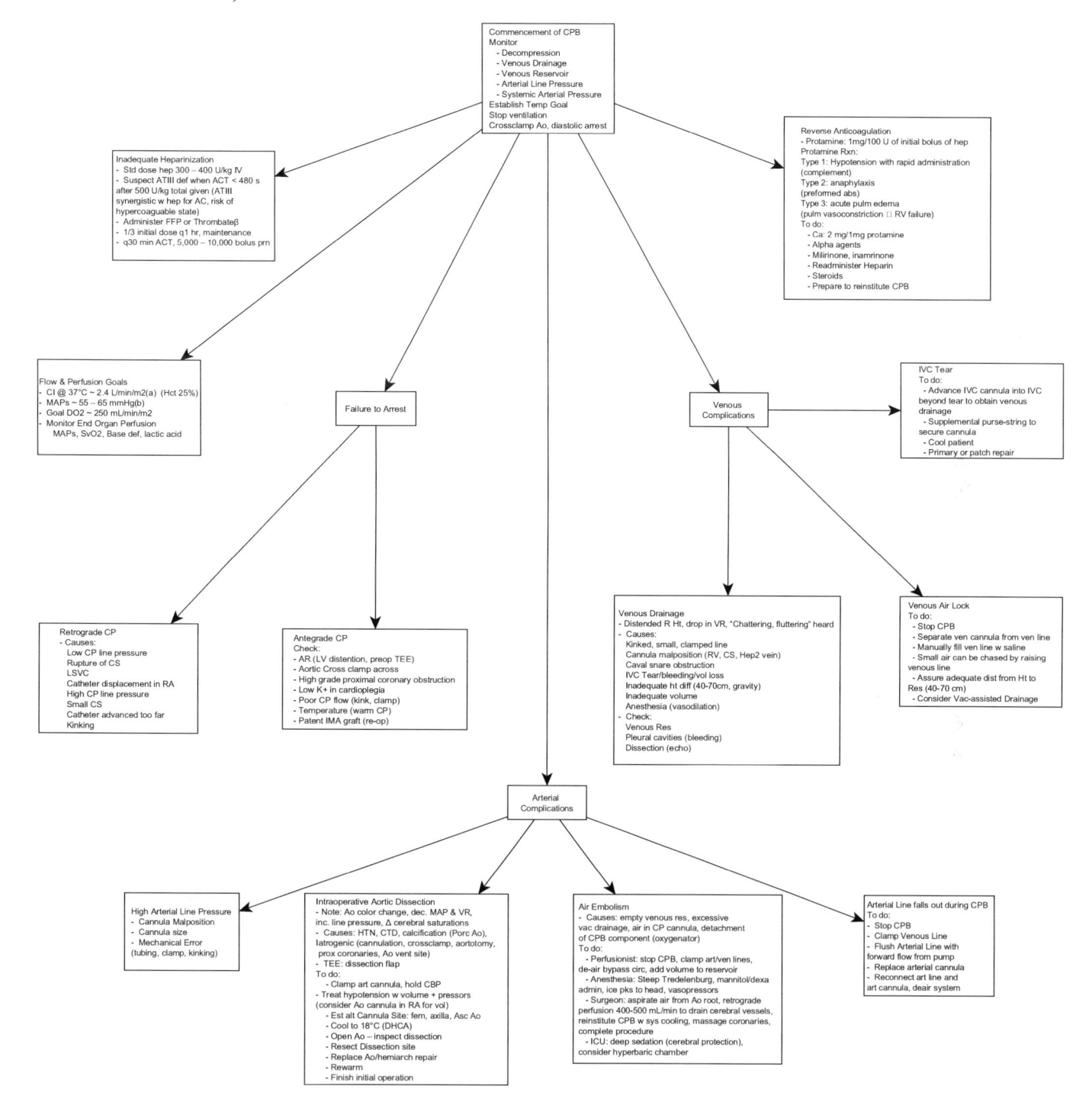

Commencement of CPB
Monitor
- Decompression
- Venous Drainage
- Venous Reservoir
- Arterial Line Pressure
- Systemic Arterial Pressure

Establish Temp Goal
Stop ventilation
Crossclamp Ao, diastolic arrest

Inadequate Heparinization
- Std dose hep 300 – 400 U/kg IV
- Suspect ATIII def when ACT < 480 s after 500 U/kg total given (ATIII synergistic w hep for AC, risk of hypercoaguable state)
- Administer FFP or Thrombateβ
- 1/3 initial dose q1 hr, maintenance
- q30 min ACT, 5,000 – 10,000 bolus prn

Reverse Anticoagulation
- Protamine: 1mg/100 U of initial bolus of hep
Protamine Rxn:
Type 1: Hypotension with rapid administration (complement)
Type 2: anaphylaxis (preformed abs)
Type 3: acute pulm edema (pulm vasoconstriction ▢ RV failure)
To do:
- Ca: 2 mg/1mg protamine
- Alpha agents
- Milrinone, inamrinone
- Readminister Heparin
- Steroids
- Prepare to reinstitute CPB

Flow & Perfusion Goals
- CI @ 37°C ~ 2.4 L/min/m2(a) (Hct 25%)
- MAPs ~ 55 – 65 mmHg(b)
- Goal DO2 ~ 250 mL/min/m2
- Monitor End Organ Perfusion
  MAPs, SvO2, Base def, lactic acid

Failure to Arrest

Venous Complications

IVC Tear
To do:
- Advance IVC cannula into IVC beyond tear to obtain venous drainage
- Supplemental purse-string to secure cannula
- Cool patient
- Primary or patch repair

Retrograde CP
- Causes:
  Low CP line pressure
  Rupture of CS
  LSVC
  Catheter displacement in RA
  High CP line pressure
  Small CS
  Catheter advanced too far
  Kinking

Antegrade CP
Check:
- AR (LV distention, preop TEE)
- Aortic Cross clamp across
- High grade proximal coronary obstruction
- Low K+ in cardioplegia
- Poor CP flow (kink, clamp)
- Temperature (warm CP)
- Patent IMA graft (re-op)

Venous Drainage
- Distended R Ht, drop in VR, "Chattering, fluttering" heard
- Causes:
  Kinked, small, clamped line
  Cannula malposition (RV, CS, Hep2 vein)
  Caval snare obstruction
  IVC Tear/bleeding/vol loss
  Inadequate ht diff (40-70cm, gravity)
  Inadequate volume
  Anesthesia (vasodilation)
- Check:
  Venous Res
  Pleural cavities (bleeding)
  Dissection (echo)

Venous Air Lock
To do:
- Stop CPB
- Separate ven cannula from ven line
- Manually fill ven line w saline
- Small air can be chased by raising venous line
- Assure adequate dist from Ht to Res (40-70 cm)
- Consider Vac-assisted Drainage

Arterial Complications

High Arterial Line Pressure
- Cannula Malposition
- Cannula size
- Mechanical Error (tubing, clamp, kinking)

Intraoperative Aortic Dissection
- Note: Ao color change, dec. MAP & VR, inc. line pressure, Δ cerebral saturations
- Causes: HTN, CTD, calcification (Porc Ao), Iatrogenic (cannulation, crossclamp, aortotomy, prox coronaries, Ao vent site)
- TEE: dissection flap
To do:
- Clamp art cannula, hold CBP
- Treat hypotension w volume + pressors (consider Ao cannula in RA for vol)
- Est alt Cannula Site: fem, axilla, Asc Ao
- Cool to 18°C (DHCA)
- Open Ao – inspect dissection
- Resect Dissection site
- Replace Ao/hemiarch repair
- Rewarm
- Finish initial operation

Air Embolism
- Causes: empty venous res, excessive vac drainage, air in CP cannula, detachment of CPB component (oxygenator)
To do:
- Perfusionist: stop CPB, clamp art/ven lines, de-air bypass circ, add volume to reservoir
- Anesthesia: Steep Tredelenburg, mannitol/dexa admin, ice pks to head, vasopressors
- Surgeon: aspirate air from Ao root, retrograde perfusion 400-500 mL/min to drain cerebral vessels, reinstitute CPB w sys cooling, massage coronaries, complete procedure
- ICU: deep sedation (cerebral protection), consider hyperbaric chamber

Arterial Line falls out during CPB
To do:
- Stop CPB
- Clamp Venous Line
- Flush Arterial Line with forward flow from pump
- Replace arterial cannula
- Reconnect art line and art cannula, deair system

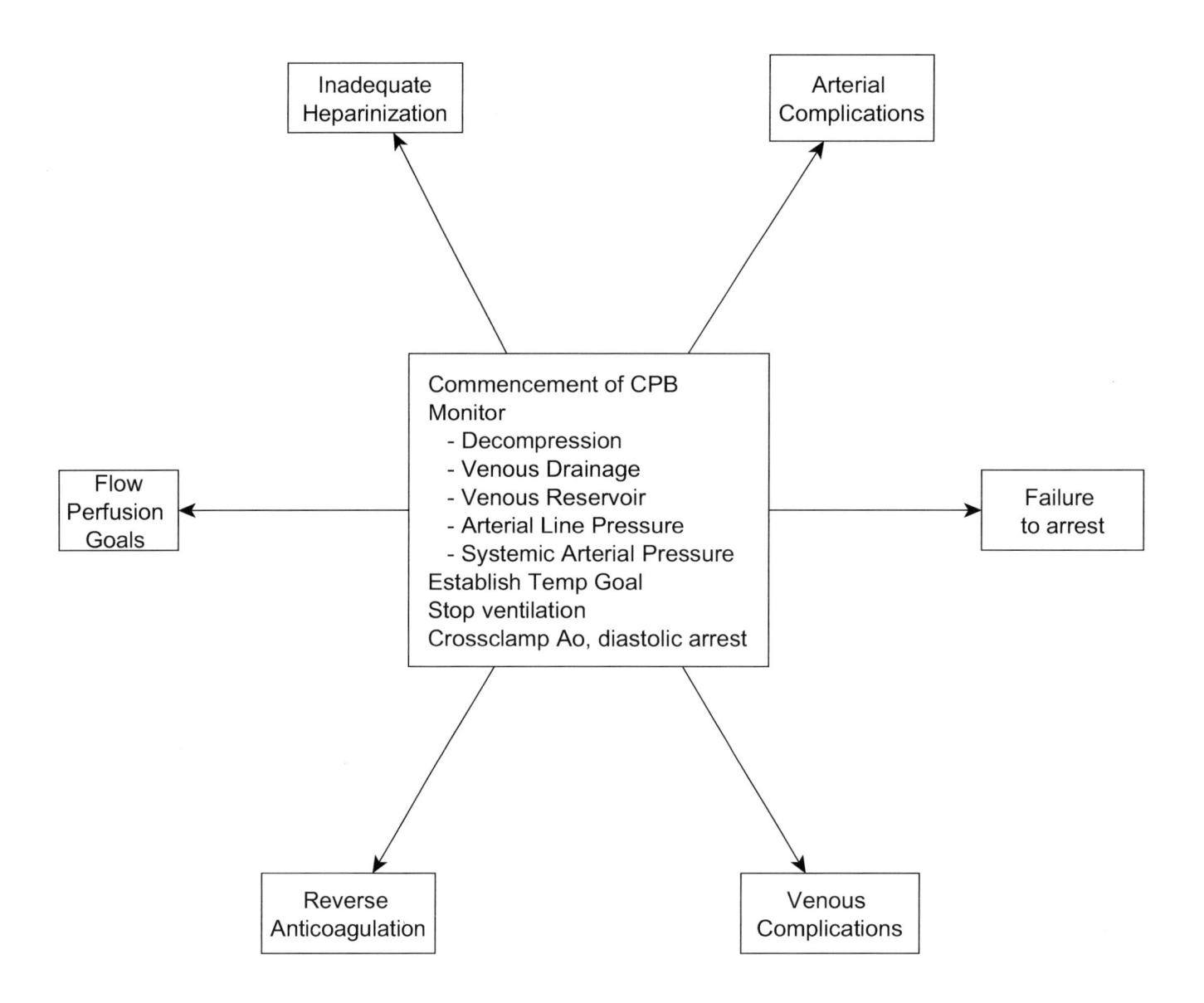

```
                    Inadequate                         Arterial
                    Heparinization                     Complications
                         ↑                                  ↑
                          \                                /
                           \                              /
                    ┌─────────────────────────────────────┐
                    │ Commencement of CPB                 │
                    │ Monitor                             │
      Flow          │    - Decompression                  │         Failure
   Perfusion   ←────│    - Venous Drainage                │────→    to arrest
     Goals          │    - Venous Reservoir               │
                    │    - Arterial Line Pressure         │
                    │    - Systemic Arterial Pressure     │
                    │ Establish Temp Goal                 │
                    │ Stop ventilation                    │
                    │ Crossclamp Ao, diastolic arrest     │
                    └─────────────────────────────────────┘
                           /                              \
                          /                                \
                         ↓                                  ↓
                    Reverse                            Venous
                    Anticoagulation                    Complications
```

Venous Complications

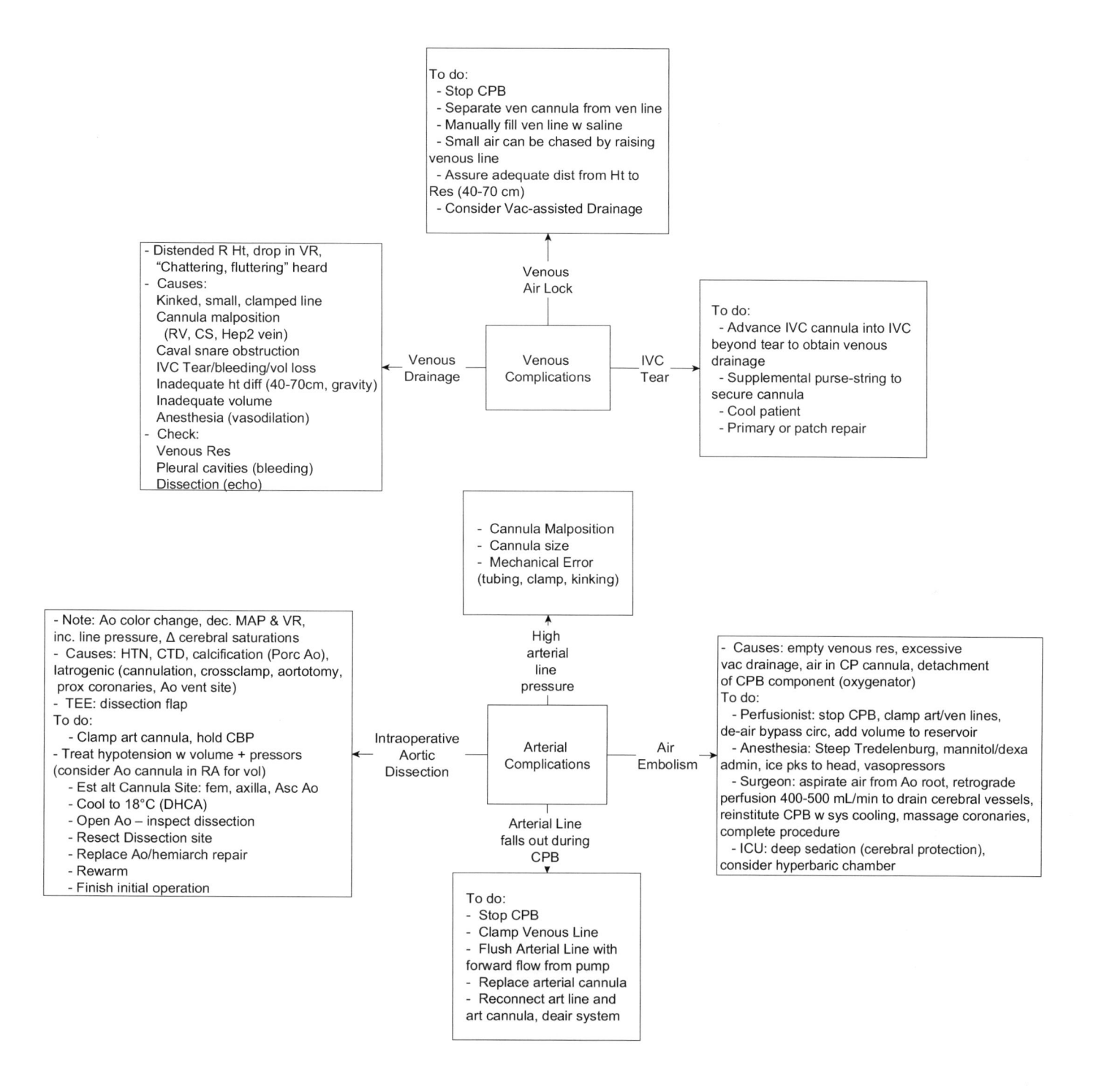

Venous Air Lock — To do:
- Stop CPB
- Separate ven cannula from ven line
- Manually fill ven line w saline
- Small air can be chased by raising venous line
- Assure adequate dist from Ht to Res (40-70 cm)
- Consider Vac-assisted Drainage

Venous Drainage:
- Distended R Ht, drop in VR, "Chattering, fluttering" heard
- Causes:
  - Kinked, small, clamped line
  - Cannula malposition (RV, CS, Hep2 vein)
  - Caval snare obstruction
  - IVC Tear/bleeding/vol loss
  - Inadequate ht diff (40-70cm, gravity)
  - Inadequate volume
  - Anesthesia (vasodilation)
- Check:
  - Venous Res
  - Pleural cavities (bleeding)
  - Dissection (echo)

IVC Tear — To do:
- Advance IVC cannula into IVC beyond tear to obtain venous drainage
- Supplemental purse-string to secure cannula
- Cool patient
- Primary or patch repair

Arterial Complications

High arterial line pressure:
- Cannula Malposition
- Cannula size
- Mechanical Error (tubing, clamp, kinking)

Intraoperative Aortic Dissection:
- Note: Ao color change, dec. MAP & VR, inc. line pressure, Δ cerebral saturations
- Causes: HTN, CTD, calcification (Porc Ao), Iatrogenic (cannulation, crossclamp, aortotomy, prox coronaries, Ao vent site)
- TEE: dissection flap
- To do:
  - Clamp art cannula, hold CBP
- Treat hypotension w volume + pressors (consider Ao cannula in RA for vol)
  - Est alt Cannula Site: fem, axilla, Asc Ao
  - Cool to 18°C (DHCA)
  - Open Ao – inspect dissection
  - Resect Dissection site
  - Replace Ao/hemiarch repair
  - Rewarm
  - Finish initial operation

Arterial Line falls out during CPB — To do:
- Stop CPB
- Clamp Venous Line
- Flush Arterial Line with forward flow from pump
- Replace arterial cannula
- Reconnect art line and art cannula, deair system

Air Embolism:
- Causes: empty venous res, excessive vac drainage, air in CP cannula, detachment of CPB component (oxygenator)
- To do:
  - Perfusionist: stop CPB, clamp art/ven lines, de-air bypass circ, add volume to reservoir
  - Anesthesia: Steep Tredelenburg, mannitol/dexa admin, ice pks to head, vasopressors
  - Surgeon: aspirate air from Ao root, retrograde perfusion 400-500 mL/min to drain cerebral vessels, reinstitute CPB w sys cooling, massage coronaries, complete procedure
  - ICU: deep sedation (cerebral protection), consider hyperbaric chamber

Flow Perfusion Goals

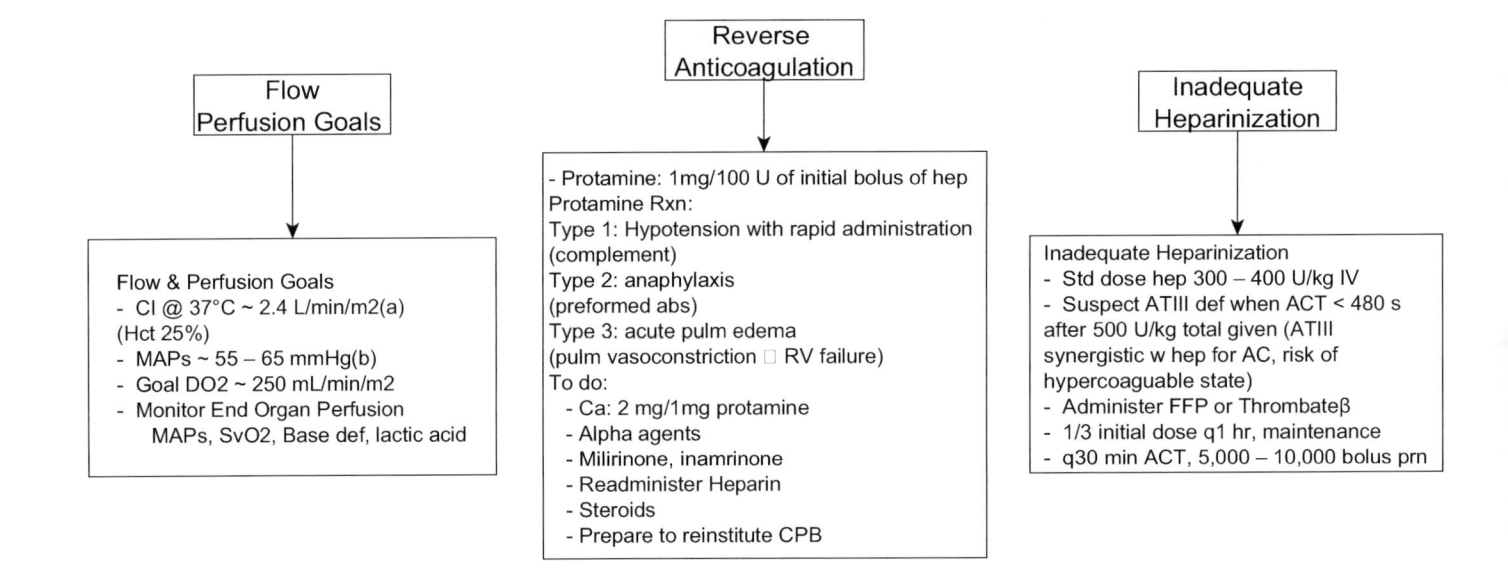

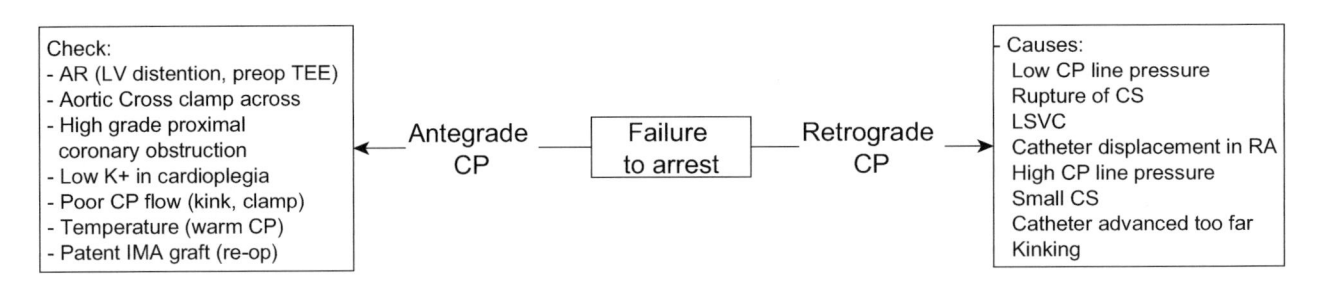

Flow & Perfusion Goals
- CI @ 37°C ~ 2.4 L/min/m2(a) (Hct 25%)
- MAPs ~ 55 – 65 mmHg(b)
- Goal DO2 ~ 250 mL/min/m2
- Monitor End Organ Perfusion
    MAPs, SvO2, Base def, lactic acid

Reverse Anticoagulation

- Protamine: 1mg/100 U of initial bolus of hep
Protamine Rxn:
Type 1: Hypotension with rapid administration (complement)
Type 2: anaphylaxis (preformed abs)
Type 3: acute pulm edema (pulm vasoconstriction → RV failure)
To do:
- Ca: 2 mg/1mg protamine
- Alpha agents
- Milirinone, inamrinone
- Readminister Heparin
- Steroids
- Prepare to reinstitute CPB

Inadequate Heparinization

Inadequate Heparinization
- Std dose hep 300 – 400 U/kg IV
- Suspect ATIII def when ACT < 480 s after 500 U/kg total given (ATIII synergistic w hep for AC, risk of hypercoaguable state)
- Administer FFP or Thrombate β
- 1/3 initial dose q1 hr, maintenance
- q30 min ACT, 5,000 – 10,000 bolus prn

Failure to arrest

Antegrade CP — Check:
- AR (LV distention, preop TEE)
- Aortic Cross clamp across
- High grade proximal coronary obstruction
- Low K+ in cardioplegia
- Poor CP flow (kink, clamp)
- Temperature (warm CP)
- Patent IMA graft (re-op)

Retrograde CP — Causes:
- Low CP line pressure
- Rupture of CS
- LSVC
- Catheter displacement in RA
- High CP line pressure
- Small CS
- Catheter advanced too far
- Kinking

[a] *Avg CI is 4.8 L/min with avg pt with BSA of 2; BSA (m^2) = [Ht (cm) x Wt (kg)/3600] x 0.5; Flow can be reduced by 7% for decrease of 1°C*

[b] *H/o HTN, carotid artery stenosis, renal disease, & elderly; higher MAP goals tolerated (65 – 75 mmHg)*

ACT, activated clotting time; admin, administration; Adv, advance; Ao, Aorta; Alt, alternative; Asc, ascending; ATIII, antithrombin III; AR, aortic regurgitation; Art, arterial; Avg, average; BP, blood pressure; CI, cardiac index; Circ; circuit; CP, cardioplegia; CPB, cardiopulmonary bypass; CS, coronary sinus; CTD, connective tissue disease; Dexa, dexamethasone; DHCA, deep hypothermic circulatory arrest; Diff, differential; Dist, distance; DO$_2$, oxygen delivery; Echo; echocardiography; EpiAo, epiaortic; Est, establish; F, French; Fem, femoral; Grd, grade; hct, hematocrit; hep, heparin; Hep^2, hepatic; ht, heart; hr, hour; HTN, hypertension; inc; increase; IV, intravenous; IVC, inferior vena cava; K+, potassium; LSVC, left superior vena cava; MAP; mean arterial pressure; Pks, packs; Porc Ao, porcelain aorta; preop, preoperative; Prox, proximal; RA, right atrium; Res, reservoir; Std, standard; SvO$_2$, mixed venous saturation of oxygen; sys, systemic; TEE; transesophageal echocardiography; US, ultrasound; Vac, vacuum-assisted; ven, venous; VR, venous return; Vol, volume; w, with; Δ, change

Difficulty Weaning from Cardiopulmonary Bypass
Ashok Venkataraman, Anthony Perez-Tamayo

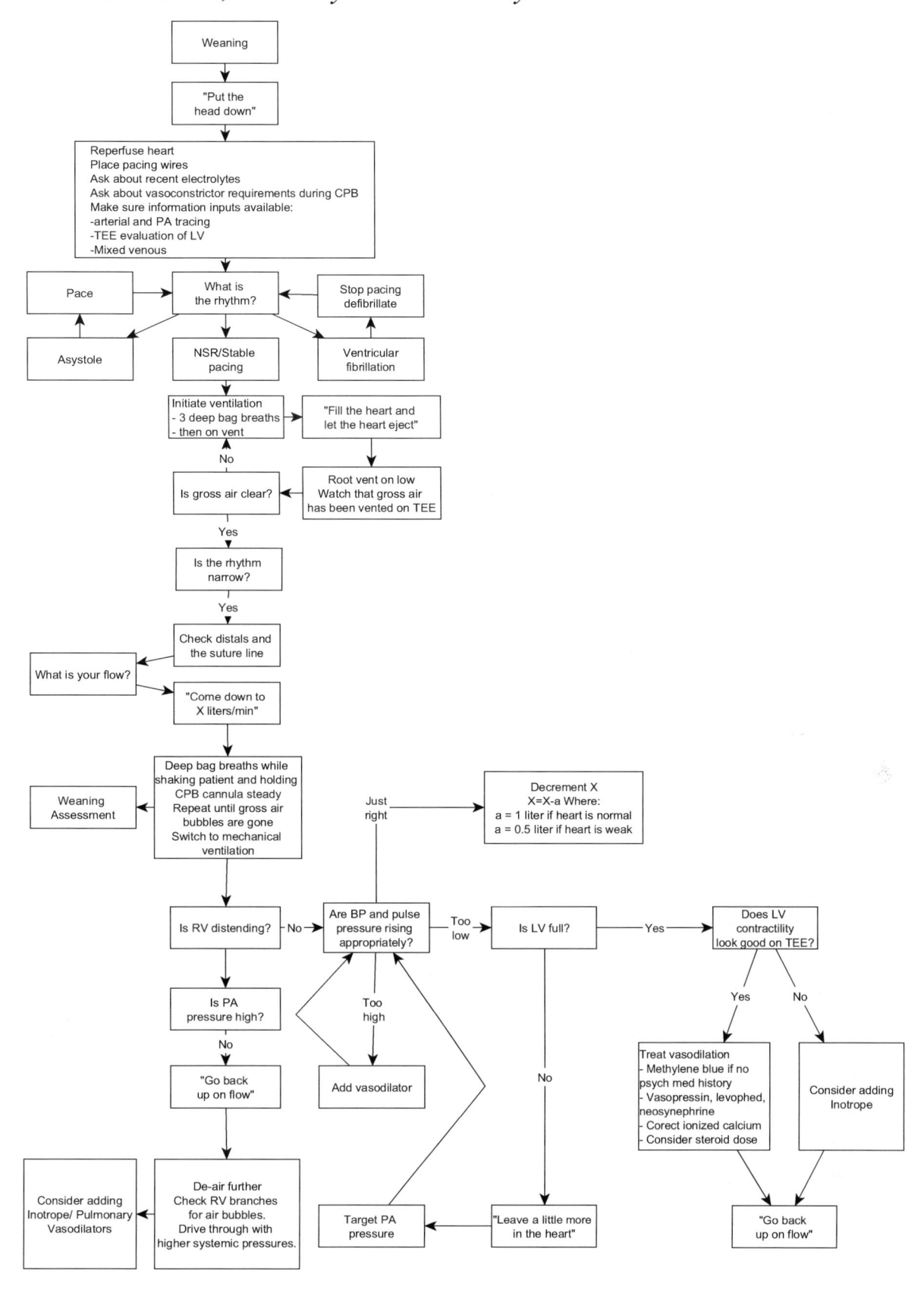

```
                    ┌─────────┐
                    │ Weaning │
                    └────┬────┘
                         ▼
                ┌──────────────┐
                │ "Put the     │
                │  head down"  │
                └──────┬───────┘
                       ▼
   ┌─────────────────────────────────────────┐
   │ Reperfuse heart                         │
   │ Place pacing wires                      │
   │ Ask about recent electrolytes           │
   │ Ask about vasoconstrictor requirements  │
   │   during CPB                            │
   │ Make sure information inputs available: │
   │  -arterial and PA tracing               │
   │  -TEE evaluation of LV                  │
   │  -Mixed venous                          │
   └─────────────────────────────────────────┘
```

- **Weaning** → "Put the head down" → Reperfuse heart, Place pacing wires, Ask about recent electrolytes, Ask about vasoconstrictor requirements during CPB, Make sure information inputs available: arterial and PA tracing, TEE evaluation of LV, Mixed venous

- **What is the rhythm?**
  - Asystole → Pace
  - Ventricular fibrillation → Stop pacing, defibrillate
  - NSR/Stable pacing → Initiate ventilation: 3 deep bag breaths, then on vent

- "Fill the heart and let the heart eject" → Root vent on low, Watch that gross air has been vented on TEE

- **Is gross air clear?**
  - No → back to root vent step
  - Yes → **Is the rhythm narrow?**
    - Yes → Check distals and the suture line → "Come down to X liters/min" (What is your flow?)

- Deep bag breaths while shaking patient and holding CPB cannula steady. Repeat until gross air bubbles are gone. Switch to mechanical ventilation. (**Weaning Assessment**)

- **Decrement X**
  - X = X − a, Where:
  - a = 1 liter if heart is normal
  - a = 0.5 liter if heart is weak

- **Is RV distending?**
  - No → **Are BP and pulse pressure rising appropriately?**
    - Just right → Decrement X
    - Too high → Add vasodilator
    - Too low → **Is LV full?**
      - Yes → **Does LV contractility look good on TEE?**
        - Yes → Treat vasodilation
          - Methylene blue if no psych med history
          - Vasopressin, levophed, neosynephrine
          - Correct ionized calcium
          - Consider steroid dose
        - No → Consider adding Inotrope
        - → "Go back up on flow"
      - No → "Leave a little more in the heart"
  - Yes → **Is PA pressure high?**
    - No → "Go back up on flow"
    - Yes → De-air further, Check RV branches for air bubbles, Drive through with higher systemic pressures → Target PA pressure
    - → Consider adding Inotrope/Pulmonary Vasodilators

35

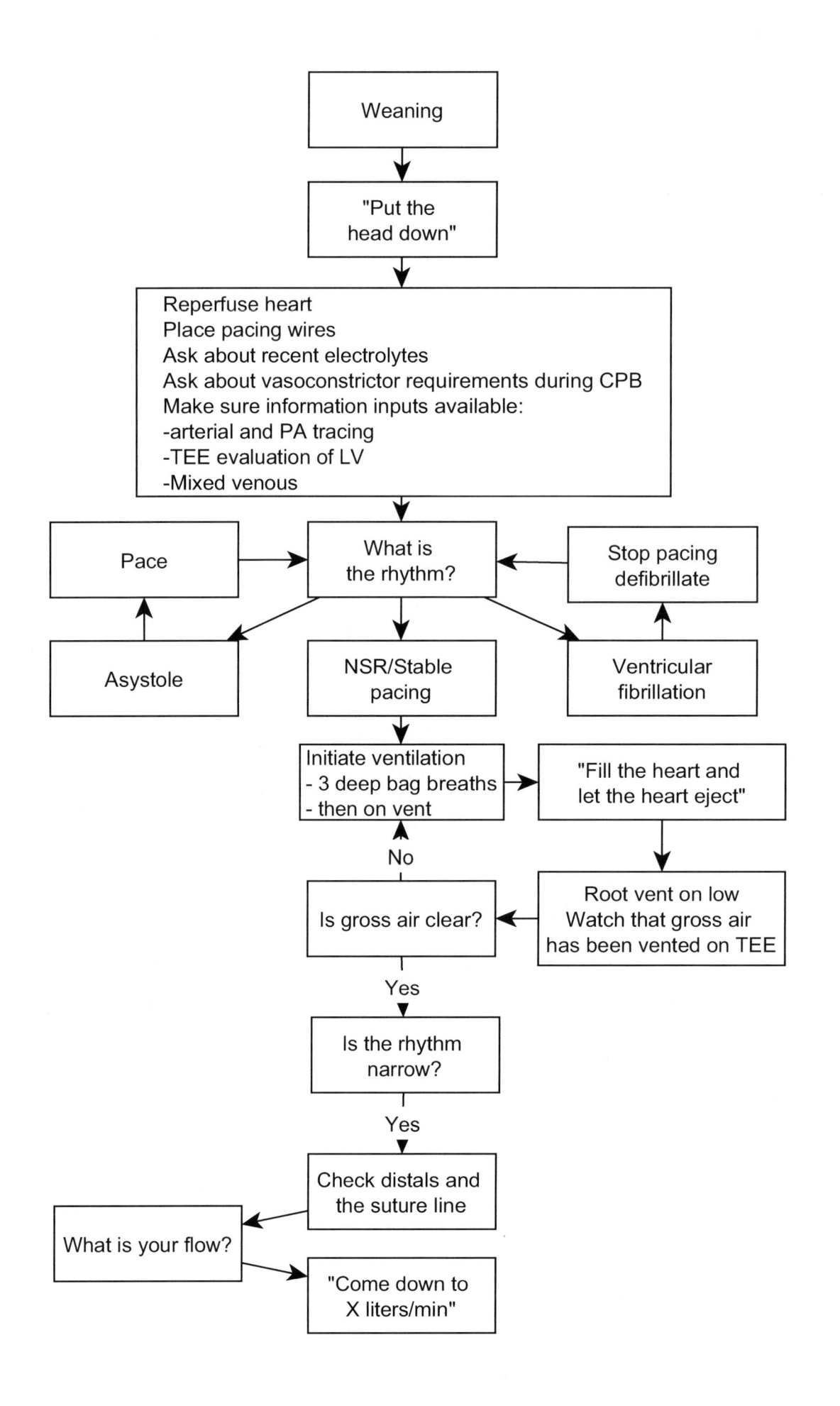

```
┌─────────────┐
│   Weaning   │
└──────┬──────┘
       ▼
┌─────────────┐
│  "Put the   │
│ head down"  │
└──────┬──────┘
       ▼
┌─────────────────────────────────────────────┐
│ Reperfuse heart                             │
│ Place pacing wires                          │
│ Ask about recent electrolytes               │
│ Ask about vasoconstrictor requirements      │
│   during CPB                                │
│ Make sure information inputs available:     │
│ -arterial and PA tracing                    │
│ -TEE evaluation of LV                       │
│ -Mixed venous                               │
└─────────────────────┬───────────────────────┘
                     ▼
```

Rhythm decision tree:

- Pace → What is the rhythm? ← Stop pacing, defibrillate
- Asystole → Pace
- What is the rhythm? → Asystole / NSR/Stable pacing / Ventricular fibrillation
- Ventricular fibrillation → Stop pacing, defibrillate

From NSR/Stable pacing:

- Initiate ventilation
  - 3 deep bag breaths
  - then on vent
- → "Fill the heart and let the heart eject"
- → Root vent on low. Watch that gross air has been vented on TEE
- → Is gross air clear?
  - No → back to Initiate ventilation
  - Yes ↓
- Is the rhythm narrow?
  - Yes ↓
- Check distals and the suture line
  - → What is your flow?
  - → "Come down to X liters/min"

36

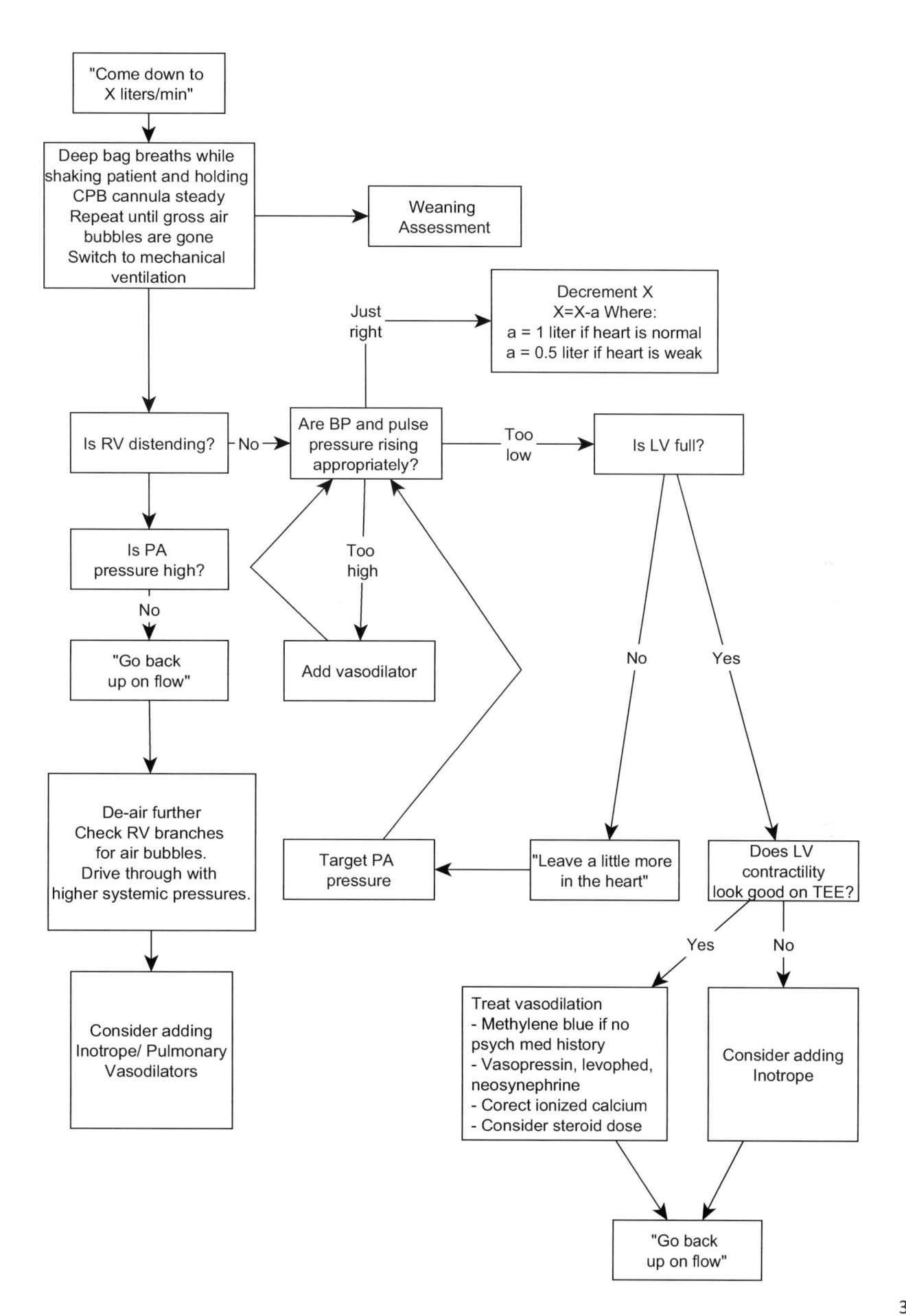

```
┌─────────────────┐
│ "Come down to   │
│  X liters/min"  │
└────────┬────────┘
         ▼
┌──────────────────────┐
│ Deep bag breaths while│      ┌──────────────┐
│ shaking patient and   │─────▶│   Weaning    │
│ holding CPB cannula   │      │  Assessment  │
│ steady. Repeat until  │      └──────────────┘
│ gross air bubbles are │
│ gone. Switch to       │
│ mechanical ventilation│
└────────┬──────────────┘
         │
         │           Just right        ┌────────────────────────────────┐
         │           ─────────────────▶│ Decrement X                    │
         │                             │ X = X − a   Where:             │
         │                             │ a = 1 liter if heart is normal │
         │                             │ a = 0.5 liter if heart is weak │
         │                             └────────────────────────────────┘
         ▼
┌────────────────┐      ┌──────────────────┐   Too low   ┌──────────────┐
│ Is RV          │─No──▶│ Are BP and pulse │────────────▶│ Is LV full?  │
│ distending?    │      │ pressure rising  │             └──────┬───────┘
└────────┬───────┘      │ appropriately?   │                    │
         │              └────────┬─────────┘                 No │ Yes
         ▼                       │ Too high
┌────────────────┐               ▼
│ Is PA          │      ┌────────────────┐
│ pressure high? │      │ Add vasodilator│
└────────┬───────┘      └────────────────┘
         │ No
         ▼
┌────────────────┐
│  "Go back      │
│  up on flow"   │
└────────┬───────┘
         │
         ▼
┌──────────────────────┐    ┌──────────────┐    ┌──────────────────┐    ┌──────────────────┐
│ De-air further       │    │  Target PA   │◀───│ "Leave a little  │    │ Does LV          │
│ Check RV branches    │    │  pressure    │    │  more in the     │    │ contractility    │
│ for air bubbles.     │    └──────────────┘    │  heart"          │    │ look good on TEE?│
│ Drive through with   │                        └──────────────────┘    └────┬────────┬────┘
│ higher systemic      │                                               Yes   │        │ No
│ pressures.           │                                                     ▼        ▼
└──────────┬───────────┘                              ┌──────────────────────┐  ┌──────────────┐
           ▼                                          │ Treat vasodilation   │  │ Consider     │
┌────────────────────┐                                │ - Methylene blue if  │  │ adding       │
│ Consider adding    │                                │   no psych med       │  │ Inotrope     │
│ Inotrope/Pulmonary │                                │   history            │  └──────┬───────┘
│ Vasodilators       │                                │ - Vasopressin,       │         │
└────────────────────┘                                │   levophed,          │         │
                                                      │   neosynephrine      │         │
                                                      │ - Corect ionized     │         │
                                                      │   calcium            │         │
                                                      │ - Consider steroid   │         │
                                                      │   dose               │         │
                                                      └──────────┬───────────┘         │
                                                                 ▼                     ▼
                                                           ┌──────────────┐
                                                           │  "Go back    │
                                                           │  up on flow" │
                                                           └──────────────┘
```

CPB, cardiopulmonary bypass; TEE, transesophageal echocardiogram; PA, pulmonary artery; LV, left ventricle; NSR, normal sinus rhythm; RV, right ventricle; BP, blood pressure

Elective evaluation for CABG
Parth Amin

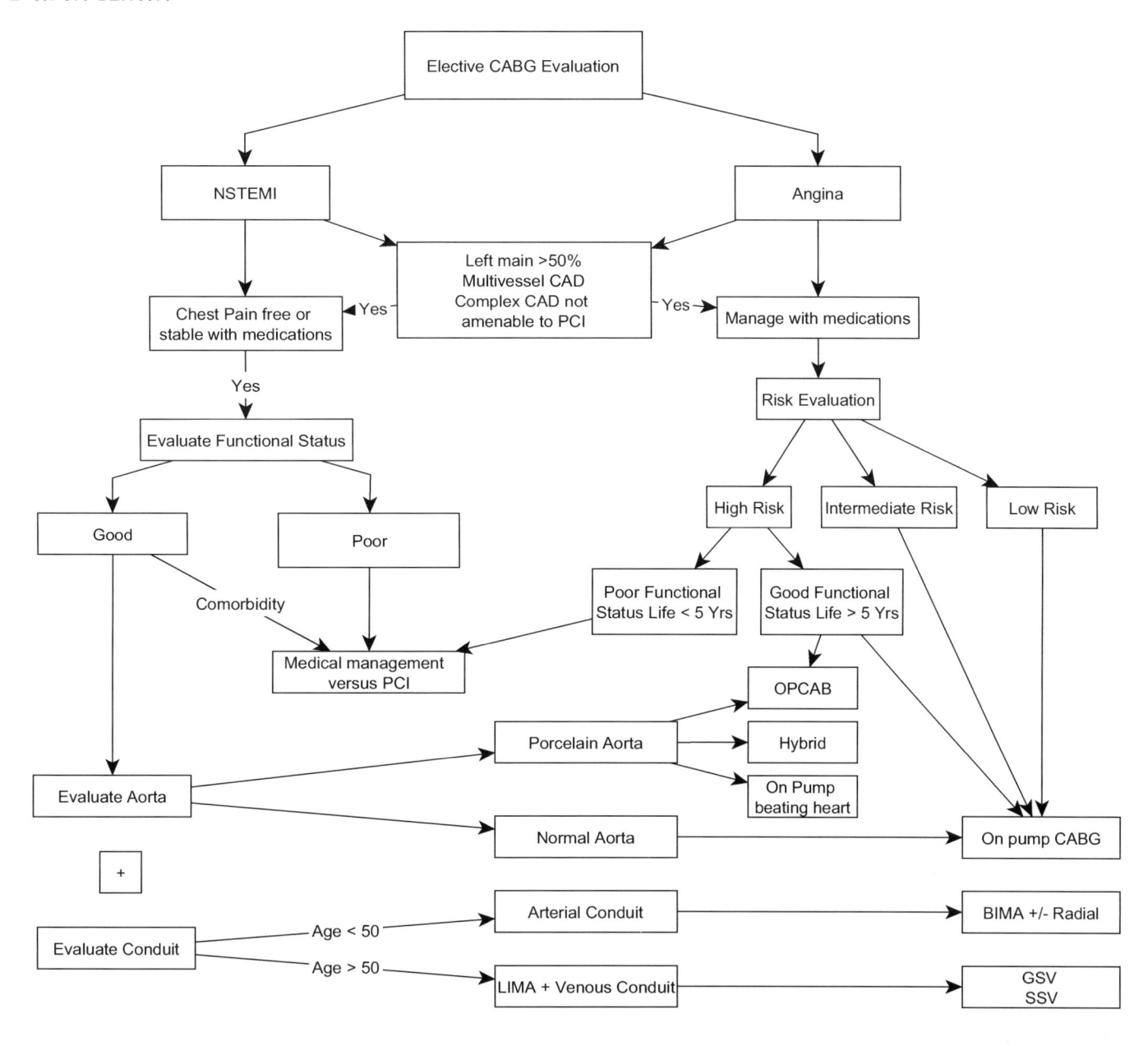

```
                        ┌─────────────────────────┐
                        │ Elective CABG Evaluation│
                        └───────────┬─────────────┘
                         ┌──────────┴──────────┐
                         ▼                     ▼
                      ┌───────┐            ┌────────┐
                      │NSTEMI │            │ Angina │
                      └───┬───┘            └────┬───┘
                          │   ┌─────────────────┐   │
                          │   │Left main >50%   │   │
                          ▼   │Multivessel CAD  │◄──┤
          ┌──────────────────┐│Complex CAD not  │   ▼
          │Chest Pain free or│◄│amenable to PCI │─Yes─►┌──────────────────┐
          │stable with meds  │ └─────────────────┘     │Manage with meds  │
          └────────┬─────────┘                         └─────────┬────────┘
                  Yes                                            ▼
                   ▼                                    ┌────────────────┐
         ┌─────────────────────┐                        │Risk Evaluation │
         │Evaluate Functional  │                        └────────┬───────┘
         │Status               │              ┌─────────────────┼─────────────┐
         └──────┬──────────────┘              ▼                 ▼             ▼
           ┌────┴────┐                   ┌─────────┐    ┌──────────────┐ ┌────────┐
           ▼         ▼                   │High Risk│    │Intermediate  │ │Low Risk│
        ┌────┐    ┌────┐                 └────┬────┘    │Risk          │ └────────┘
        │Good│    │Poor│                      │         └──────────────┘
        └─┬──┘    └─┬──┘              ┌───────┴────────┐
          │Comorbidity                ▼                ▼
          │         ▼          ┌──────────────┐ ┌──────────────┐
          │   ┌──────────────┐ │Poor Functional│ │Good Functional│
          │   │Medical mgmt  │◄│Status Life<5Y │ │Status Life>5Y │
          │   │versus PCI    │ └──────────────┘ └───────┬──────┘
          │   └──────────────┘                          ▼
          ▼                                       ┌────────┐
  ┌──────────────┐      ┌──────────────┐         │ OPCAB  │
  │Evaluate Aorta│─────►│Porcelain Aorta│────────►└────────┘
  └──────┬───────┘      └──────────────┘         ┌────────┐
         │                                       │ Hybrid │
         │                                       └────────┘
         │                                       ┌──────────┐
         │                                       │On Pump   │
         │                                       │beating   │
         │                                       │heart     │
         │                                       └──────────┘
         └─────────────►┌────────────┐           ┌──────────────┐
                        │Normal Aorta│──────────►│On pump CABG  │
                        └────────────┘           └──────────────┘
    +
  ┌────────────────┐  Age<50  ┌──────────────┐  ┌──────────────┐
  │Evaluate Conduit│─────────►│Arterial Conduit│►│BIMA +/- Radial│
  └────────────────┘  Age>50  └──────────────┘  └──────────────┘
                     ─────────►┌──────────────────┐ ┌────────┐
                              │LIMA+Venous Conduit│►│GSV SSV │
                              └──────────────────┘ └────────┘
```

CAD, coronary artery disease; NSTEMI, Non-ST segment myocardial infarction; PCI, percutaneous coronary intervention; BIMA, bilateral internal mammary arteries; LIMA, left internal mammary artery; GSV, greater saphenous vein; SSV, small saphenous vein

ST Elevation Myocardial Infarction (STEMI)
William S. Ragalie MD, Clauden Louis MD, Peyman Banharash MD

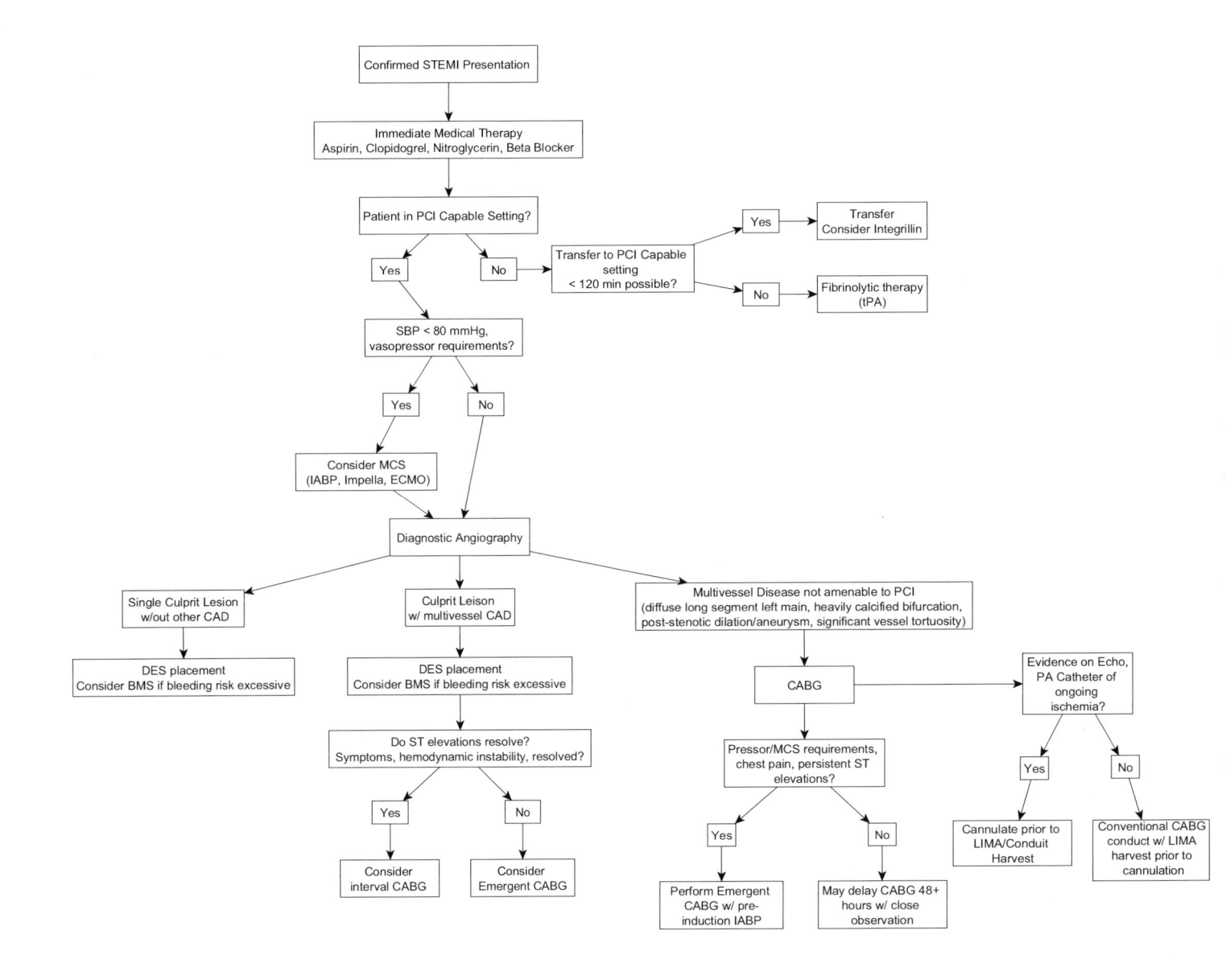

```
                    ┌─────────────────────────────┐
                    │ Confirmed STEMI Presentation│
                    └──────────────┬──────────────┘
                                   ↓
                    ┌─────────────────────────────────┐
                    │    Immediate Medical Therapy    │
                    │ Aspirin, Clopidogrel,           │
                    │ Nitroglycerin, Beta Blocker     │
                    └──────────────┬──────────────────┘
                                   ↓
                    ┌─────────────────────────────┐                                   ┌──────────────┐
                    │ Patient in PCI Capable      │                              Yes →│  Transfer    │
                    │         Setting?            │                                   │  Consider    │
                    └──┬────────────────────────┬─┘                                   │  Integrillin │
                       │                        │                                     └──────────────┘
                     Yes                       No                                          ↑
                       ↓                        ↓                                          │
                       │           ┌─────────────────────────┐                             │
                       │           │ Transfer to PCI Capable │─────────────────────────────┘
                       │           │         setting         │
                       │           │   < 120 min possible?   │──── No ──→ ┌──────────────┐
                       │           └─────────────────────────┘            │ Fibrinolytic │
                       │                                                  │ therapy (tPA)│
                       │                                                  └──────────────┘
                       ↓
         ┌──────────────────────────────┐
         │   SBP < 80 mmHg,             │
         │ vasopressor requirements?    │
         └──┬─────────────────────┬─────┘
          Yes                    No
            ↓                     │
    ┌──────────────────┐          │
    │  Consider MCS    │          │
    │(IABP, Impella,   │          │
    │     ECMO)        │          │
    └────────┬─────────┘          │
             ↓                    ↓
         ┌──────────────────────────┐
         │   Diagnostic Angiography │
         └──┬──────────┬──────────┬─┘
            ↓          ↓          ↓
```

- Single Culprit Lesion w/out other CAD → **DES placement** / Consider BMS if bleeding risk excessive
- Culprit Leison w/ multivessel CAD → **DES placement** / Consider BMS if bleeding risk excessive → Do ST elevations resolve? Symptoms, hemodynamic instability, resolved?
  - Yes → Consider interval CABG
  - No → Consider Emergent CABG
- Multivessel Disease not amenable to PCI (diffuse long segment left main, heavily calcified bifurcation, post-stenotic dilation/aneurysm, significant vessel tortuosity) → **CABG** → Pressor/MCS requirements, chest pain, persistent ST elevations?
  - Yes → Perform Emergent CABG w/ pre-induction IABP
  - No → May delay CABG 48+ hours w/ close observation

Evidence on Echo, PA Catheter of ongoing ischemia?
- Yes → Cannulate prior to LIMA/Conduit Harvest
- No → Conventional CABG conduct w/ LIMA harvest prior to cannulation

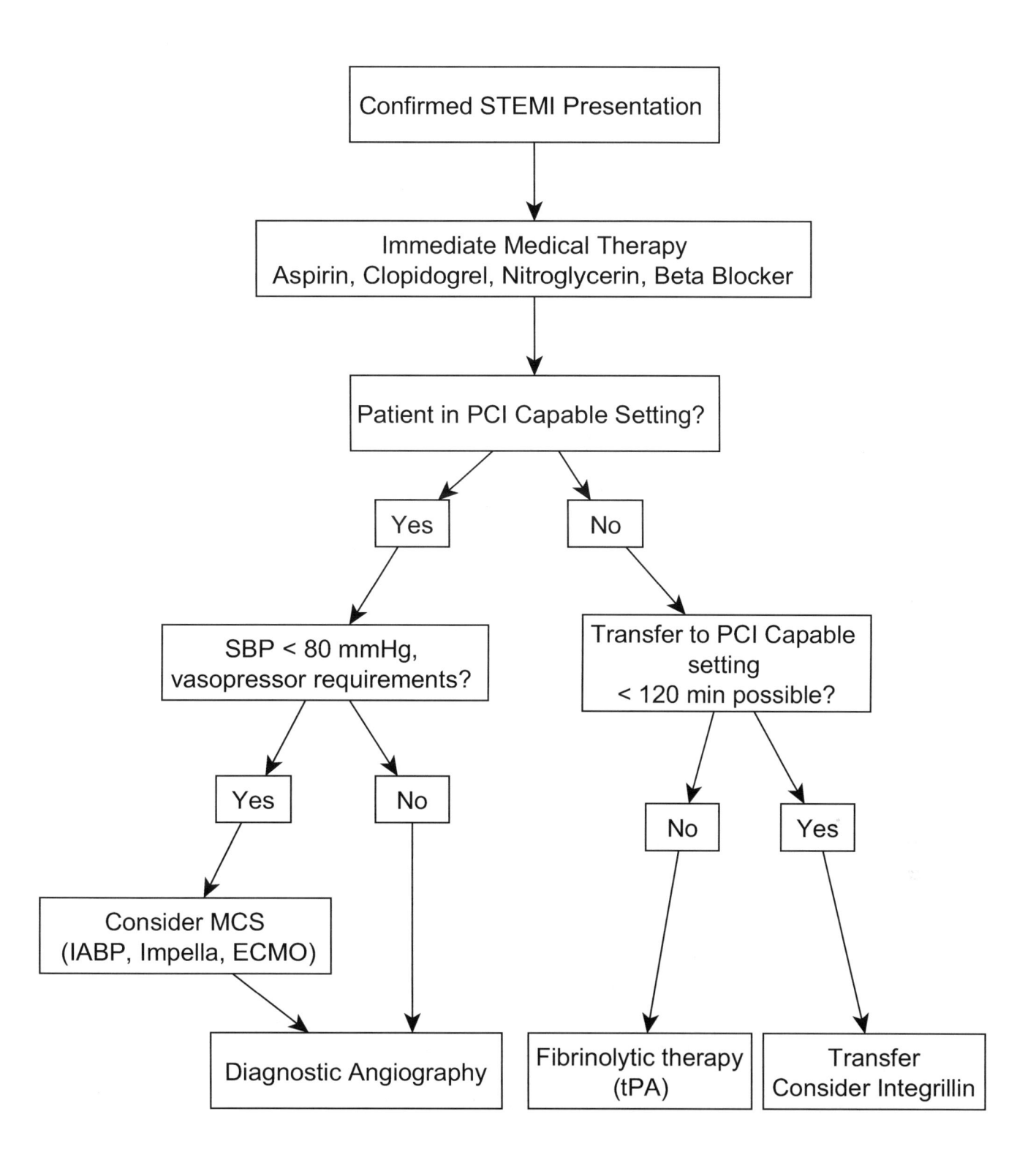

```
┌─────────────────────────────┐
│ Confirmed STEMI Presentation │
└─────────────────────────────┘
              │
              ▼
┌──────────────────────────────────────────────────┐
│           Immediate Medical Therapy              │
│ Aspirin, Clopidogrel, Nitroglycerin, Beta Blocker│
└──────────────────────────────────────────────────┘
              │
              ▼
┌─────────────────────────────┐
│ Patient in PCI Capable Setting? │
└─────────────────────────────┘
        │             │
       Yes            No
        │             │
        ▼             ▼
┌──────────────────┐   ┌──────────────────────┐
│ SBP < 80 mmHg,   │   │ Transfer to PCI Capable │
│ vasopressor      │   │      setting            │
│ requirements?    │   │  < 120 min possible?    │
└──────────────────┘   └──────────────────────┘
    │        │              │           │
   Yes       No             No         Yes
    │        │              │           │
    ▼        │              ▼           ▼
┌──────────────┐      ┌──────────────┐  ┌──────────────┐
│ Consider MCS │      │ Fibrinolytic │  │   Transfer   │
│ (IABP,       │      │   therapy    │  │   Consider   │
│ Impella,     │      │    (tPA)     │  │  Integrillin │
│ ECMO)        │      └──────────────┘  └──────────────┘
└──────────────┘
    │        │
    ▼        ▼
┌──────────────────────┐
│ Diagnostic Angiography │
└──────────────────────┘
```

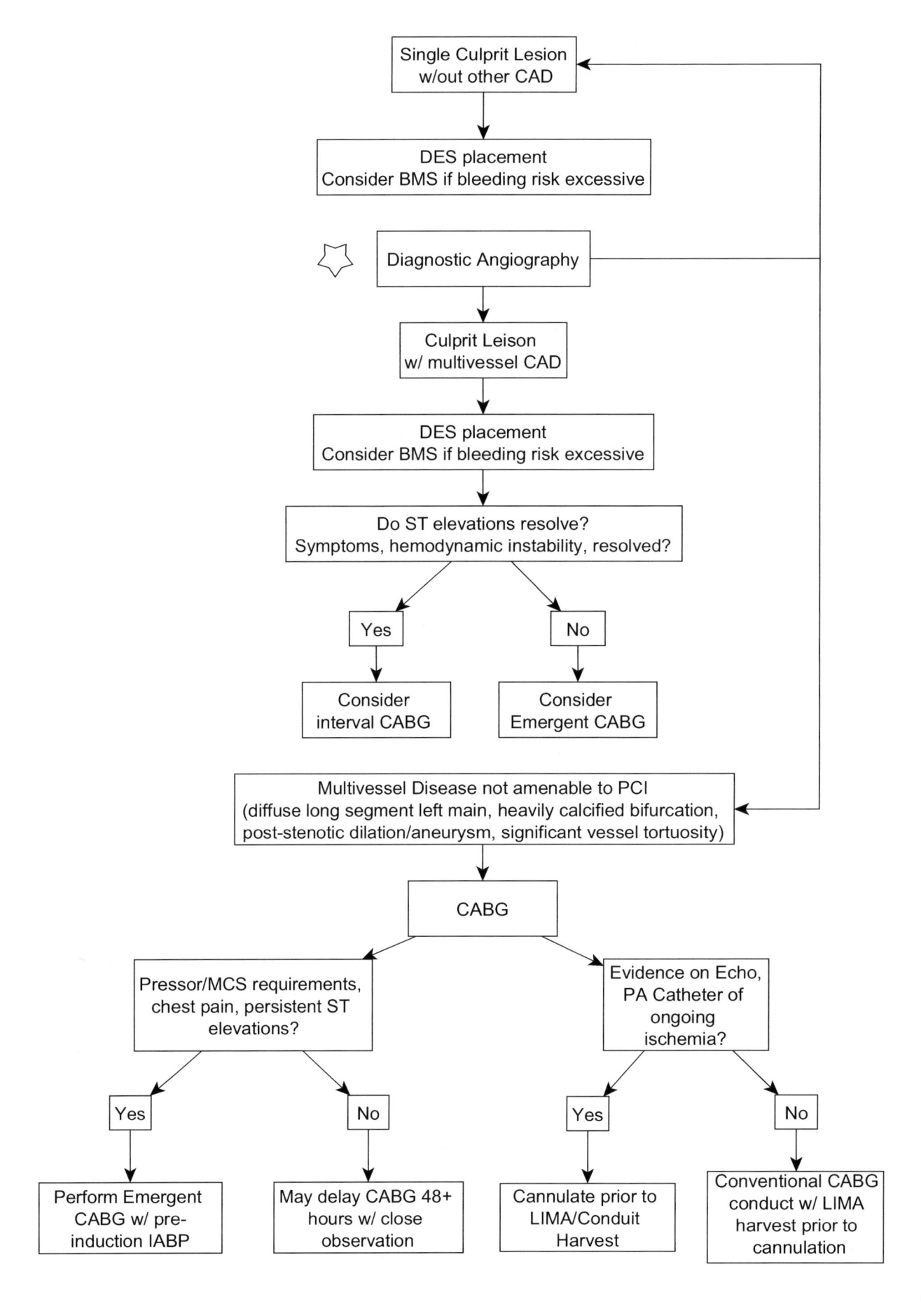

```
                    ┌─────────────────────────┐
                    │ Single Culprit Lesion   │◄─────────┐
                    │   w/out other CAD       │          │
                    └───────────┬─────────────┘          │
                                ▼                        │
                    ┌─────────────────────────────────┐  │
                    │ DES placement                   │  │
                    │ Consider BMS if bleeding risk   │  │
                    │ excessive                       │  │
                    └─────────────────────────────────┘  │
                                                         │
          ☆         ┌─────────────────────────┐          │
                    │ Diagnostic Angiography  │──────────┤
                    └───────────┬─────────────┘          │
                                ▼                        │
                    ┌─────────────────────────┐          │
                    │ Culprit Leison          │          │
                    │ w/ multivessel CAD      │          │
                    └───────────┬─────────────┘          │
                                ▼                        │
                    ┌─────────────────────────────────┐  │
                    │ DES placement                   │  │
                    │ Consider BMS if bleeding risk   │  │
                    │ excessive                       │  │
                    └───────────┬─────────────────────┘  │
                                ▼                        │
                    ┌─────────────────────────────────┐  │
                    │ Do ST elevations resolve?       │  │
                    │ Symptoms, hemodynamic           │  │
                    │ instability, resolved?          │  │
                    └─────┬─────────────────────┬─────┘  │
                      Yes │                     │ No     │
                          ▼                     ▼        │
                    ┌──────────┐          ┌──────────┐   │
                    │ Consider │          │ Consider │   │
                    │ interval │          │ Emergent │   │
                    │  CABG    │          │  CABG    │   │
                    └──────────┘          └──────────┘   │
                                                         │
          ┌──────────────────────────────────────────┐   │
          │ Multivessel Disease not amenable to PCI  │◄──┘
          │ (diffuse long segment left main, heavily │
          │ calcified bifurcation, post-stenotic     │
          │ dilation/aneurysm, significant vessel    │
          │ tortuosity)                              │
          └─────────────────┬────────────────────────┘
                            ▼
                       ┌─────────┐
                       │  CABG   │
                       └────┬────┘
              ┌─────────────┴─────────────┐
              ▼                           ▼
    ┌──────────────────┐         ┌──────────────────┐
    │ Pressor/MCS      │         │ Evidence on Echo,│
    │ requirements,    │         │ PA Catheter of   │
    │ chest pain,      │         │ ongoing          │
    │ persistent ST    │         │ ischemia?        │
    │ elevations?      │         │                  │
    └──┬────────────┬──┘         └──┬────────────┬──┘
   Yes │            │ No         Yes│            │ No
       ▼            ▼               ▼            ▼
  ┌─────────┐  ┌──────────┐   ┌──────────┐  ┌──────────┐
  │ Perform │  │ May delay│   │ Cannulate│  │Conventional│
  │ Emergent│  │ CABG 48+ │   │ prior to │  │ CABG     │
  │ CABG w/ │  │ hours w/ │   │ LIMA/    │  │ conduct  │
  │ pre-    │  │ close    │   │ Conduit  │  │ w/ LIMA  │
  │induction│  │observation│  │ Harvest  │  │ harvest  │
  │  IABP   │  │          │   │          │  │ prior to │
  │         │  │          │   │          │  │cannulation│
  └─────────┘  └──────────┘   └──────────┘  └──────────┘
```

*IMA harvest reasonable if harvest can be performed expeditiously/concomitant w/ vein harvest

BMS, Bare Metal Stent. CAD, Coronary Artery Disease. CABG, Coronary Artery Bypass Graft. DES, Drug Eluting Stent. ECMO, Extracorporeal Membrane Oxygenation. IABP, Intra-aortic Balloon Pump. LIMA, Left Internal Mammary Artery. PA, Pulmonary Artery. PCI, Percutaneous Coronary Intervention. SBP, Systolic Blood Pressure. STEMI, ST Elevation Myocardial Infarction. TPA, Tissue Plasminogen Activator.

Cardiogenic Shock Post STEMI
Clauden Louis, Jessica G.Y Luc, Sunil Prasad

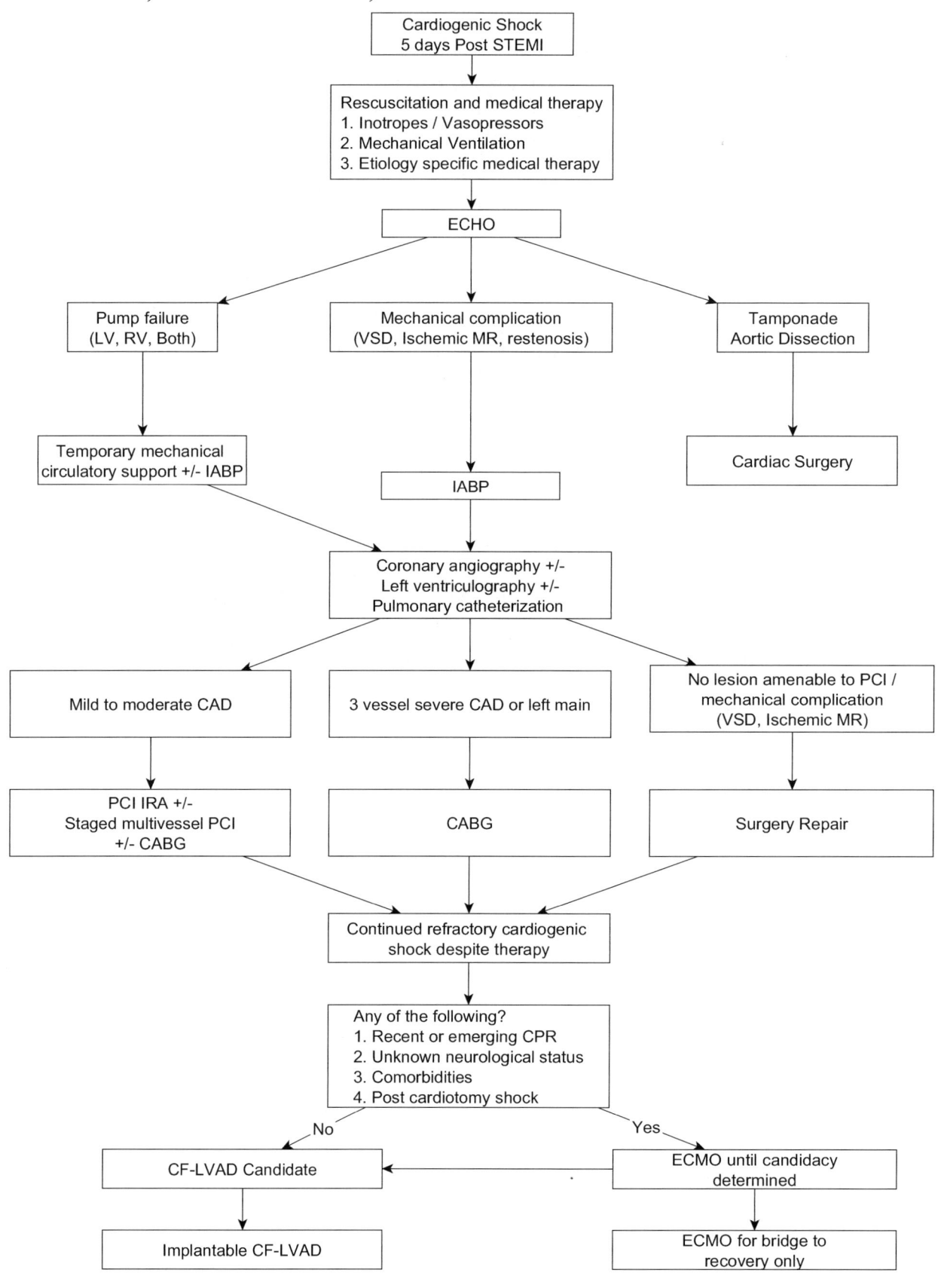

```
┌─────────────────────────┐
│   Cardiogenic Shock     │
│   5 days Post STEMI     │
└───────────┬─────────────┘
            ▼
┌─────────────────────────────────────┐
│ Rescuscitation and medical therapy  │
│ 1. Inotropes / Vasopressors         │
│ 2. Mechanical Ventilation           │
│ 3. Etiology specific medical therapy│
└───────────┬─────────────────────────┘
            ▼
         ┌──────┐
         │ ECHO │
         └──┬───┘
    ┌───────┼────────────────┐
    ▼       ▼                ▼
┌────────┐ ┌──────────────────┐ ┌──────────────┐
│ Pump   │ │ Mechanical       │ │ Tamponade    │
│ failure│ │ complication     │ │ Aortic       │
│(LV, RV,│ │(VSD, Ischemic MR,│ │ Dissection   │
│ Both)  │ │ restenosis)      │ │              │
└───┬────┘ └────────┬─────────┘ └──────┬───────┘
    ▼               ▼                  ▼
┌─────────────┐  ┌──────┐      ┌───────────────┐
│ Temporary   │  │ IABP │      │Cardiac Surgery│
│ mechanical  │  └──┬───┘      └───────────────┘
│ circulatory │     │
│ support +/- │     │
│ IABP        │     │
└──────┬──────┘     │
       └─────┬──────┘
             ▼
┌───────────────────────────┐
│ Coronary angiography +/-  │
│ Left ventriculography +/- │
│ Pulmonary catheterization │
└────┬──────────┬──────────┬┘
     ▼          ▼          ▼
┌─────────┐ ┌──────────┐ ┌──────────────────┐
│ Mild to │ │3 vessel  │ │No lesion amenable│
│moderate │ │severe CAD│ │to PCI / mechanical│
│ CAD     │ │or left   │ │complication      │
│         │ │main      │ │(VSD, Ischemic MR)│
└────┬────┘ └────┬─────┘ └────────┬─────────┘
     ▼           ▼                ▼
┌──────────┐ ┌──────┐      ┌──────────────┐
│PCI IRA +/│ │ CABG │      │Surgery Repair│
│- Staged  │ └──┬───┘      └──────┬───────┘
│multivess.│    │                 │
│PCI +/-   │    │                 │
│CABG      │    │                 │
└────┬─────┘    │                 │
     └──────────┴─────────┬───────┘
                          ▼
            ┌──────────────────────────┐
            │Continued refractory      │
            │cardiogenic shock despite │
            │therapy                   │
            └────────────┬─────────────┘
                         ▼
            ┌──────────────────────────┐
            │Any of the following?     │
            │1. Recent or emerging CPR │
            │2. Unknown neurological   │
            │   status                 │
            │3. Comorbidities          │
            │4. Post cardiotomy shock  │
            └──────┬────────────┬──────┘
                 No│            │Yes
                   ▼            ▼
           ┌─────────────┐ ┌─────────────────┐
           │CF-LVAD      │◄│ECMO until       │
           │Candidate    │ │candidacy        │
           └──────┬──────┘ │determined       │
                  ▼        └────────┬────────┘
           ┌─────────────┐          ▼
           │Implantable  │ ┌─────────────────┐
           │CF-LVAD      │ │ECMO for bridge  │
           └─────────────┘ │to recovery only │
                           └─────────────────┘
```

```
┌─────────────────────────┐
│   Cardiogenic Shock     │
│   5 days Post STEMI     │
└───────────┬─────────────┘
            ▼
┌─────────────────────────────────────┐
│ Rescuscitation and medical therapy  │
│ 1. Inotropes / Vasopressors         │
│ 2. Mechanical Ventilation           │
│ 3. Etiology specific medical therapy│
└───────────┬─────────────────────────┘
            ▼
        ┌───────┐
        │ ECHO  │
        └───┬───┘
```

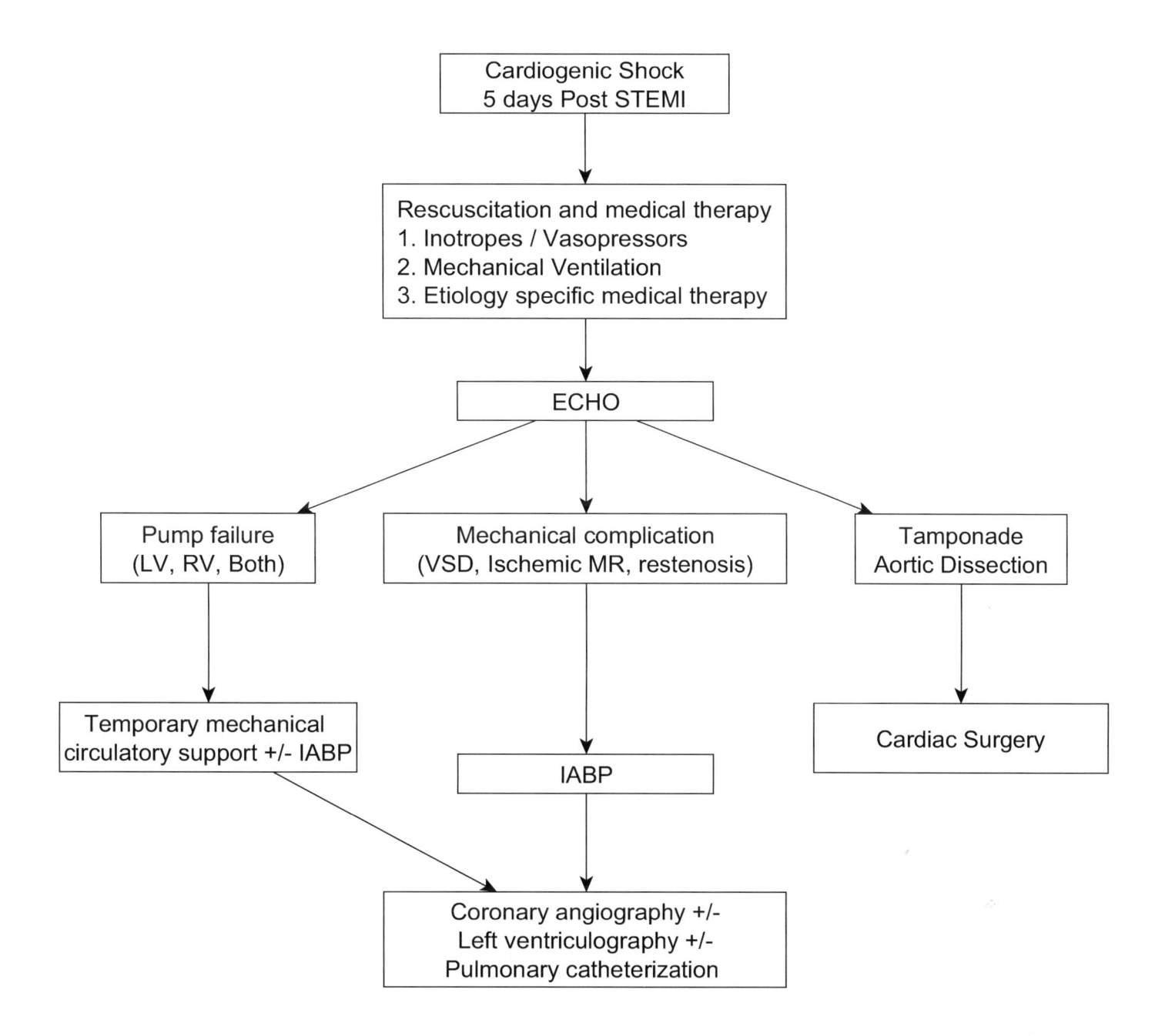

- Pump failure (LV, RV, Both) → Temporary mechanical circulatory support +/- IABP
- Mechanical complication (VSD, Ischemic MR, restenosis) → IABP
- Tamponade / Aortic Dissection → Cardiac Surgery

Pump failure and Mechanical complication pathways → Coronary angiography +/- Left ventriculography +/- Pulmonary catheterization

```
┌─────────────────────────────┐
│   Coronary angiography +/-  │
│  Left ventriculography +/-  │
│   Pulmonary catheterization │
└─────────────────────────────┘
         │         │         │
         ▼         ▼         ▼
```

- Mild to moderate CAD
- 3 vessel severe CAD or left main
- No lesion amenable to PCI / mechanical complication (VSD, Ischemic MR)

↓ ↓ ↓

- PCI IRA +/- Staged multivessel PCI +/- CABG
- CABG
- Surgery Repair

↓

Continued refractory cardiogenic shock despite therapy

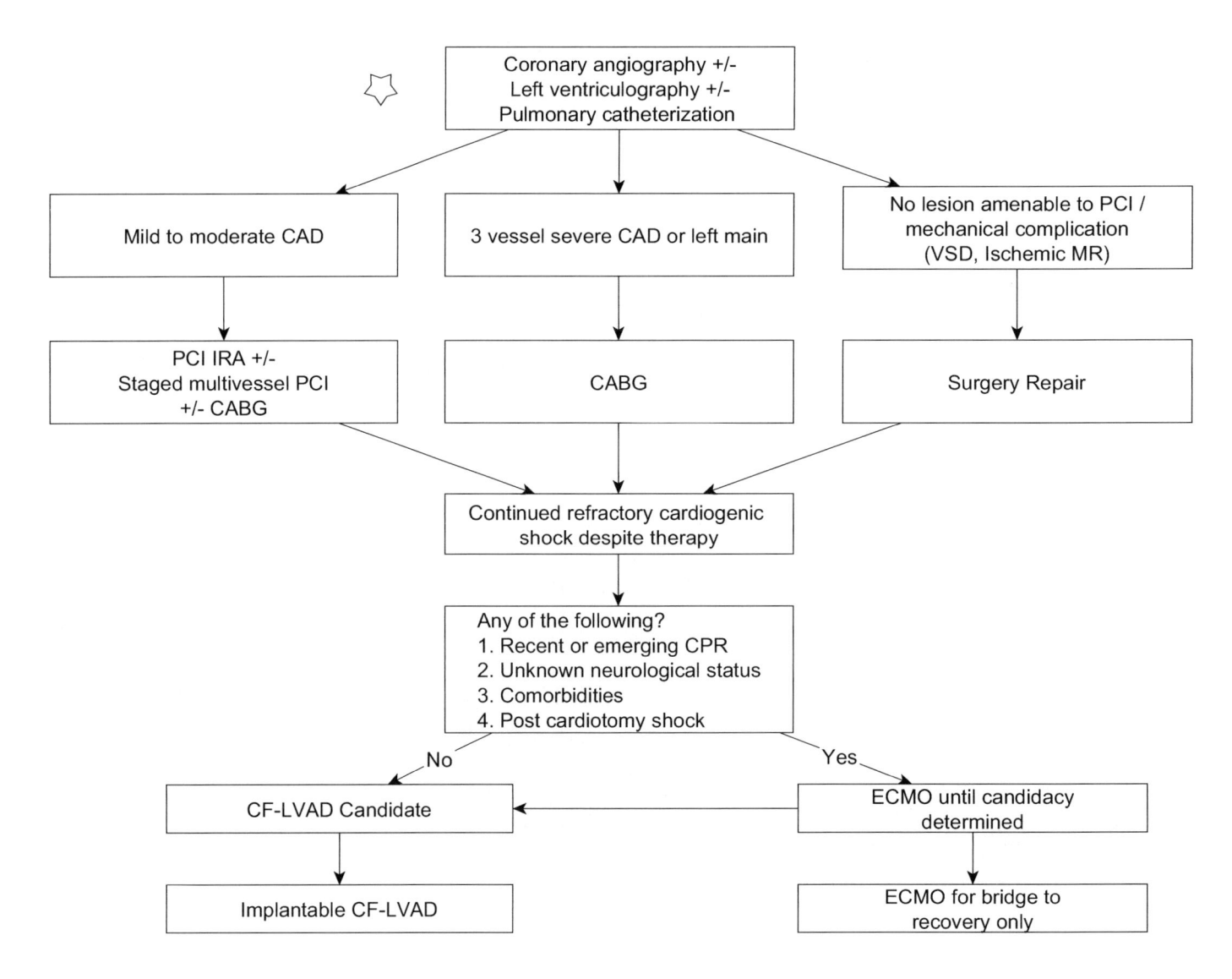

↓

Any of the following?
1. Recent or emerging CPR
2. Unknown neurological status
3. Comorbidities
4. Post cardiotomy shock

No → **CF-LVAD Candidate** → Implantable CF-LVAD

Yes → **ECMO until candidacy determined** → ECMO for bridge to recovery only

CABG, Coronary Artery Bypass Surgery; CAD, coronary artery disease; CF-LVAD, continuous-flow left ventricular assist device; ECHO, echocardiography; ECMO, extracorporeal membrane oxygenation; IRA, infarct-related artery; LBBB, left bundle branch block; MR, mitral regurgitation; PCI, Percutaneous Coronary Intervention; VSD, ventricular septal defect

Intraoperative management of ascending atheroma in CABG
Jared P. Beller, Leora T. Yarboro

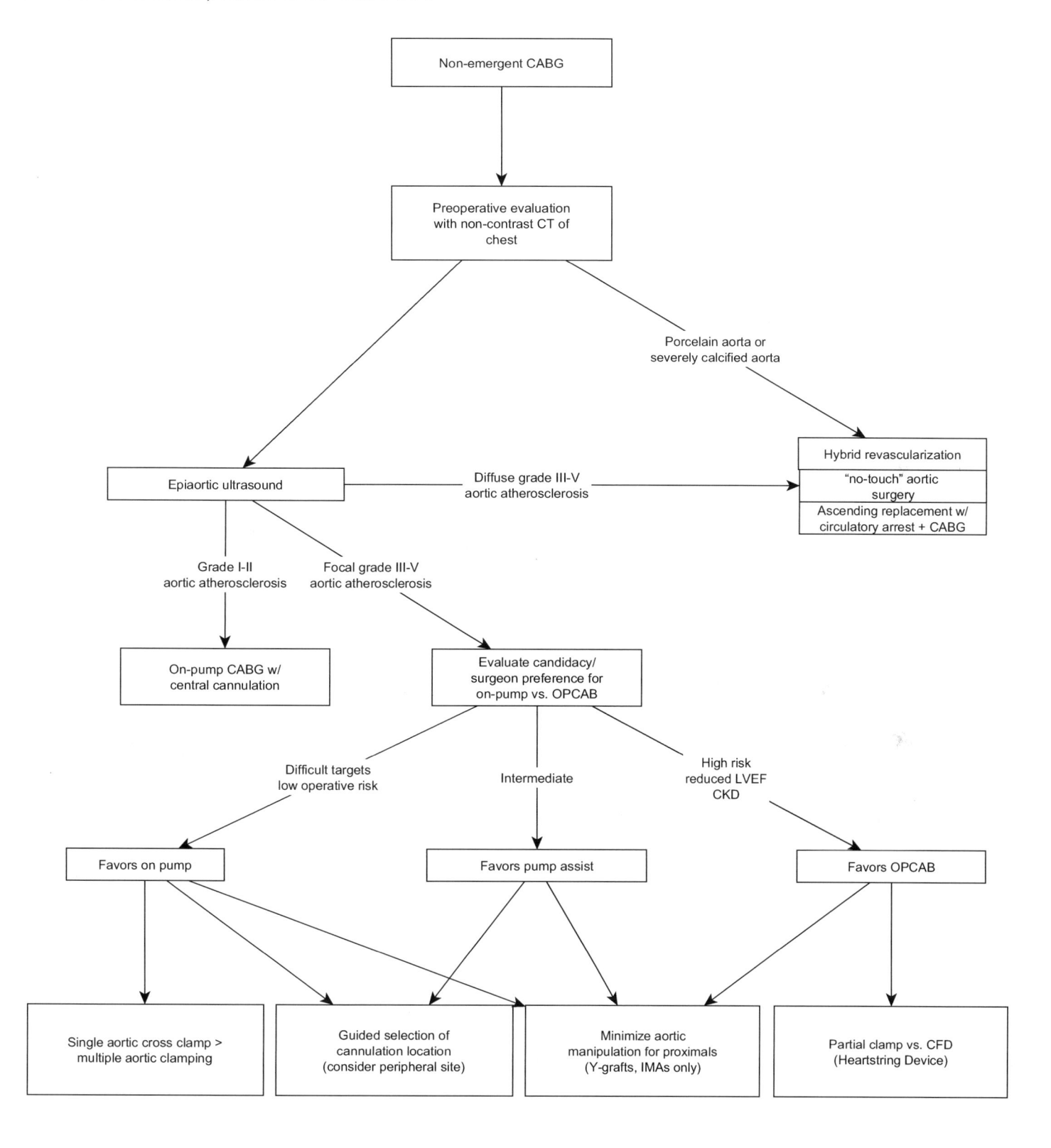

```
                    ┌─────────────────────┐
                    │ Non-emergent CABG   │
                    └──────────┬──────────┘
                               │
                    ┌──────────▼──────────┐
                    │ Preoperative        │
                    │ evaluation with     │
                    │ non-contrast CT of  │
                    │ chest               │
                    └──┬────────────────┬─┘
                       │                │ Porcelain aorta or
                       │                │ severely calcified aorta
                       │                ▼
                       │      ┌──────────────────────────┐
                       │      │ Hybrid revascularization │
                       │      │ "no-touch" aortic        │
                       │      │   surgery                │
                       │      │ Ascending replacement w/ │
                       │      │ circulatory arrest + CABG│
                       │      └──────────────────────────┘
                       ▼
           ┌──────────────────────┐   Diffuse grade III-V
           │ Epiaortic ultrasound │───aortic atherosclerosis──▲
           └──┬───────────────┬───┘
     Grade I-II          Focal grade III-V
   aortic athero.       aortic atherosclerosis
              │                │
              ▼                ▼
     ┌──────────────┐   ┌─────────────────────┐
     │ On-pump CABG │   │ Evaluate candidacy/ │
     │ w/ central   │   │ surgeon preference  │
     │ cannulation  │   │ for on-pump vs OPCAB│
     └──────────────┘   └─┬────────┬────────┬─┘
              Difficult targets  Intermediate  High risk
              low operative risk               reduced LVEF
                                               CKD
                       ▼         ▼          ▼
              ┌──────────┐ ┌──────────┐ ┌──────────┐
              │ Favors   │ │ Favors   │ │ Favors   │
              │ on pump  │ │ pump     │ │ OPCAB    │
              │          │ │ assist   │ │          │
              └──────────┘ └──────────┘ └──────────┘
```

- Single aortic cross clamp > multiple aortic clamping
- Guided selection of cannulation location (consider peripheral site)
- Minimize aortic manipulation for proximals (Y-grafts, IMAs only)
- Partial clamp vs. CFD (Heartstring Device)

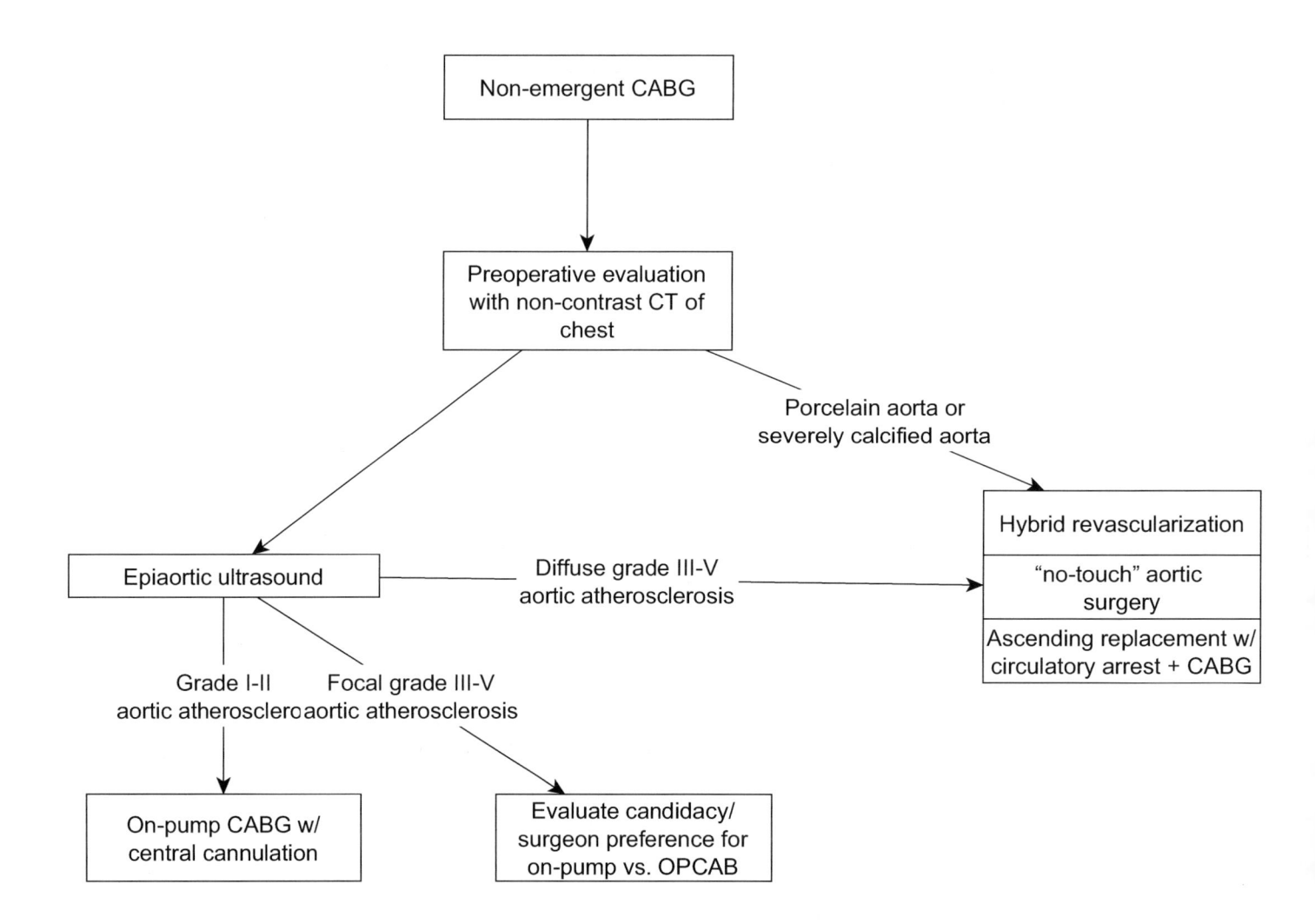

```
┌─────────────────────┐
│  Non-emergent CABG  │
└──────────┬──────────┘
           │
           ▼
┌─────────────────────┐
│ Preoperative evaluation │
│ with non-contrast CT of │
│        chest        │
└──────┬──────────────┴──────────┐
       │                Porcelain aorta or
       │              severely calcified aorta
       ▼                          │
┌─────────────────────┐           │
│ Epiaortic ultrasound │──────────┼──────┐
└──┬──────────┬───────┘  Diffuse grade III-V │
   │          │         aortic atherosclerosis │
Grade I-II  Focal grade III-V                  ▼
aortic       aortic atherosclerosis  ┌──────────────────────┐
atherosclerosis                      │ Hybrid revascularization │
   │          │                      ├──────────────────────┤
   ▼          ▼                      │  "no-touch" aortic    │
┌─────────┐ ┌──────────────┐         │      surgery          │
│On-pump  │ │Evaluate candidacy/│    ├──────────────────────┤
│CABG w/  │ │surgeon preference for│ │Ascending replacement w/│
│central  │ │on-pump vs. OPCAB │    │ circulatory arrest + CABG│
│cannulation│└──────────────┘        └──────────────────────┘
└─────────┘
```

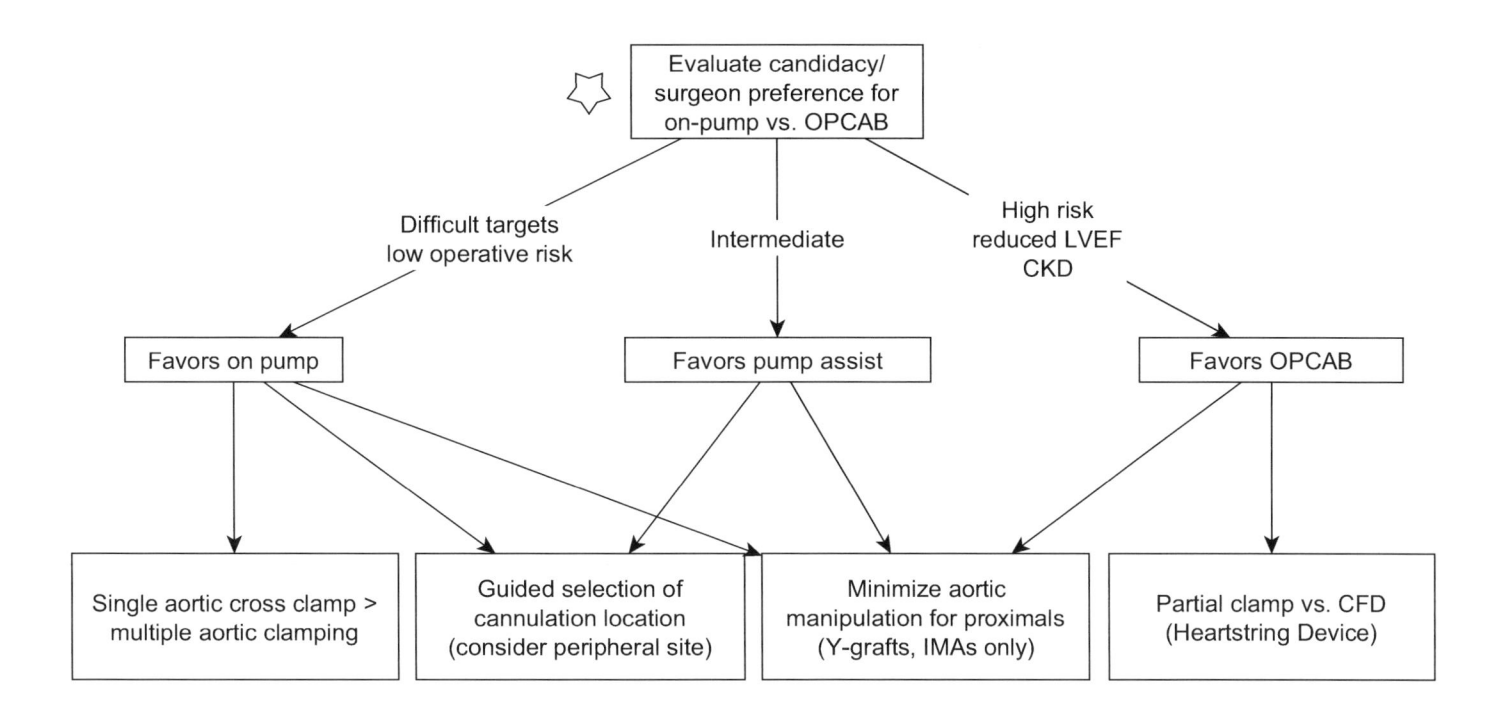

```
                    ┌─────────────────────┐
                    │ Evaluate candidacy/ │
              ☆     │ surgeon preference for│
                    │  on-pump vs. OPCAB  │
                    └─────────────────────┘
                 /            |            \
     Difficult targets    Intermediate    High risk
     low operative risk                   reduced LVEF
                                          CKD
            ↓               ↓                 ↓
    ┌──────────────┐  ┌──────────────┐  ┌──────────────┐
    │Favors on pump│  │Favors pump   │  │Favors OPCAB  │
    │              │  │   assist     │  │              │
    └──────────────┘  └──────────────┘  └──────────────┘
```

| Single aortic cross clamp > multiple aortic clamping | Guided selection of cannulation location (consider peripheral site) | Minimize aortic manipulation for proximals (Y-grafts, IMAs only) | Partial clamp vs. CFD (Heartstring Device) |

CABG, Coronary Artery Bypass Grafting; CT, Computed Tomography; TEE, Transesophogeal Echocardiography; OPCAB, Off-pump coronary artery bypass; IMA, internal mammary artery; LVEF, Left Ventricular Ejection Fraction; CKD, Chronic Kidney Disease; CFD, Clampless facilitating device

Management of combined Coronary Artery Bypass Grafting and Carotid Endarterectomy

Sandeep Sainathan, Luigi Lagazzi

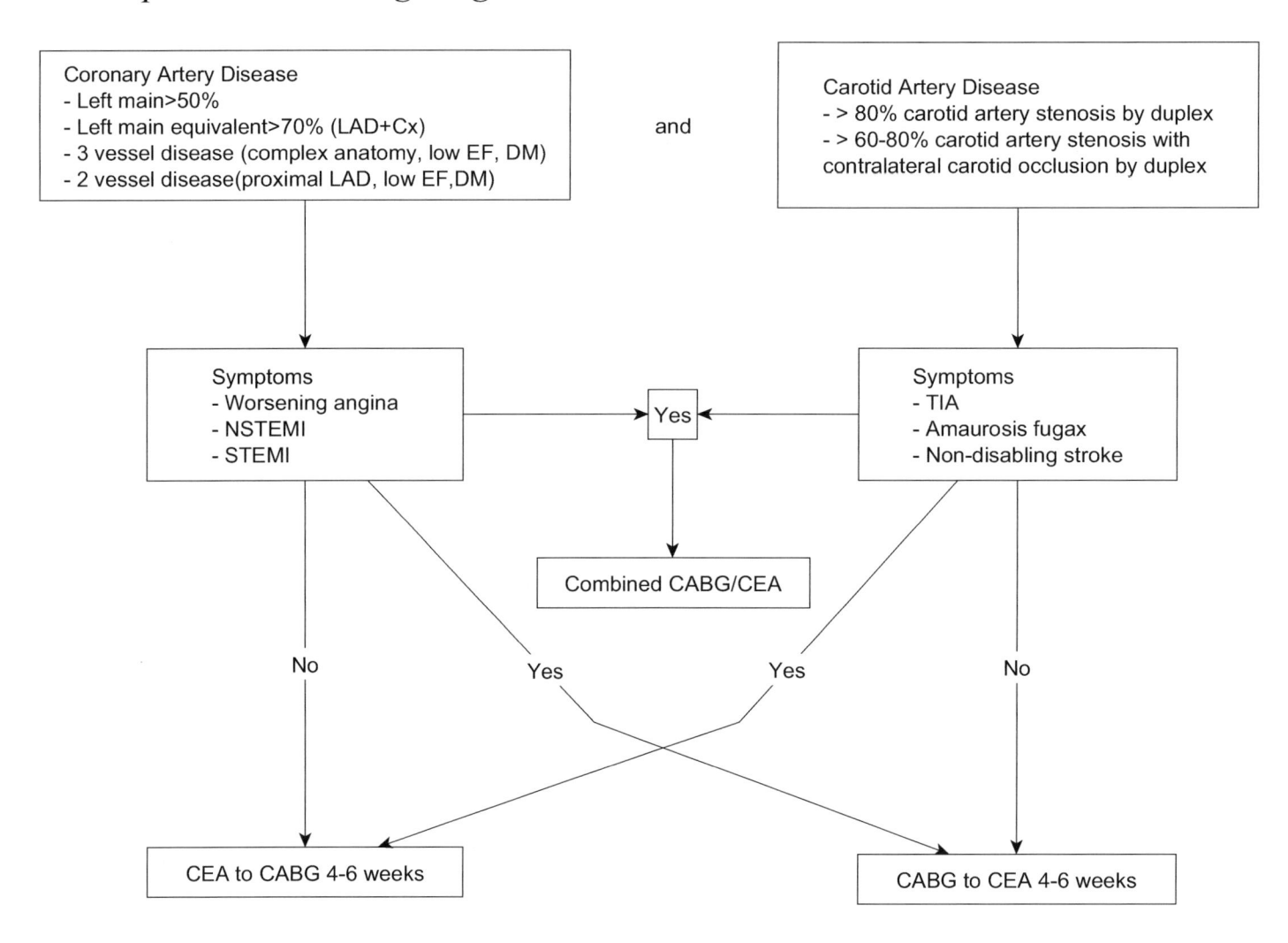

```
┌─────────────────────────────────────────┐                    ┌─────────────────────────────────────────┐
│ Coronary Artery Disease                 │                    │ Carotid Artery Disease                  │
│ - Left main>50%                         │                    │ - > 80% carotid artery stenosis by duplex│
│ - Left main equivalent>70% (LAD+Cx)     │        and         │ - > 60-80% carotid artery stenosis with │
│ - 3 vessel disease (complex anatomy,    │                    │   contralateral carotid occlusion by duplex│
│   low EF, DM)                           │                    │                                         │
│ - 2 vessel disease (proximal LAD,       │                    │                                         │
│   low EF, DM)                           │                    │                                         │
└─────────────────────────────────────────┘                    └─────────────────────────────────────────┘
                    │                                                              │
                    ▼                                                              ▼
        ┌──────────────────────┐                                      ┌──────────────────────┐
        │ Symptoms             │                                      │ Symptoms             │
        │ - Worsening angina   │────────►  Yes  ◄──────────────       │ - TIA                │
        │ - NSTEMI             │                                      │ - Amaurosis fugax    │
        │ - STEMI              │                                      │ - Non-disabling stroke│
        └──────────────────────┘             │                        └──────────────────────┘
              │         │                    ▼                              │         │
              │         │           ┌──────────────────┐                    │         │
              │         │           │ Combined CABG/CEA│                    │         │
              │         │           └──────────────────┘                    │         │
           No │     Yes │                                               Yes │      No │
              ▼         ▼                                                   ▼         ▼
        ┌──────────────────────┐                                      ┌──────────────────────┐
        │ CEA to CABG 4-6 weeks│                                      │ CABG to CEA 4-6 weeks│
        └──────────────────────┘                                      └──────────────────────┘
```

LAD, Left Anterior Descending artery; Cx, Circumflex coronary artery; EF, Ejection Fraction; DM, Diabetes Mellitus; NSTEMI, Non ST Elevation Myocardial Infarction; STEMI, ST Elevation Myocardial Infarction; TIA, Transient Ischemic Attacks; CABG, Coronary Artery Bypass Grafting; CEA, Carotid Endarterectomy

Intraoperative Decision Making for OPCAB
Michael O. Kayatta, Omar M. Lattouf

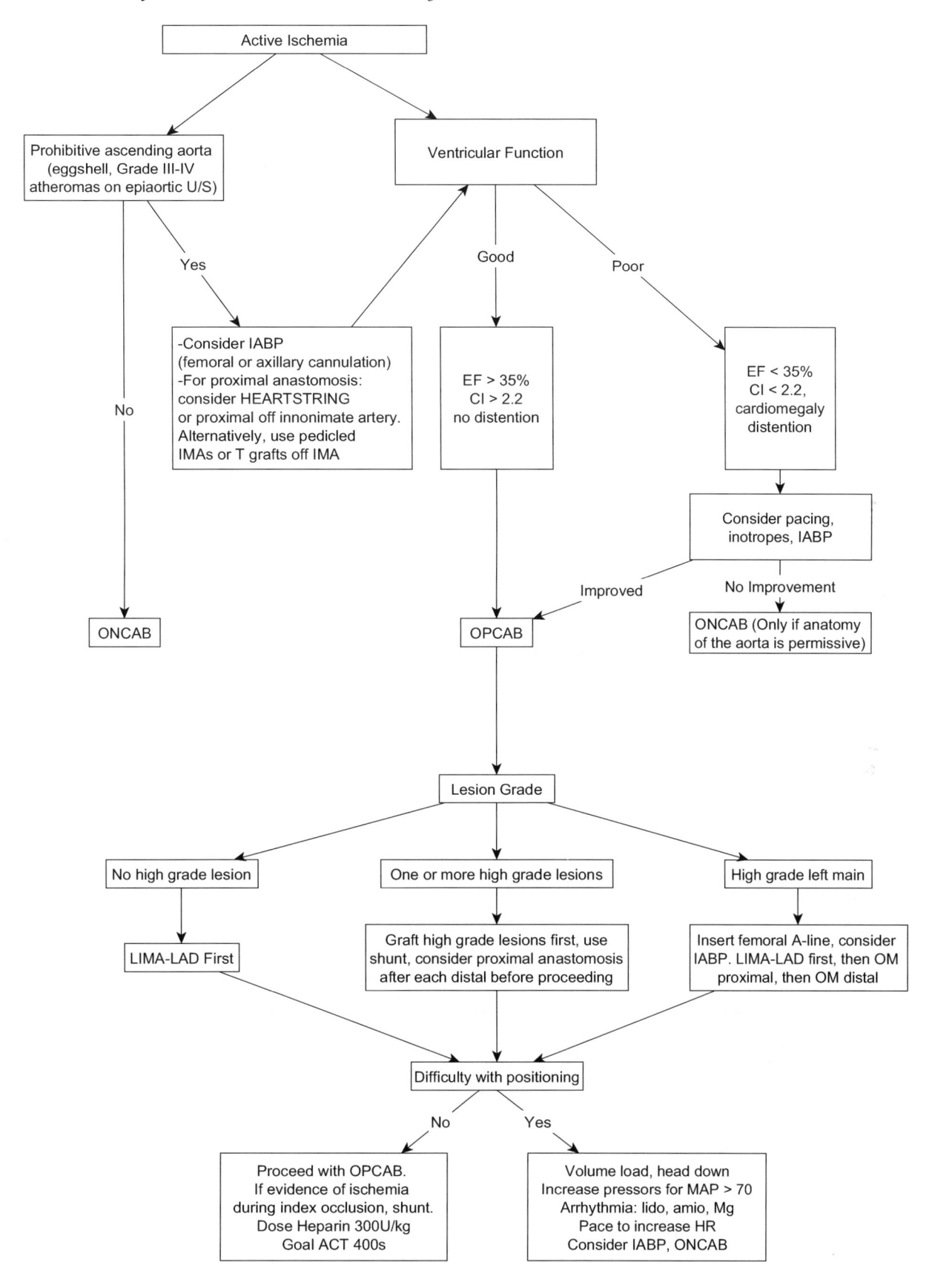

```
                        Active Ischemia
                       /              \
        Prohibitive ascending aorta    Ventricular Function
        (eggshell, Grade III-IV       /        |         \
        atheromas on epiaortic U/S)  Good              Poor
           |         |
          Yes        →  -Consider IABP
           |            (femoral or axillary cannulation)
           |            -For proximal anastomosis:
           |            consider HEARTSTRING
          No            or proximal off innonimate artery.
           |            Alternatively, use pedicled
           |            IMAs or T grafts off IMA
         ONCAB
```

- EF > 35%, CI > 2.2, no distention → OPCAB
- EF < 35%, CI < 2.2, cardiomegaly distention → Consider pacing, inotropes, IABP
  - Improved → OPCAB
  - No Improvement → ONCAB (Only if anatomy of the aorta is permissive)

Lesion Grade

- **No high grade lesion**: LIMA-LAD First
- **One or more high grade lesions**: Graft high grade lesions first, use shunt, consider proximal anastomosis after each distal before proceeding
- **High grade left main**: Insert femoral A-line, consider IABP. LIMA-LAD first, then OM proximal, then OM distal

Difficulty with positioning

- **No**: Proceed with OPCAB. If evidence of ischemia during index occlusion, shunt. Dose Heparin 300U/kg. Goal ACT 400s
- **Yes**: Volume load, head down. Increase pressors for MAP > 70. Arrhythmia: lido, amio, Mg. Pace to increase HR. Consider IABP, ONCAB

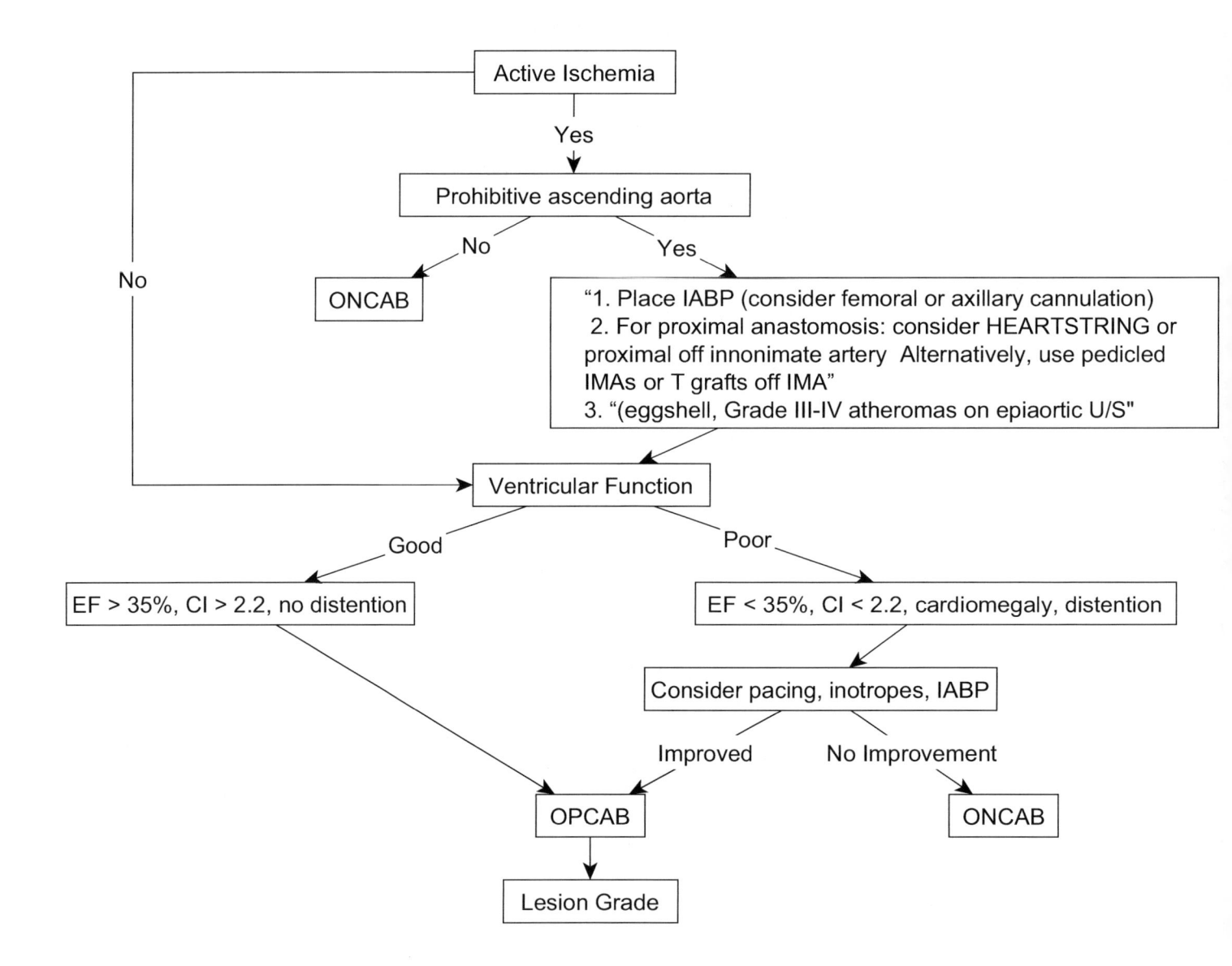

```
                        ┌─────────────────┐
                        │ Active Ischemia │
                        └─────────────────┘
                                │ Yes
                                ▼
                    ┌───────────────────────────┐
                    │ Prohibitive ascending aorta│
                    └───────────────────────────┘
                        No  │       │  Yes
                            ▼       ▼
                         ONCAB   [IABP / HEARTSTRING box]
```

- Active Ischemia → No → Ventricular Function
- Active Ischemia → Yes → Prohibitive ascending aorta
  - No → ONCAB
  - Yes →
    1. Place IABP (consider femoral or axillary cannulation)
    2. For proximal anastomosis: consider HEARTSTRING or proximal off innominate artery Alternatively, use pedicled IMAs or T grafts off IMA
    3. "(eggshell, Grade III-IV atheromas on epiaortic U/S"
  - → Ventricular Function

Ventricular Function
- Good → EF > 35%, CI > 2.2, no distention → OPCAB → Lesion Grade
- Poor → EF < 35%, CI < 2.2, cardiomegaly, distention → Consider pacing, inotropes, IABP
  - Improved → OPCAB
  - No Improvement → ONCAB

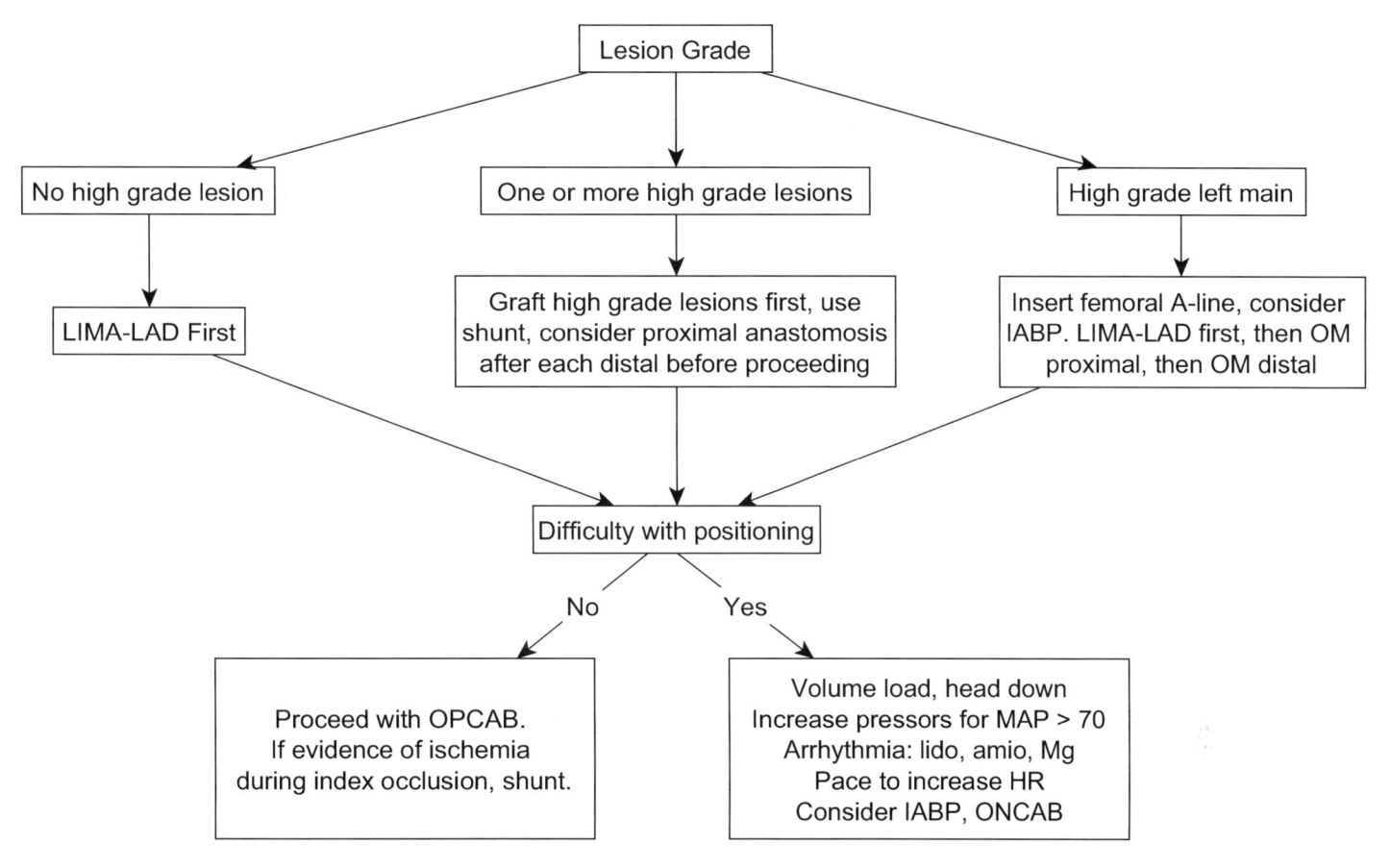

```
                        ┌─────────────┐
                        │ Lesion Grade │
                        └─────────────┘
              ↙                 ↓                  ↘
┌──────────────────┐  ┌──────────────────────┐  ┌─────────────────┐
│ No high grade    │  │ One or more high     │  │ High grade      │
│ lesion           │  │ grade lesions        │  │ left main       │
└──────────────────┘  └──────────────────────┘  └─────────────────┘
         ↓                     ↓                         ↓
┌──────────────────┐  ┌──────────────────────┐  ┌─────────────────────┐
│ LIMA-LAD First   │  │ Graft high grade     │  │ Insert femoral      │
└──────────────────┘  │ lesions first, use   │  │ A-line, consider    │
                      │ shunt, consider      │  │ IABP. LIMA-LAD      │
                      │ proximal anastomosis │  │ first, then OM      │
                      │ after each distal    │  │ proximal, then      │
                      │ before proceeding    │  │ OM distal           │
                      └──────────────────────┘  └─────────────────────┘
```

```
                    ┌──────────────────────────┐
                    │ Difficulty with positioning │
                    └──────────────────────────┘
                       No              Yes
              ↙                               ↘
┌──────────────────────────┐      ┌──────────────────────────────┐
│ Proceed with OPCAB.      │      │ Volume load, head down       │
│ If evidence of ischemia  │      │ Increase pressors for MAP > 70│
│ during index occlusion,  │      │ Arrhythmia: lido, amio, Mg   │
│ shunt.                   │      │ Pace to increase HR          │
└──────────────────────────┘      │ Consider IABP, ONCAB         │
                                  └──────────────────────────────┘
```

CI, cardiac index; EF, ejection fraction; HR, heart rate; IABP, intra-aortic balloon pump; IMA, internal mammary artery; LAD, left anterior descending artery; MAP, mean arterial pressure; ONCAB, on-pump coronary artery bypass grafting; OM, obtuse marginal artery; OPCAB, off-pump coronary artery bypass grafting

Moderate and Severe Aortic Stenosis
Gregory Pattakos, Joseph Coselli

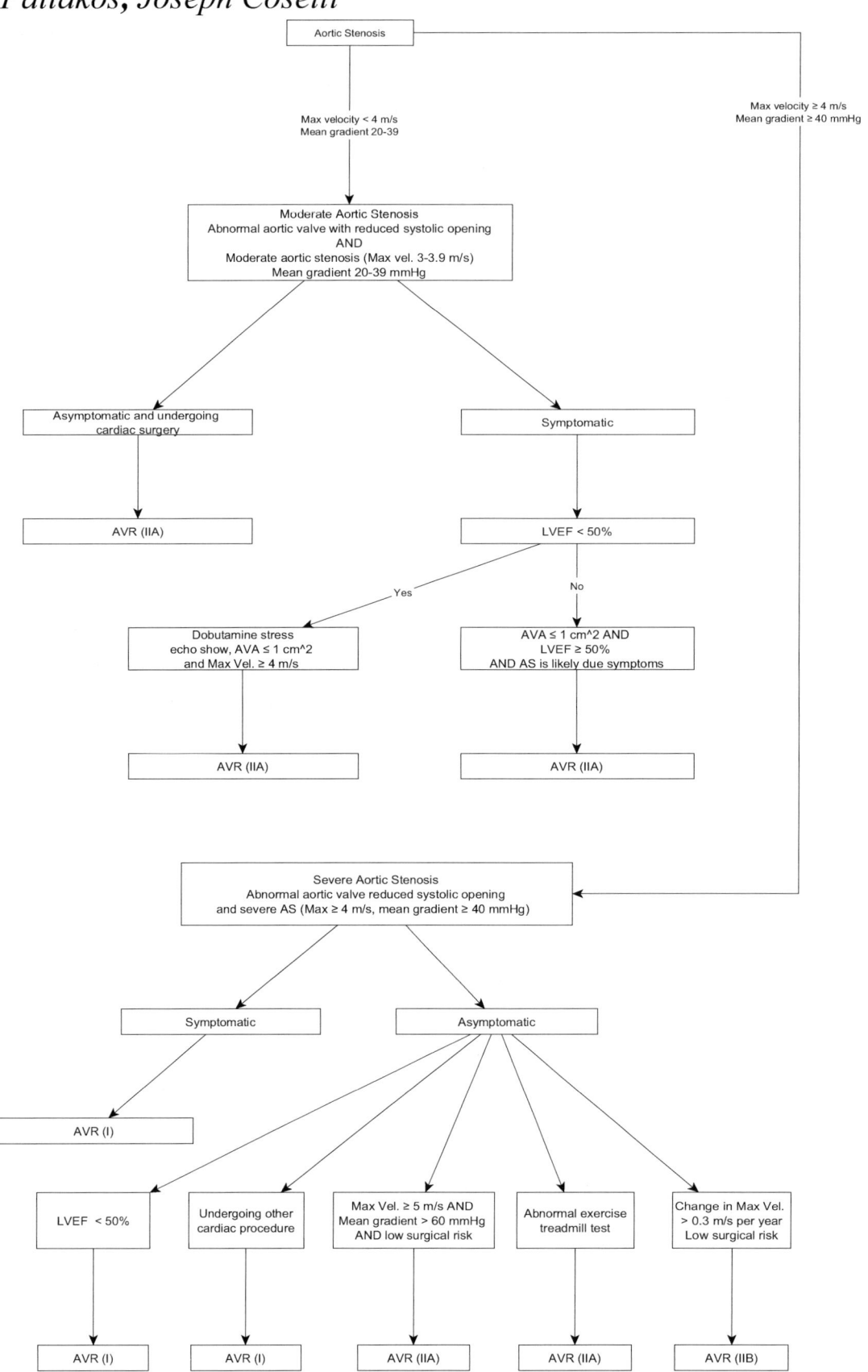

```
                          ┌──────────────────┐
                          │ Aortic Stenosis  │
                          └──────────────────┘
           Max velocity < 4 m/s         Max velocity ≥ 4 m/s
           Mean gradient 20-39          Mean gradient ≥ 40 mmHg
                    │                              │
                    ▼                              │
   ┌─────────────────────────────────────────┐     │
   │ Moderate Aortic Stenosis                │     │
   │ Abnormal aortic valve with reduced      │     │
   │ systolic opening                        │     │
   │ AND                                     │     │
   │ Moderate aortic stenosis (Max vel.      │     │
   │ 3-3.9 m/s)                              │     │
   │ Mean gradient 20-39 mmHg                │     │
   └─────────────────────────────────────────┘     │
           │                      │                │
           ▼                      ▼                │
   ┌──────────────────┐   ┌──────────────┐         │
   │ Asymptomatic and │   │ Symptomatic  │         │
   │ undergoing       │   └──────────────┘         │
   │ cardiac surgery  │          │                 │
   └──────────────────┘          ▼                 │
           │              ┌──────────────┐         │
           ▼              │  LVEF < 50%  │         │
   ┌──────────────┐       └──────────────┘         │
   │   AVR (IIA)  │       Yes │      │ No          │
   └──────────────┘           ▼      ▼             │
              ┌─────────────────┐  ┌─────────────────────┐
              │ Dobutamine      │  │ AVA ≤ 1 cm^2 AND    │
              │ stress echo     │  │ LVEF ≥ 50%          │
              │ show, AVA ≤ 1   │  │ AND AS is likely    │
              │ cm^2 and Max    │  │ due symptoms        │
              │ Vel. ≥ 4 m/s    │  │                     │
              └─────────────────┘  └─────────────────────┘
                      │                    │
                      ▼                    ▼
              ┌──────────────┐      ┌──────────────┐
              │  AVR (IIA)   │      │  AVR (IIA)   │
              └──────────────┘      └──────────────┘

   ┌────────────────────────────────────────────────┐
   │ Severe Aortic Stenosis                         │◄──
   │ Abnormal aortic valve reduced systolic opening │
   │ and severe AS (Max ≥ 4 m/s, mean gradient      │
   │ ≥ 40 mmHg)                                     │
   └────────────────────────────────────────────────┘
              │                    │
              ▼                    ▼
      ┌──────────────┐     ┌──────────────┐
      │ Symptomatic  │     │ Asymptomatic │
      └──────────────┘     └──────────────┘
              │           ┌─────┬─────┬─────┬─────┐
              ▼           ▼     ▼     ▼     ▼     ▼
      ┌────────────┐
      │  AVR (I)   │
      └────────────┘
   ┌──────────┐ ┌──────────┐ ┌──────────────┐ ┌──────────┐ ┌──────────────┐
   │ LVEF     │ │Undergoing│ │Max Vel.≥5m/s │ │Abnormal  │ │Change in Max │
   │ < 50%    │ │ other    │ │AND Mean      │ │exercise  │ │Vel. > 0.3    │
   │          │ │ cardiac  │ │gradient > 60 │ │treadmill │ │m/s per year  │
   │          │ │procedure │ │mmHg AND low  │ │test      │ │Low surgical  │
   │          │ │          │ │surgical risk │ │          │ │risk          │
   └──────────┘ └──────────┘ └──────────────┘ └──────────┘ └──────────────┘
       │            │             │               │              │
       ▼            ▼             ▼               ▼              ▼
   ┌────────┐  ┌────────┐   ┌──────────┐    ┌──────────┐   ┌──────────┐
   │AVR (I) │  │AVR (I) │   │AVR (IIA) │    │AVR (IIA) │   │AVR (IIB) │
   └────────┘  └────────┘   └──────────┘    └──────────┘   └──────────┘
```

```
                        ┌─────────────────┐
                        │ Aortic Stenosis │──────────────────────┐
                        └─────────────────┘                      │
                               │                                 │
         Max velocity < 4 m/s  │                                 │  Max velocity ≥ 4 m/s
         Mean gradient 20-39   │                                 │  Mean gradient ≥ 40 mmHg
                               ▼                                 │
        ┌────────────────────────────────────────────┐           │
        │ Moderate Aortic Stenosis                   │           │
        │ Abnormal aortic valve with reduced systolic│           │
        │ opening AND                                │           │
        │ Moderate aortic stenosis (Max vel. 3-3.9   │           │
        │ m/s) Mean gradient 20-39 mmHg              │           │
        └────────────────────────────────────────────┘           │
              │                              │                   │
              ▼                              ▼                   │
   ┌─────────────────────┐        ┌─────────────────┐            │
   │ Asymptomatic and    │        │   Symptomatic   │            │
   │ undergoing cardiac  │        └─────────────────┘            │
   │ surgery             │                 │                     │
   └─────────────────────┘                 ▼                     │
              │                  ┌─────────────────┐             │
              ▼                  │   LVEF < 50%    │             │
        ┌───────────┐            └─────────────────┘             │
        │ AVR (IIA) │              Yes │      │ No               │
        └───────────┘                  ▼      ▼                  │
                          ┌──────────────┐  ┌──────────────────┐ │
                          │ Dobutamine   │  │ AVA ≤ 1 cm^2 AND │ │
                          │ stress echo  │  │ LVEF ≥ 50%       │ │
                          │ show, AVA ≤  │  │ AND AS is likely │ │
                          │ 1 cm^2 and   │  │ due symptoms     │ │
                          │ Max Vel.≥4m/s│  └──────────────────┘ │
                          └──────────────┘           │           │
                                 │                   ▼           │
                                 ▼             ┌───────────┐     │
                           ┌───────────┐       │ AVR (IIA) │     │
                           │ AVR (IIA) │       └───────────┘     │
                           └───────────┘                         │
                                                                 │
              ┌──────────────────────────────────────────┐       │
              │ Severe Aortic Stenosis                   │◄──────┘
              │ Abnormal aortic valve reduced systolic   │
              │ opening and severe AS (Max ≥ 4 m/s,      │
              │ mean gradient ≥ 40 mmHg)                 │
              └──────────────────────────────────────────┘
```

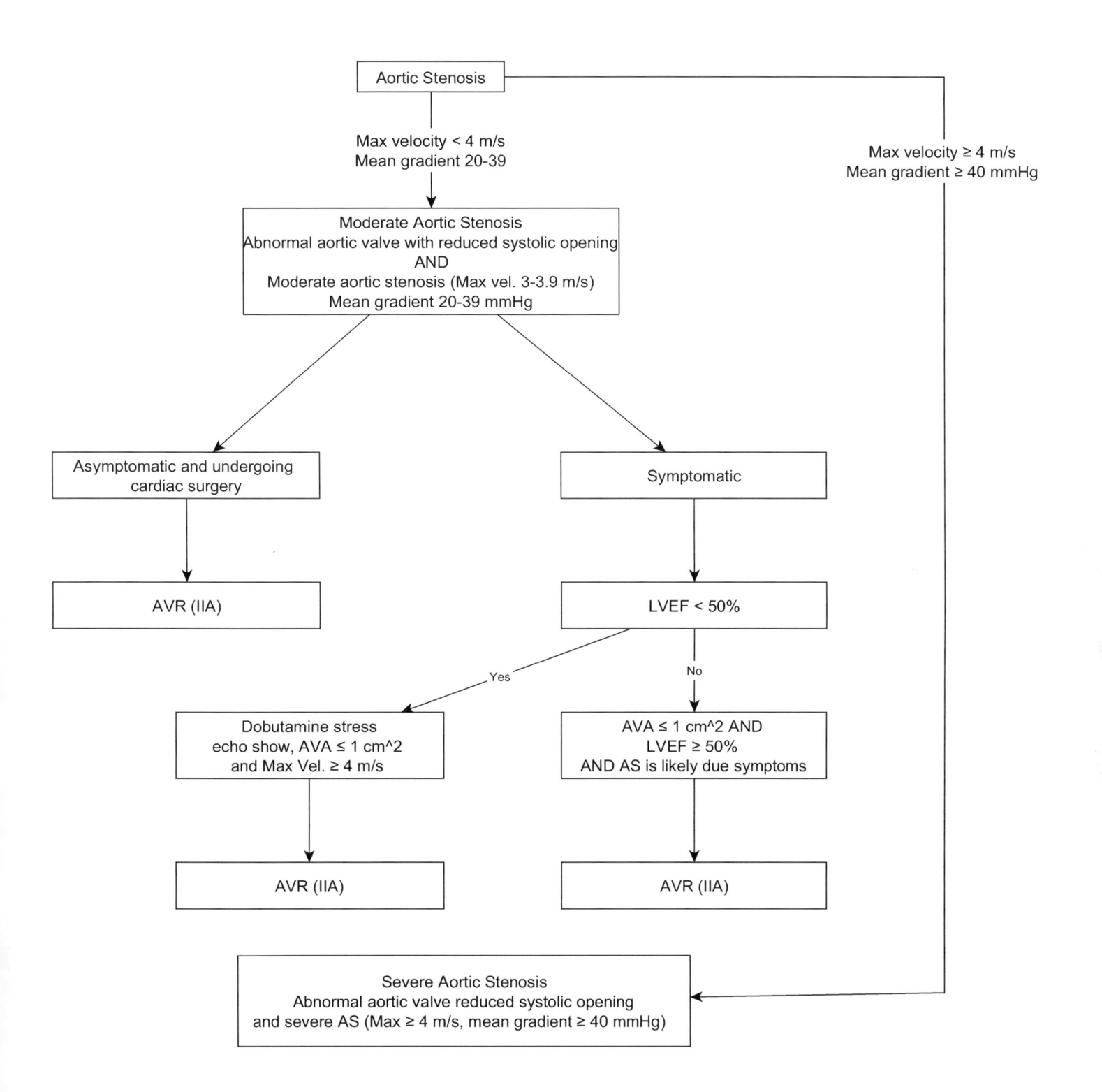

```
                    Severe Aortic Stenosis
            Abnormal aortic valve reduced systolic opening
         and severe AS (Max ≥ 4 m/s, mean gradient ≥ 40 mmHg)
                    /                    \
              Symptomatic              Asymptomatic
                  |
               AVR (I)
```

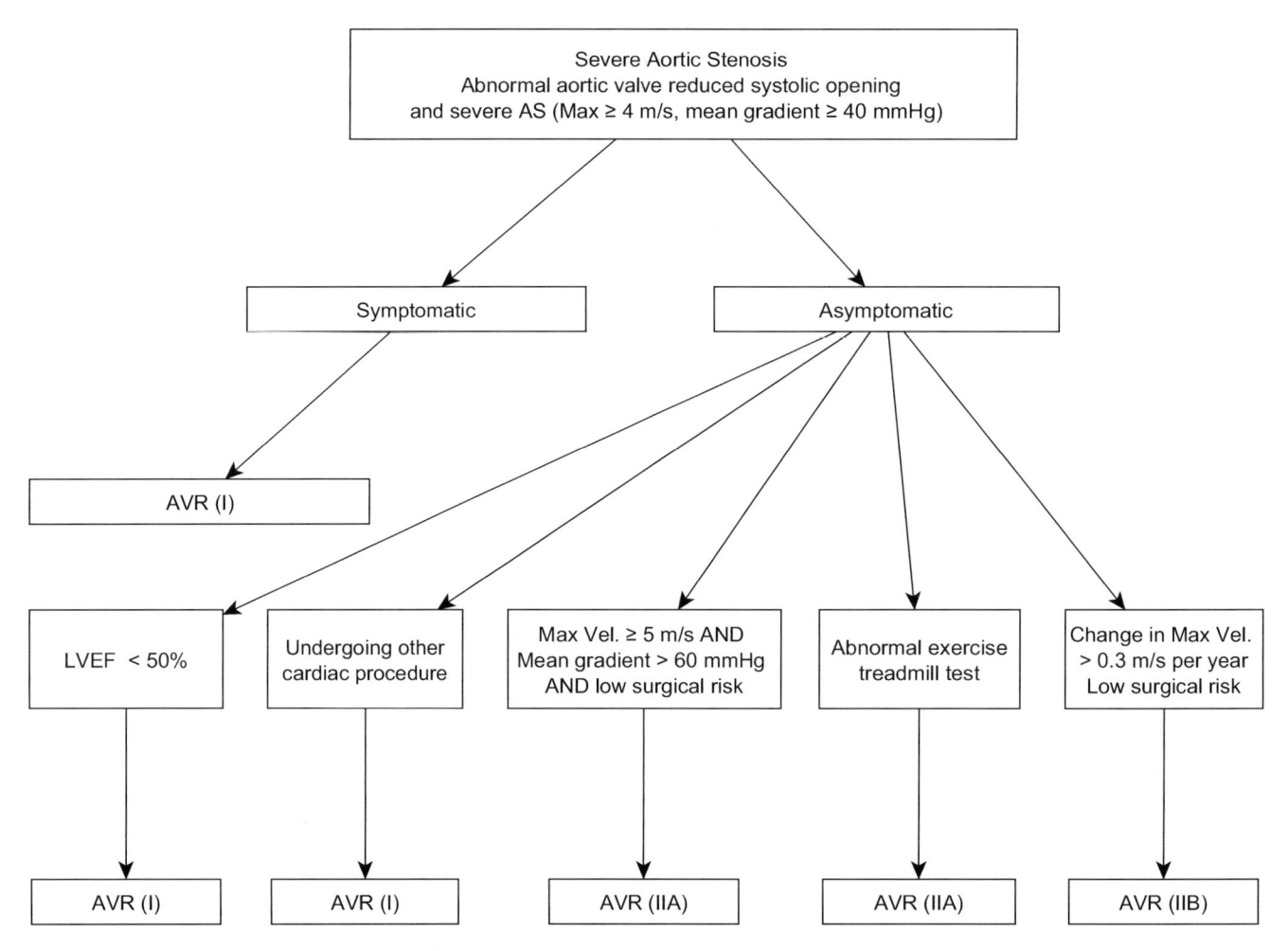

LVEF < 50%	Undergoing other cardiac procedure	Max Vel. ≥ 5 m/s AND Mean gradient > 60 mmHg AND low surgical risk	Abnormal exercise treadmill test	Change in Max Vel. > 0.3 m/s per year Low surgical risk
AVR (I)	AVR (I)	AVR (IIA)	AVR (IIA)	AVR (IIB)

AS, Aortic stenosis; AVR, Aortic Valve Replacement; LVEF, Left Ventricular Ejection Fraction; AVA, Aortic valve area; Vel, Velocity

Transcatheter Aortic Valve Replacement
Michael Kayatta, Vinod Thourani

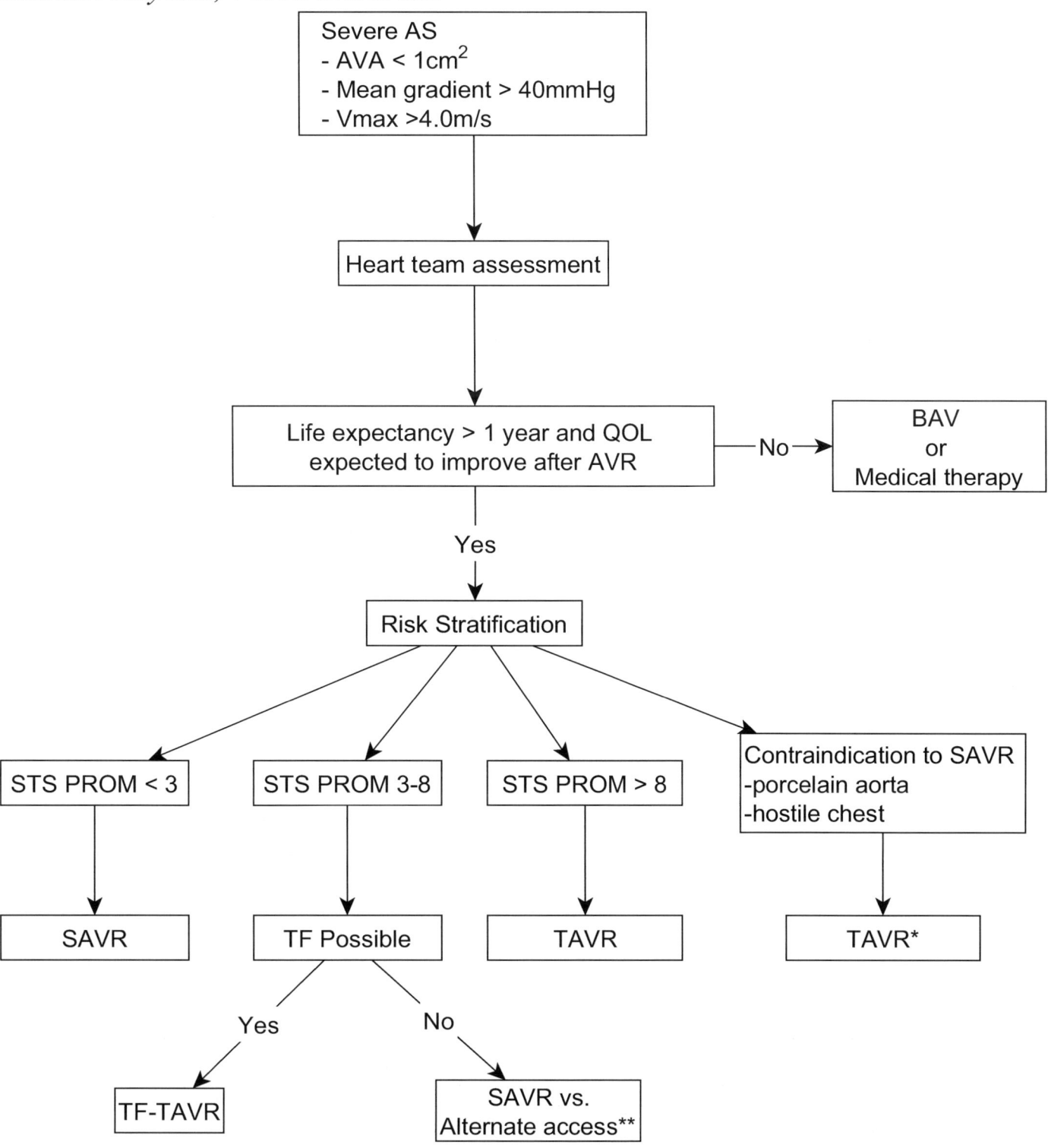

```
┌─────────────────────────┐
│ Severe AS               │
│  - AVA < 1cm²           │
│  - Mean gradient > 40mmHg│
│  - Vmax >4.0m/s         │
└───────────┬─────────────┘
            ▼
┌─────────────────────────┐
│ Heart team assessment   │
└───────────┬─────────────┘
            ▼
┌─────────────────────────────────┐       ┌──────────────┐
│ Life expectancy > 1 year and QOL│─ No ─▶│ BAV          │
│ expected to improve after AVR   │       │ or           │
└───────────┬─────────────────────┘       │ Medical therapy│
           Yes                            └──────────────┘
            ▼
┌─────────────────────────┐
│ Risk Stratification     │
└─┬────────┬─────────┬────┴─────┐
  ▼        ▼         ▼          ▼
┌──────┐ ┌────────┐ ┌────────┐ ┌──────────────────────┐
│STS   │ │STS PROM│ │STS PROM│ │Contraindication to SAVR│
│PROM<3│ │ 3-8    │ │ > 8    │ │ -porcelain aorta     │
└──┬───┘ └───┬────┘ └───┬────┘ │ -hostile chest       │
   ▼         ▼          ▼      └──────────┬───────────┘
┌──────┐ ┌──────────┐ ┌──────┐            ▼
│ SAVR │ │TF Possible│ │ TAVR │         ┌──────┐
└──────┘ └─┬──────┬─┘ └──────┘         │TAVR* │
         Yes     No                     └──────┘
           ▼      ▼
      ┌───────┐ ┌─────────────────┐
      │TF-TAVR│ │ SAVR vs.        │
      └───────┘ │ Alternate access**│
                └─────────────────┘
```

57

TAVR may be performed in low risk patients as part of a clinical trial.

*Anatomic criteria (eg: low coronaries, bicuspid valve) or other patient-specific factors may make SAVR more appropriate for some patients compared to TAVR.

**Transfemoral access is the preferred access route and is used in >90% of cases. Alternative access including aortic, apical, subclavian, carotid, or caval should be chosen on a case by case basis.

AS, aortic stenosis; AVA, aortic valve area; AVR, aortic valve replacement; BAV, balloon aortic valvuloplasty; QOL, quality of life; SAVR, surgical aortic valve replacement; STS PROM, Society of Thoracic Surgeons predicted risk of mortality; TAVR, transcatheter aortic valve replacement; TF, transfemoral

Aortic Insufficiency
Yogesh Patel, Philip Hess

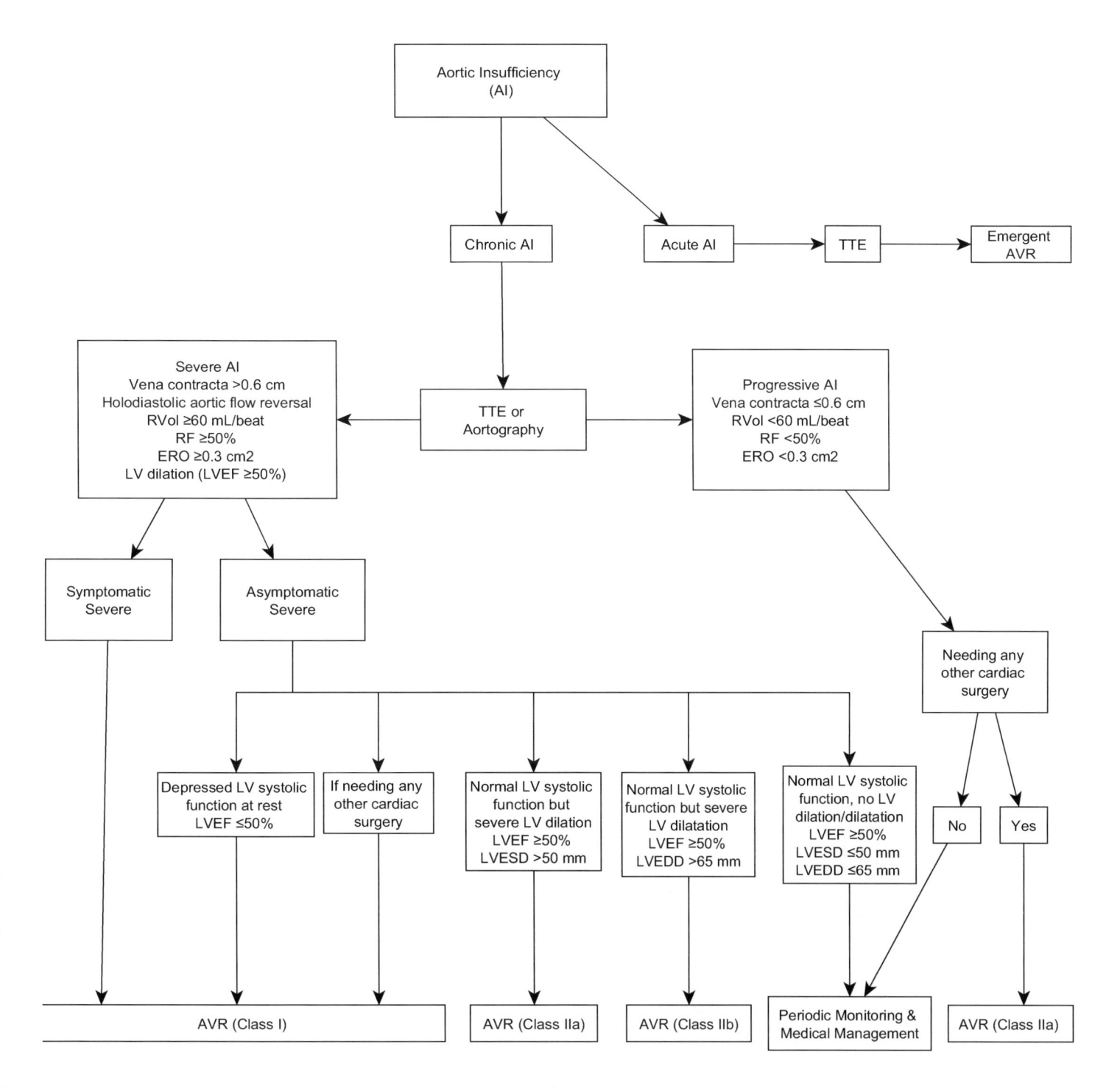

```
                    ┌─────────────────────┐
                    │ Aortic Insufficiency│
                    │        (AI)         │
                    └──────────┬──────────┘
                               │
              ┌────────────────┼────────────────┐
              ▼                                 ▼
        ┌──────────┐                      ┌──────────┐      ┌─────┐      ┌──────────┐
        │Chronic AI│                      │ Acute AI │ ───▶ │ TTE │ ───▶ │ Emergent │
        └────┬─────┘                      └──────────┘      └─────┘      │   AVR    │
             │                                                           └──────────┘
             ▼
        ┌──────────────┐
        │ TTE or       │
        │ Aortography  │
        └──────────────┘
```

Severe AI
- Vena contracta >0.6 cm
- Holodiastolic aortic flow reversal
- RVol ≥60 mL/beat
- RF ≥50%
- ERO ≥0.3 cm2
- LV dilation (LVEF ≥50%)

  → Symptomatic Severe
  → Asymptomatic Severe

Progressive AI
- Vena contracta ≤0.6 cm
- RVol <60 mL/beat
- RF <50%
- ERO <0.3 cm2

  → Needing any other cardiac surgery (No / Yes)

Symptomatic Severe → AVR (Class I)

Asymptomatic Severe:
- Depressed LV systolic function at rest LVEF ≤50% → AVR (Class I)
- If needing any other cardiac surgery → AVR (Class I)
- Normal LV systolic function but severe LV dilation LVEF ≥50% LVESD >50 mm → AVR (Class IIa)
- Normal LV systolic function but severe LV dilatation LVEF ≥50% LVEDD >65 mm → AVR (Class IIb)
- Normal LV systolic function, no LV dilation/dilatation LVEF ≥50% LVESD ≤50 mm LVEDD ≤65 mm → Periodic Monitoring & Medical Management

Progressive AI:
- No → Periodic Monitoring & Medical Management
- Yes → AVR (Class IIa)

Levels of recommendation are noted in parentheses
AI, Aortic Insufficiency; AVR, Aortic Valve Replacement; LVEF, Left ventricular ejection fraction; LVESD, Left ventricular end-systolic dimension; LVEDD, Left ventricular end-diastolic dimension; RF, Regurgitant fraction; RVol, Regurgitant volume; ERO, Effective regurgitant orifice

Management of Small Aortic Root
Carlo Maria Rosati, Christopher Lau

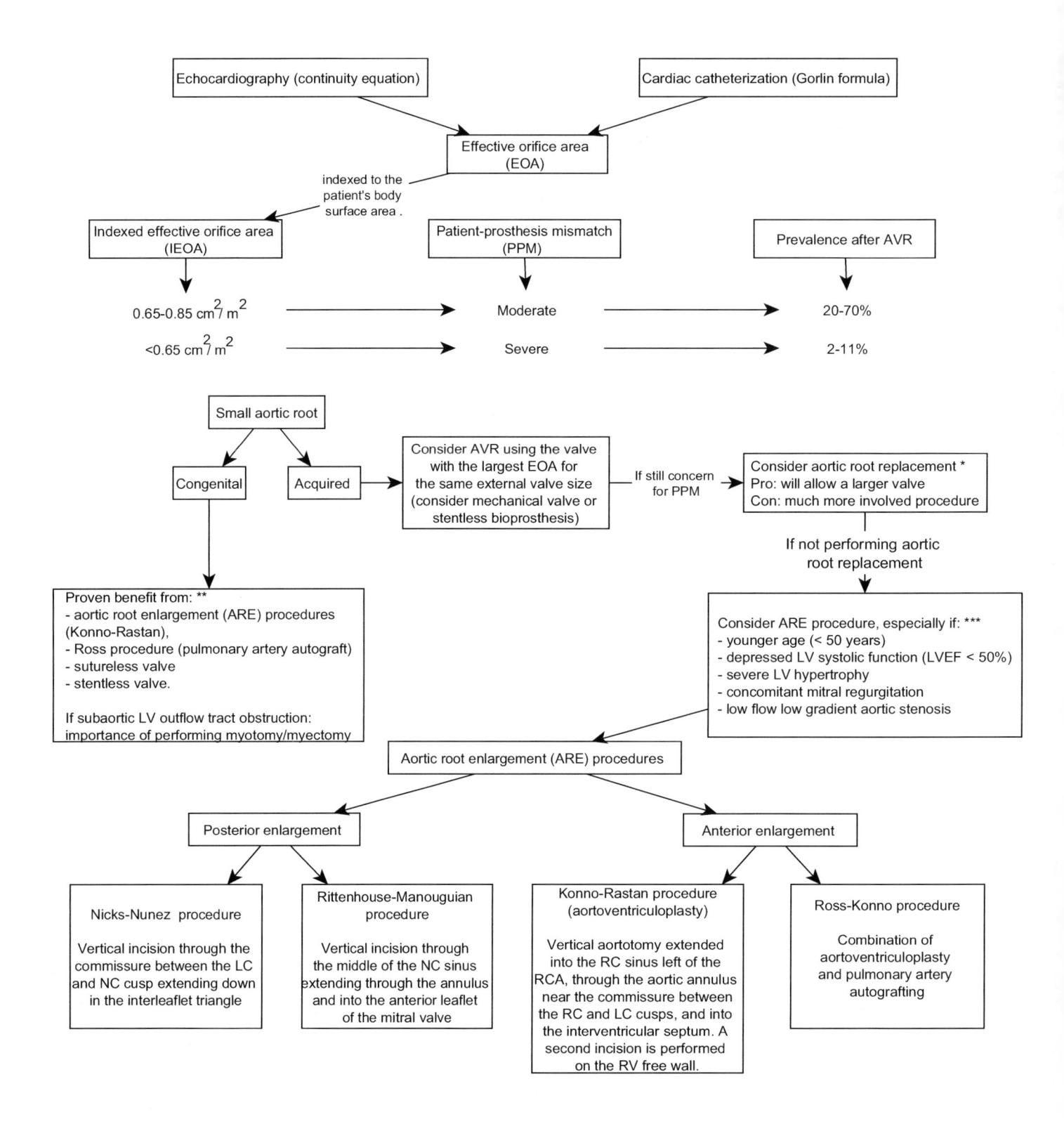

```
        Echocardiography (continuity equation)         Cardiac catheterization (Gorlin formula)
                            \                           /
                             → Effective orifice area ←
                                      (EOA)
              indexed to the  /
              patient's body
              surface area
         ↓
Indexed effective orifice area        Patient-prosthesis mismatch           Prevalence after AVR
         (IEOA)                                 (PPM)
           ↓                                      ↓                               ↓
   0.65-0.85 cm²/m²        →              Moderate             →              20-70%

     <0.65 cm²/m²          →              Severe               →              2-11%
```

```
                   Small aortic root
                    /          \
              Congenital      Acquired  →  Consider AVR using the valve      If still concern    Consider aortic root replacement *
                                            with the largest EOA for          for PPM      →    Pro: will allow a larger valve
                                            the same external valve size                         Con: much more involved procedure
                                            (consider mechanical valve or
                                            stentless bioprosthesis)
                                                                                                  If not performing aortic
                                                                                                    root replacement
                                                                                                           ↓
       ↓                                                                            Consider ARE procedure, especially if: ***
Proven benefit from: **                                                             - younger age (< 50 years)
 - aortic root enlargement (ARE)                                                    - depressed LV systolic function (LVEF < 50%)
   procedures (Konno-Rastan),                                                       - severe LV hypertrophy
 - Ross procedure (pulmonary artery autograft)                                      - concomitant mitral regurgitation
 - sutureless valve                                                                 - low flow low gradient aortic stenosis
 - stentless valve.

If subaortic LV outflow tract obstruction:
importance of performing myotomy/myectomy
                                                            ↓
                                         Aortic root enlargement (ARE) procedures
                                              /                            \
                                 Posterior enlargement              Anterior enlargement
                                  /           \                       /              \
                        Nicks-Nunez       Rittenhouse-       Konno-Rastan procedure     Ross-Konno procedure
                         procedure         Manouguian        (aortoventriculoplasty)
                                           procedure
                     Vertical incision    Vertical incision  Vertical aortotomy extended   Combination of
                     through the         through the         into the RC sinus left of the  aortoventriculoplasty
                     commissure between  middle of the NC    RCA, through the aortic annulus and pulmonary artery
                     the LC and NC cusp  sinus extending     near the commissure between    autografting
                     extending down      through the annulus the RC and LC cusps, and into
                     in the interleaflet and into the anterior the interventricular septum. A
                     triangle            leaflet of the      second incision is performed
                                         mitral valve        on the RV free wall.
```

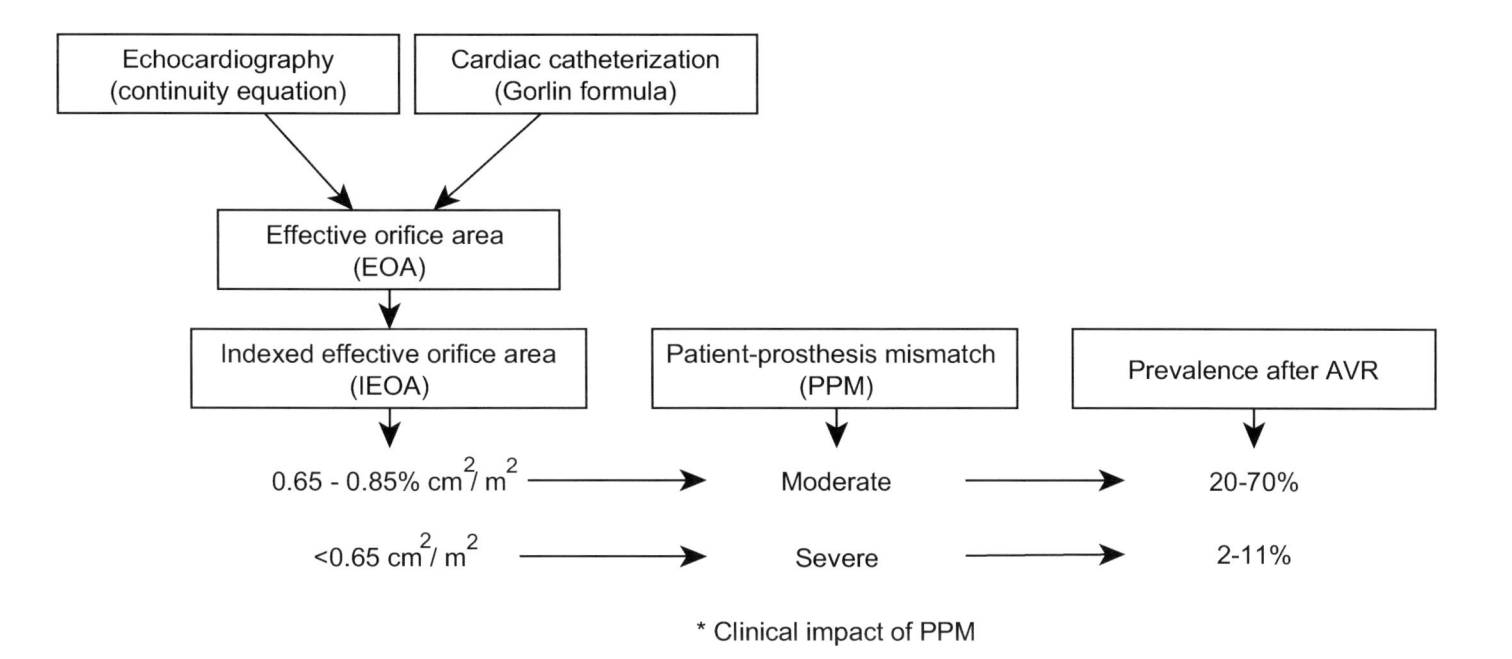

```
┌─────────────────────────┐   ┌─────────────────────────┐
│   Echocardiography      │   │  Cardiac catheterization│
│  (continuity equation)  │   │     (Gorlin formula)    │
└───────────┬─────────────┘   └───────────┬─────────────┘
            │                             │
            └──────────────┬──────────────┘
                           ▼
            ┌──────────────────────────┐
            │  Effective orifice area  │
            │          (EOA)           │
            └──────────────┬───────────┘
                           ▼
┌──────────────────────────┐   ┌─────────────────────────┐   ┌─────────────────────────┐
│ Indexed effective orifice│   │Patient-prosthesis mismatch│  │  Prevalence after AVR   │
│        area (IEOA)       │   │          (PPM)          │   │                         │
└──────────────┬───────────┘   └───────────┬─────────────┘   └───────────┬─────────────┘
               ▼                           ▼                             ▼
```

0.65 - 0.85% cm^2/m^2 ⟶ Moderate ⟶ 20-70%

<0.65 cm^2/m^2 ⟶ Severe ⟶ 2-11%

* Clinical impact of PPM

```
┌─────────────────┐
│ Small Aortic Root│
└────────┬────────┘
    ┌────┴────┐
    ▼         ▼
┌────────┐ ┌────────┐      ┌──────────────────────┐                      ┌──────────────────────┐
│Congenital│ │Acquired│ ──▶ │Consider AVR using the│ If concern for PPM  │Consider aortic root  │
└────┬───┘ └────────┘      │valve with the largest│ ──────────────────▶ │replacement*          │
     │                     │EOA for the same extent│                     └──────────┬───────────┘
     │                     │valve size (consider   │                                │
     │                     │mechanical valve or    │                                │ If not performing
     │                     │stentless bioprosthesis)│                               │ aortic root replacement
     │                     └──────────────────────┘                                 ▼
     ▼                                                               ┌──────────────────────────────┐
┌──────────────────────────────┐                                     │Consider ARE procedure,       │
│Proven benefit from: **       │                                     │especially if:***             │
│- aortic root enlargement(ARE)│                                     │- Younger age (<50 years)     │
│  procedures (Konno-Rastan)   │                                     │- depressed LV systolic       │
│- Ross procedure (pulmonary   │                                     │  function (LVEF < 50%)       │
│  artery autograft)           │                                     │- severe LV hypertrophy       │
│- Sutureless valve            │                                     │- concomitant mitral          │
│- Stentless valve             │                                     │  regurgitation               │
└──────────────┬───────────────┘                                     │- low flow low gradient       │
               │                                                     │  aortic stenosis             │
               │                                                     └──────────────┬───────────────┘
               └──────────────────────┬──────────────────────────────────────────────┘
                                      ▼
                         ┌──────────────────────────┐
                         │Aortic root enlargement   │
                         │(ARE) procedures          │
                         └────────────┬─────────────┘
                        ┌─────────────┴─────────────┐
                        ▼                           ▼
              ┌──────────────────┐       ┌──────────────────┐
              │Posterior         │       │Anterior          │
              │enlargement       │       │enlargement       │
              └─────────┬────────┘       └─────────┬────────┘
                ┌───────┴───────┐           ┌──────┴───────┐
                ▼               ▼           ▼              ▼
         ┌────────────┐ ┌──────────────┐ ┌──────────────┐ ┌──────────┐
         │Nicks-Nunez │ │Rittenhouse-  │ │Konno-Rastan  │ │Ross-Konno│
         │procedure   │ │Manouguian    │ │procedure     │ │procedure │
         │            │ │procedure     │ │(aortoventri- │ │          │
         │            │ │              │ │culoplasty)   │ │          │
         └────────────┘ └──────────────┘ └──────────────┘ └──────────┘
```

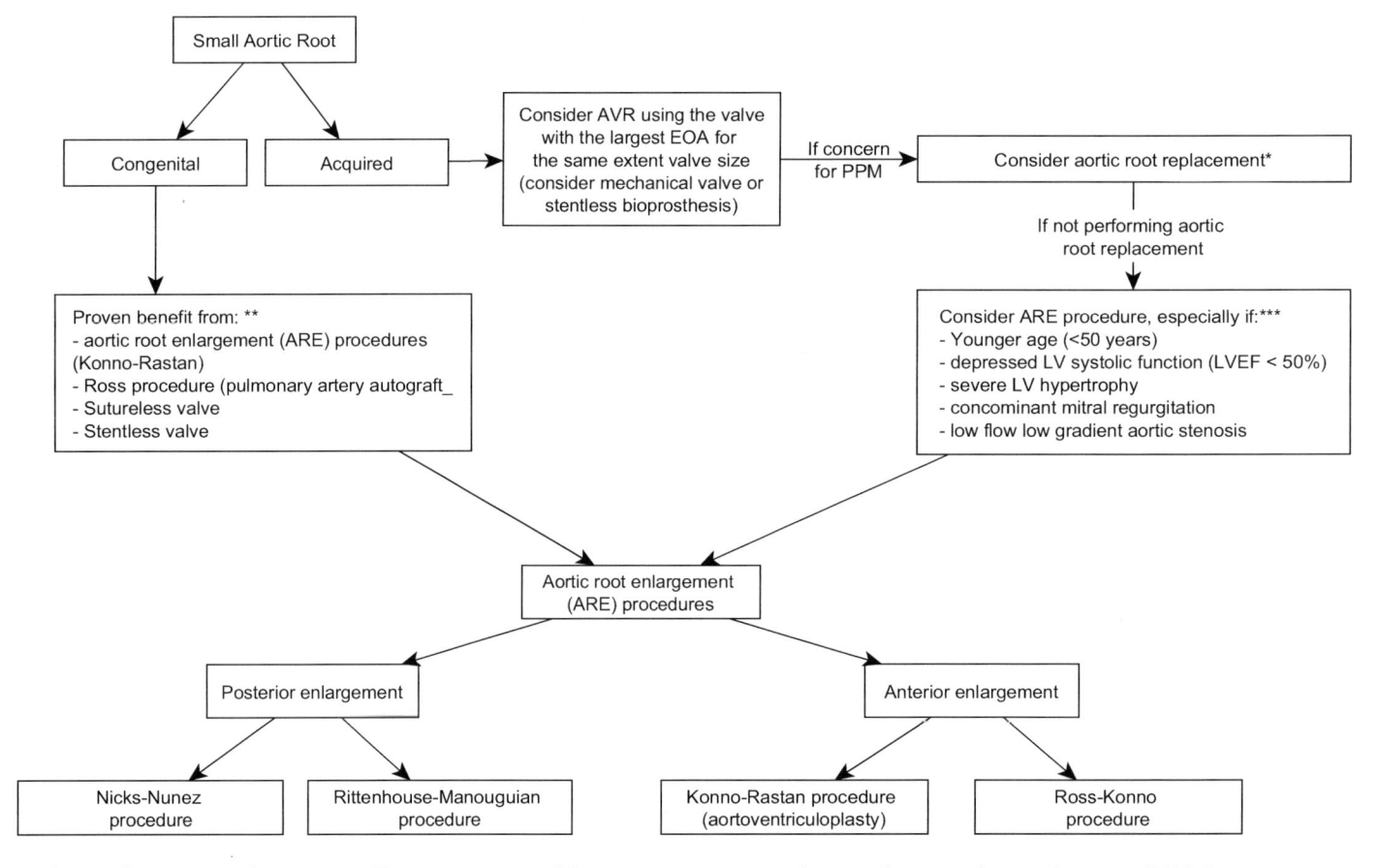

*Clinical impact of PPM- still controversial but increasing evidence that moderate/severe PPM is associated with less improvement in functional status, less regression of LV hypertrophy, higher risk of heart failure, redo AVR, and increased long-term mortality.

** Pro: will allow a larger valve. Con: Much more involved procedure.

** If subaortic LV outflow tract obstruction: importance of performing myotomy/myectomy.

*** Pros: larger neo-aortic annulus, less PPM. Cons: unclear evidence of long-term overall survival or functional status advantage; longer operative and cross clamp times; possible increase in perioperative morbidity and mortality

ARE, aortic root enlargement; AVR, aortic valve replacement; EOA, effective orifice area; IEOA, indexed effective orifice area; LC, left coronary; LV, left ventricle; NC, noncoronary; PPM, patient-prosthesis mismatch; RC, right coronary; RV, right ventricle

Non-cardiac surgery and aortic valve endocarditis
Parth Amin, Ryan Plichta

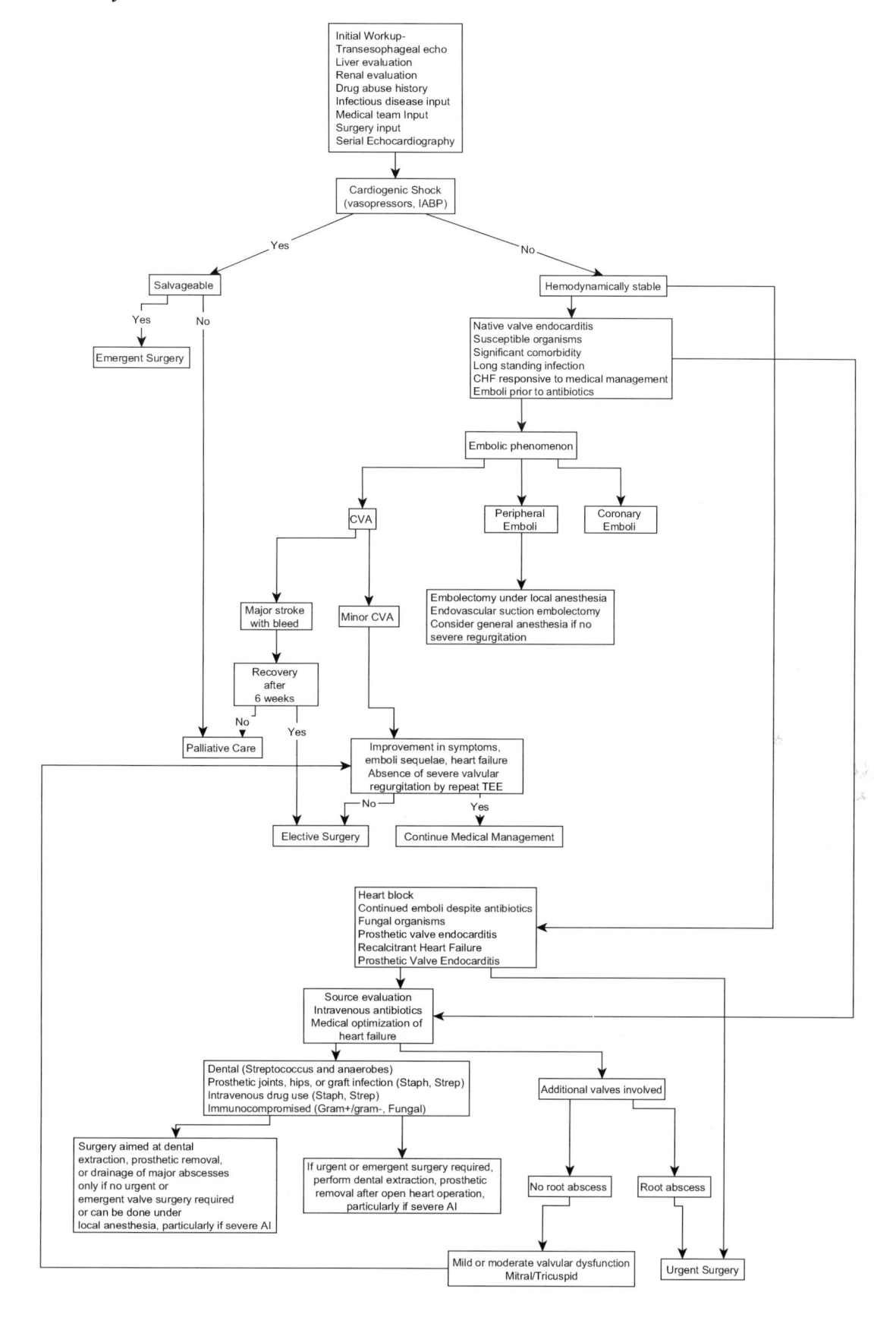

```
┌─────────────────────────┐
│ Initial Workup-         │
│ Transesophageal echo    │
│ Liver evaluation        │
│ Renal evaluation        │
│ Drug abuse history      │
│ Infectious disease input│
│ Medical team Input      │
│ Surgery input           │
│ Serial Echocardiography │
└─────────────────────────┘
              │
              ▼
   ┌──────────────────────┐
   │ Cardiogenic Shock    │
   │ (vasopressors, IABP) │
   └──────────────────────┘
       Yes ↙        ↘ No
   ┌──────────┐   ┌─────────────────────┐
   │Salvageable│  │Hemodynamically stable│
   └──────────┘   └─────────────────────┘
   Yes ↙  ↘ No              │
 ┌────────┐                  ▼
 │Emergent│        ┌──────────────────────────────┐
 │Surgery │        │ Native valve endocarditis    │
 └────────┘        │ Susceptible organisms        │
                   │ Significant comorbidity      │
                   │ Long standing infection      │
                   │ CHF responsive to medical mgmt│
                   │ Emboli prior to antibiotics  │
                   └──────────────────────────────┘
                                │
                                ▼
                   ┌──────────────────┐
                   │Embolic phenomenon│
                   └──────────────────┘
                    ↙       ↓        ↘
                ┌─────┐ ┌──────────┐ ┌────────┐
                │ CVA │ │Peripheral│ │Coronary│
                └─────┘ │  Emboli  │ │ Emboli │
                  ↙ ↘   └──────────┘ └────────┘
        ┌──────────┐ ┌─────────┐
        │Major     │ │Minor CVA│    ┌────────────────────────────────┐
        │stroke    │ └─────────┘    │Embolectomy under local anesthesia│
        │with bleed│                │Endovascular suction embolectomy │
        └──────────┘                │Consider general anesthesia if no│
              │                     │severe regurgitation             │
              ▼                     └────────────────────────────────┘
        ┌─────────┐
        │Recovery │
        │after    │
        │6 weeks  │
        └─────────┘
        No ↙  ↘ Yes
    ┌──────────┐    ┌──────────────────────────────┐
    │Palliative│    │Improvement in symptoms,      │
    │  Care    │    │emboli sequelae, heart failure│
    └──────────┘    │Absence of severe valvular    │
         │          │regurgitation by repeat TEE   │
         ▼          └──────────────────────────────┘
    ┌────────┐           No ↙        ↘ Yes
    │  Next  │    ┌─────────────┐  ┌──────────────────────┐
    │  Page  │    │Elective     │  │Continue Medical      │
    └────────┘    │Surgery      │  │Management            │
                  └─────────────┘  └──────────────────────┘

                                           Next Page   Next Page
```

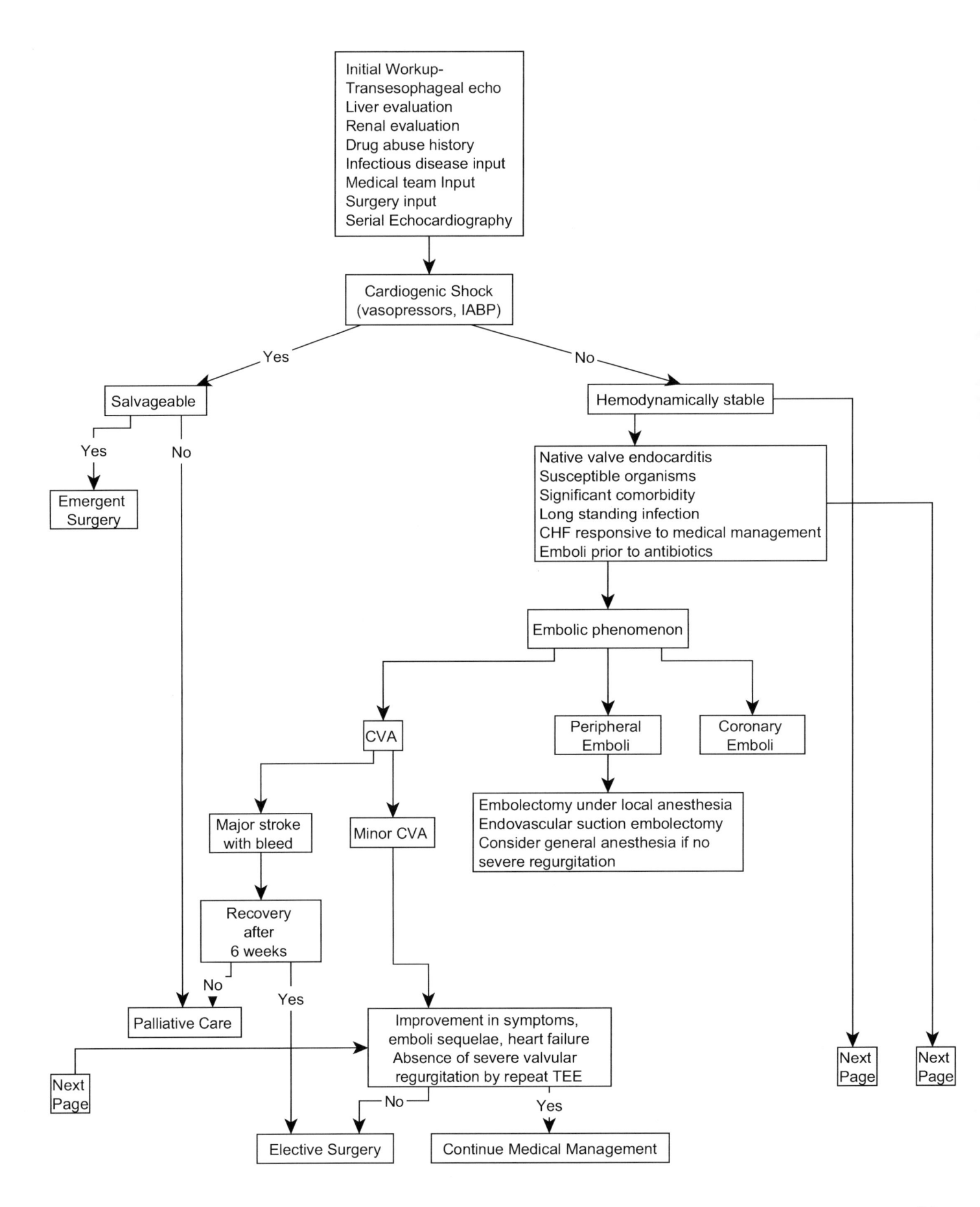

64

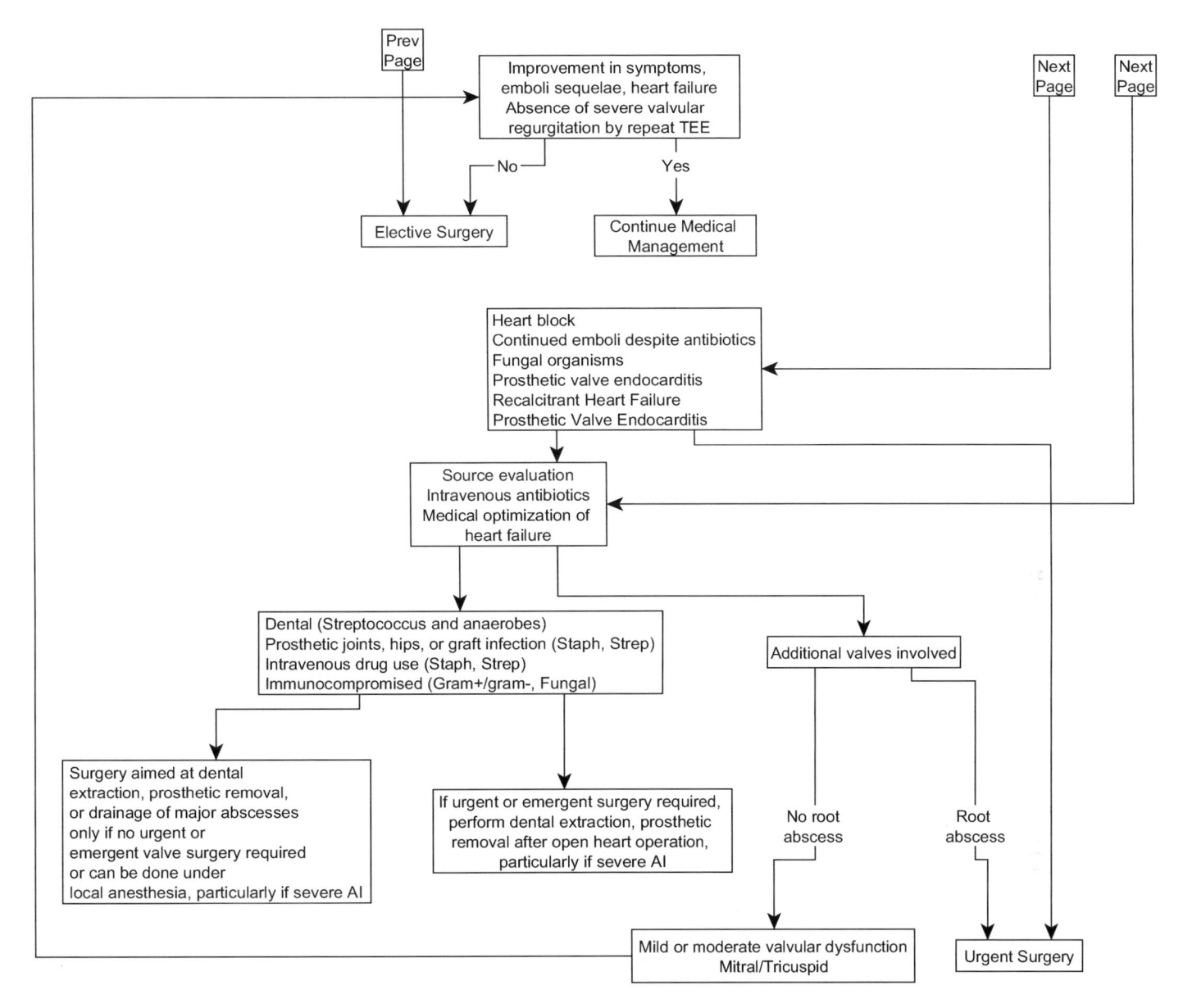

```
[Prev Page] → Improvement in symptoms,
              emboli sequelae, heart failure
              Absence of severe valvular
              regurgitation by repeat TEE
                    │          │
                   No         Yes
                    ↓          ↓
              Elective Surgery    Continue Medical
                                  Management

[Next Page] → Heart block
              Continued emboli despite antibiotics
              Fungal organisms
              Prosthetic valve endocarditis
              Recalcitrant Heart Failure
              Prosthetic Valve Endocarditis
                    ↓
[Next Page] → Source evaluation
              Intravenous antibiotics
              Medical optimization of
              heart failure
                    ↓
              Dental (Streptococcus and anaerobes)
              Prosthetic joints, hips, or graft infection (Staph, Strep)
              Intravenous drug use (Staph, Strep)
              Immunocompromised (Gram+/gram-, Fungal)
                                                     Additional valves involved
                    ↓                                    │         │
  Surgery aimed at dental      If urgent or emergent   No root    Root
  extraction, prosthetic       surgery required,       abscess    abscess
  removal, or drainage of      perform dental
  major abscesses only if      extraction, prosthetic
  no urgent or emergent        removal after open
  valve surgery required       heart operation,
  or can be done under         particularly if severe AI
  local anesthesia,
  particularly if severe AI
                               Mild or moderate valvular dysfunction
                               Mitral/Tricuspid              Urgent Surgery
```

CVA, cerebrovascular accident; TEE, transesophageal echocardiography; TTE, transthoracic echocardiography

Indications for Surgical Intervention in the Treatment of Tricuspid Disease at the Time of Operation for Left-Sided Valvular Disease

Rahul R. Handa, MD, Spencer J. Melby, MD

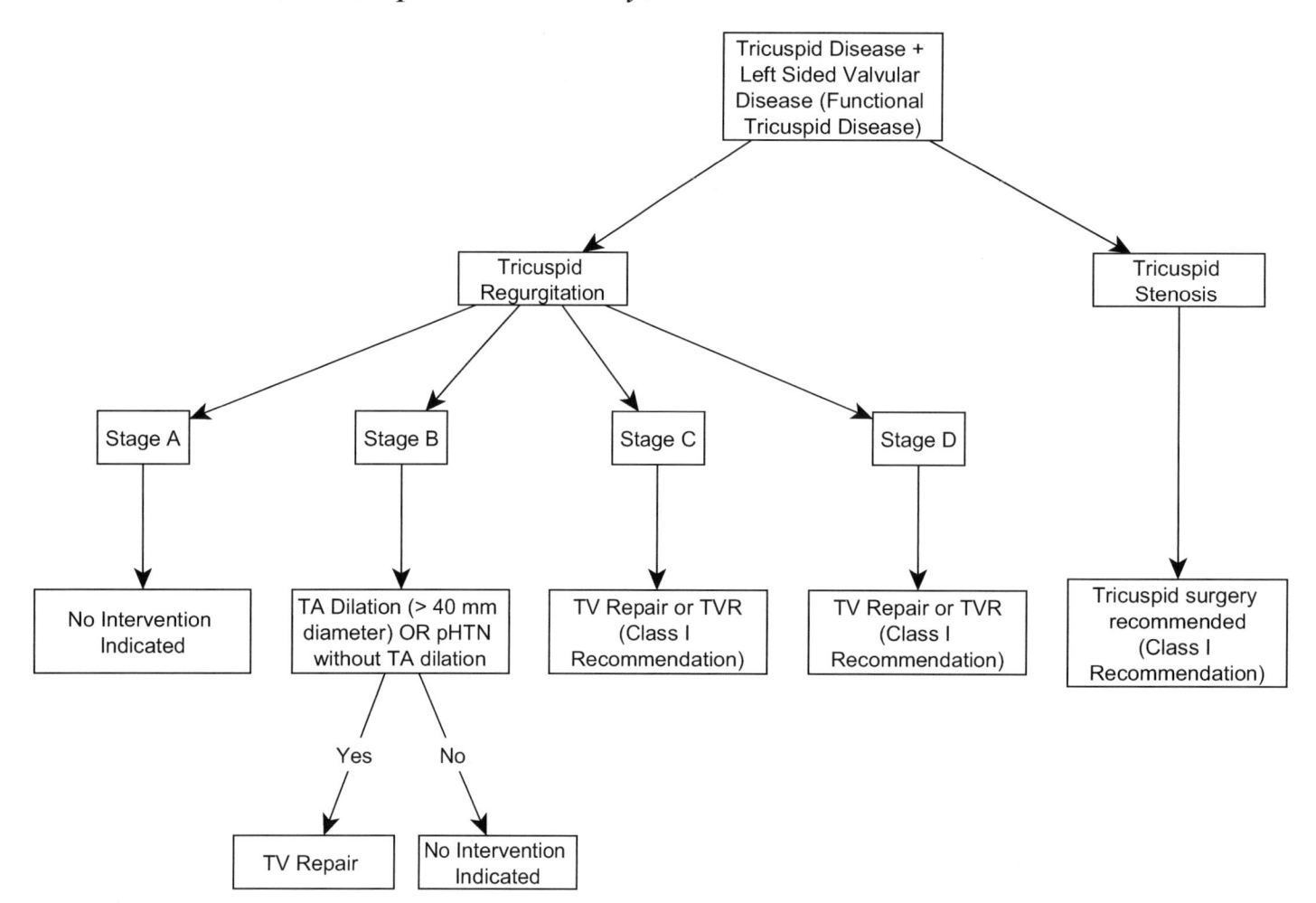

```
                    Tricuspid Disease +
                    Left Sided Valvular
                    Disease (Functional
                    Tricuspid Disease)
                   /                    \
        Tricuspid Regurgitation        Tricuspid Stenosis
        /      |        |      \              |
   Stage A  Stage B  Stage C  Stage D    Tricuspid surgery
      |        |        |        |        recommended
      |        |        |        |        (Class I
      |        |        |        |        Recommendation)
 No Intervention  TA Dilation   TV Repair or TVR   TV Repair or TVR
    Indicated    (> 40 mm       (Class I           (Class I
                 diameter) OR   Recommendation)    Recommendation)
                 pHTN without
                 TA dilation
                    /    \
                  Yes    No
                   |      |
                TV Repair  No Intervention
                           Indicated
```

66

Stages of Tricuspid Regurgitation

Stage	Degree of TR	Hemodynamic Consequences				Symptoms
		RV size	RA Size	IVC Size	RA Pressure	
Stage A	Trace TR	Normal				None, or in relation to other valvular disease
Stage B	Mild TR	
(Progressive)	Moderate TR	Normal	Normal or mildly enlarged	Normal or mildly enlarged	Normal	
Stage C (Severe, Asymptomatic)	Severe TR	Dilated	Dilated	Dilated	Elevated with "c-V" Wave	
Stage D (Severe, Symptomatic)						Fatigue, palpitations, dyspnea, bloating, anorexia, edema

Stage	Degree of TR	Valve Hemodynamics			
		Central Jet Area (cm²)	Vena Contracta Width (cm)	CW Jet Density and Contour	Hepatic Vein Flow
Stage A	Trace TR	< 5	< .7	Soft, parabolic	Systolic dominance
Stage B	Mild TR				
(Progressive)	Moderate TR	10-May		Dense, variable contour	Systolic blunting
Stage C (Severe, Asymptomatic)	Severe TR	> 10	> .7	Dense, triangular w/ early peak	Systolic Reversal
Stage D (Severe, Symptomatic)					

Mitral regurgitation – Valve reconstruction options
Sudhan Nagarajan, Percy Boateng

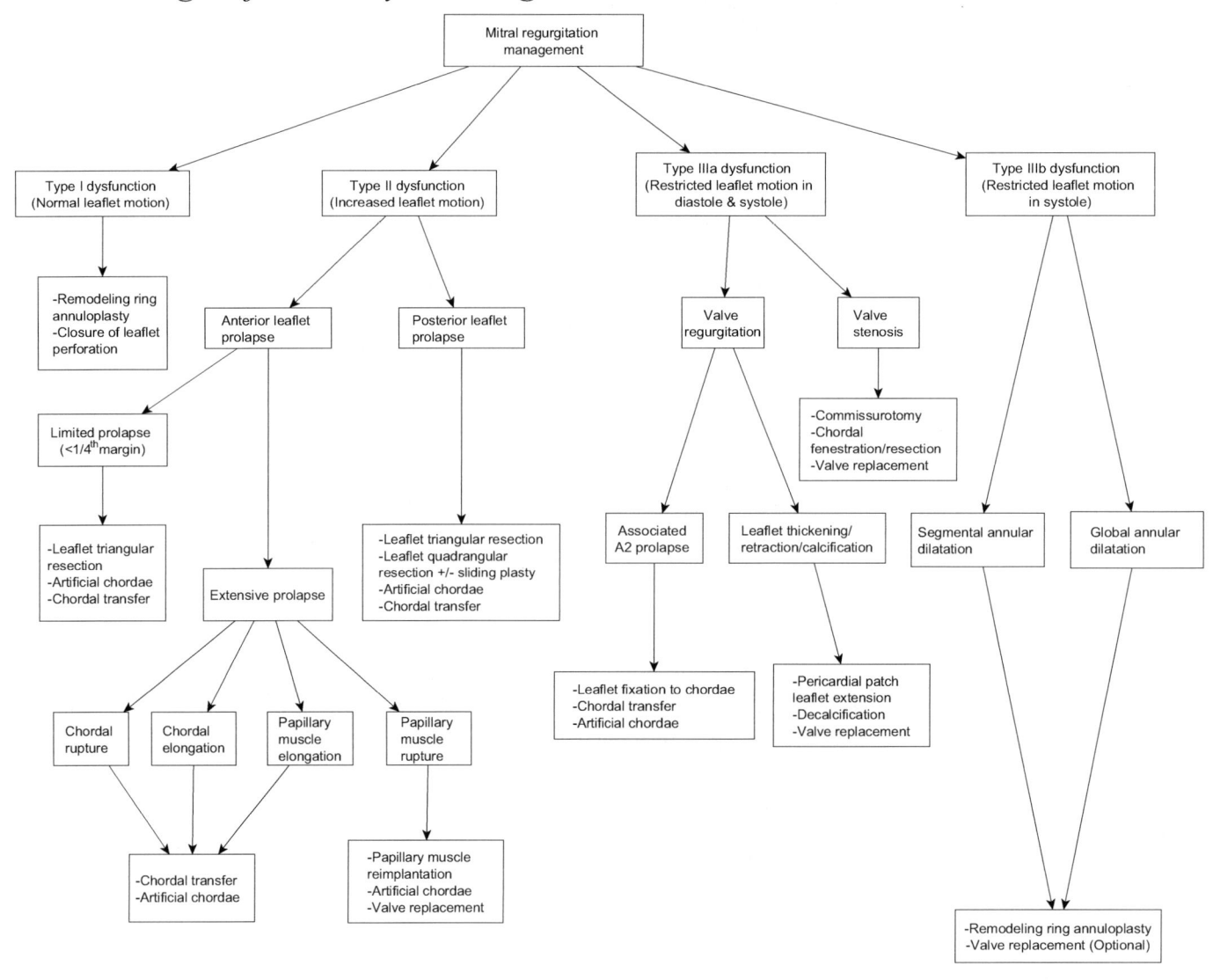

```
                            Mitral regurgitation
                                management
         ┌──────────────────┬────────────────────┬──────────────────┐
         ▼                  ▼                    ▼                  ▼
  Type I dysfunction   Type II dysfunction   Type IIIa dysfunction   Type IIIb dysfunction
  (Normal leaflet      (Increased leaflet    (Restricted leaflet     (Restricted leaflet
   motion)              motion)               motion in diastole      motion in systole)
                                              & systole)
         │                  │                    │                  │
         ▼                  │                    │                  │
  -Remodeling ring     ┌────┴────┐          ┌────┴────┐        ┌────┴────┐
   annuloplasty        ▼         ▼          ▼         ▼        ▼         ▼
  -Closure of leaflet  Anterior  Posterior  Valve     Valve    Segmental Global
   perforation         leaflet   leaflet    regurgi-  stenosis annular   annular
                       prolapse  prolapse   tation             dilatation dilatation
                          │         │         │         │
                          ▼         ▼         │         ▼
                    Limited    -Leaflet       │    -Commissurotomy
                    prolapse    triangular    │    -Chordal
                    (<1/4th     resection     │     fenestration/resection
                    margin)    -Leaflet       │    -Valve replacement
                       │        quadrangular  │
                       ▼        resection     │
                    -Leaflet    +/- sliding   │
                     triangular plasty        │
                     resection -Artificial    │
                    -Artificial chordae       │
                     chordae   -Chordal       │
                    -Chordal    transfer      │
                     transfer                 │
                          │                ┌──┴──┐
                          ▼                ▼     ▼
                    Extensive         Associated  Leaflet thickening/
                    prolapse          A2 prolapse retraction/calcification
              ┌────┬────┬────┐             │           │
              ▼    ▼    ▼    ▼             ▼           ▼
           Chordal Chordal Papillary Papillary  -Leaflet fixation  -Pericardial patch
           rupture elonga- muscle    muscle      to chordae         leaflet extension
                   tion    elonga-   rupture    -Chordal transfer  -Decalcification
                           tion                 -Artificial chordae -Valve replacement
              │    │    │    │
              ▼    ▼    ▼    ▼
           -Chordal transfer  -Papillary muscle
           -Artificial chordae  reimplantation
                               -Artificial chordae
                               -Valve replacement

                                              -Remodeling ring annuloplasty
                                              -Valve replacement (Optional)
```

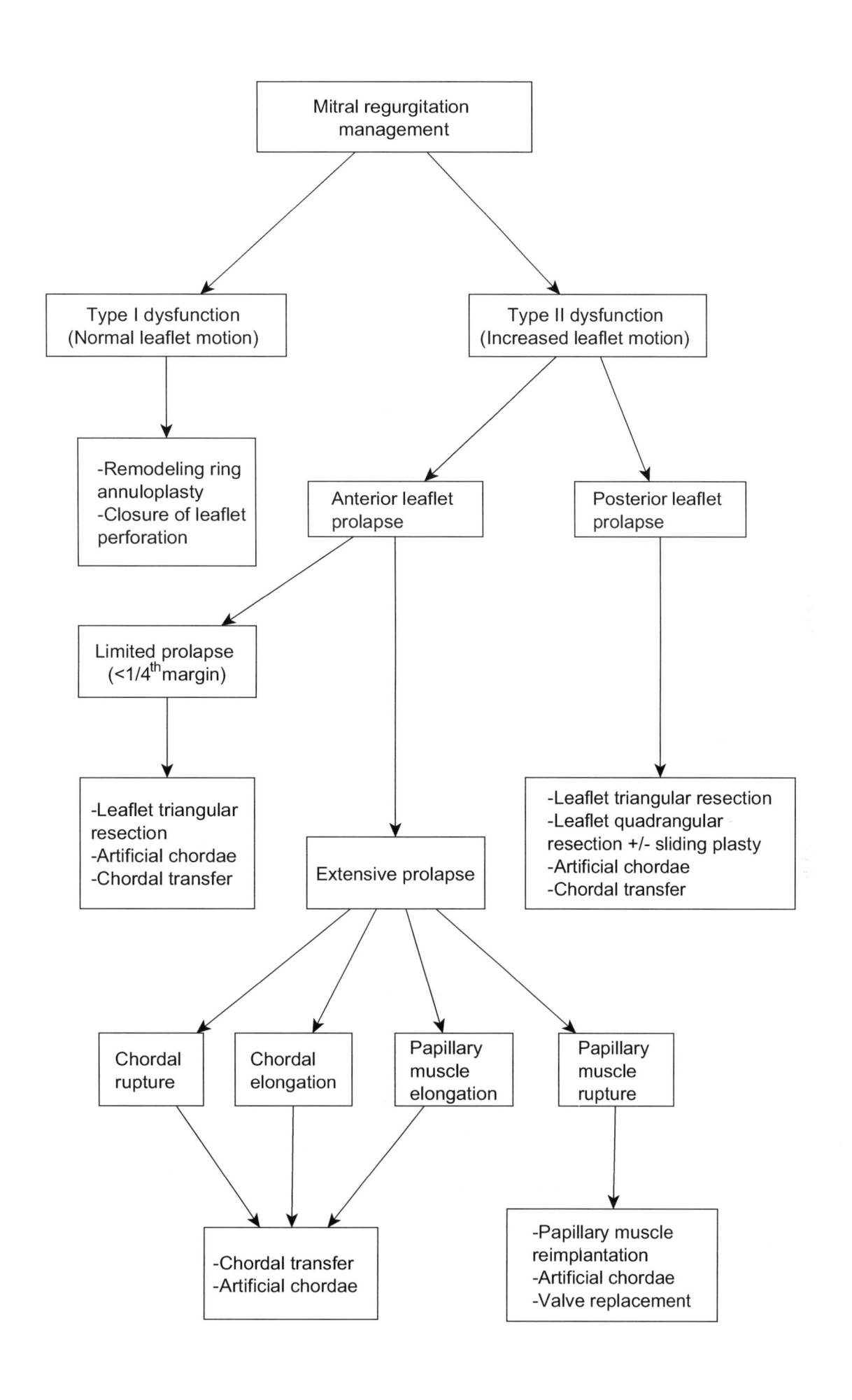

```
                    ┌─────────────────────┐
                    │ Mitral regurgitation│
                    │     management      │
                    └──────────┬──────────┘
                               │
              ┌────────────────┴────────────────┐
              ▼                                 ▼
  ┌─────────────────────┐           ┌─────────────────────┐
  │  Type I dysfunction │           │ Type II dysfunction │
  │(Normal leaflet motion)│         │(Increased leaflet motion)│
  └──────────┬──────────┘           └──────────┬──────────┘
             │                                 │
             ▼                     ┌───────────┴───────────┐
  ┌─────────────────────┐          ▼                       ▼
  │ -Remodeling ring    │  ┌───────────────┐      ┌───────────────┐
  │  annuloplasty       │  │Anterior leaflet│     │Posterior leaflet│
  │ -Closure of leaflet │  │   prolapse    │      │   prolapse    │
  │  perforation        │  └───────┬───────┘      └───────┬───────┘
  └─────────────────────┘          │                      │
                                   │                      │
                    ┌──────────────┤                      │
                    ▼              │                      ▼
         ┌─────────────────┐       │           ┌─────────────────────┐
         │ Limited prolapse│       │           │-Leaflet triangular resection│
         │  (<1/4th margin)│       │           │-Leaflet quadrangular│
         └────────┬────────┘       │           │ resection +/- sliding plasty│
                  ▼                ▼           │-Artificial chordae  │
         ┌─────────────────┐  ┌──────────┐     │-Chordal transfer    │
         │-Leaflet triangular│ │Extensive │    └─────────────────────┘
         │ resection       │  │ prolapse │
         │-Artificial chordae│ └────┬─────┘
         │-Chordal transfer│       │
         └─────────────────┘   ┌───┼───┬────────┐
                               ▼   ▼   ▼        ▼
                           ┌──────┐┌──────┐┌────────┐┌──────────┐
                           │Chordal││Chordal││Papillary││Papillary│
                           │rupture││elongation││muscle ││muscle   │
                           │      ││      ││elongation││rupture  │
                           └──┬───┘└──┬───┘└────┬───┘└────┬─────┘
                              │       │        │         │
                              └───────┴────────┘         ▼
                                      ▼         ┌─────────────────┐
                           ┌─────────────────┐  │-Papillary muscle│
                           │-Chordal transfer│  │ reimplantation  │
                           │-Artificial chordae│ │-Artificial chordae│
                           └─────────────────┘  │-Valve replacement│
                                                └─────────────────┘
```

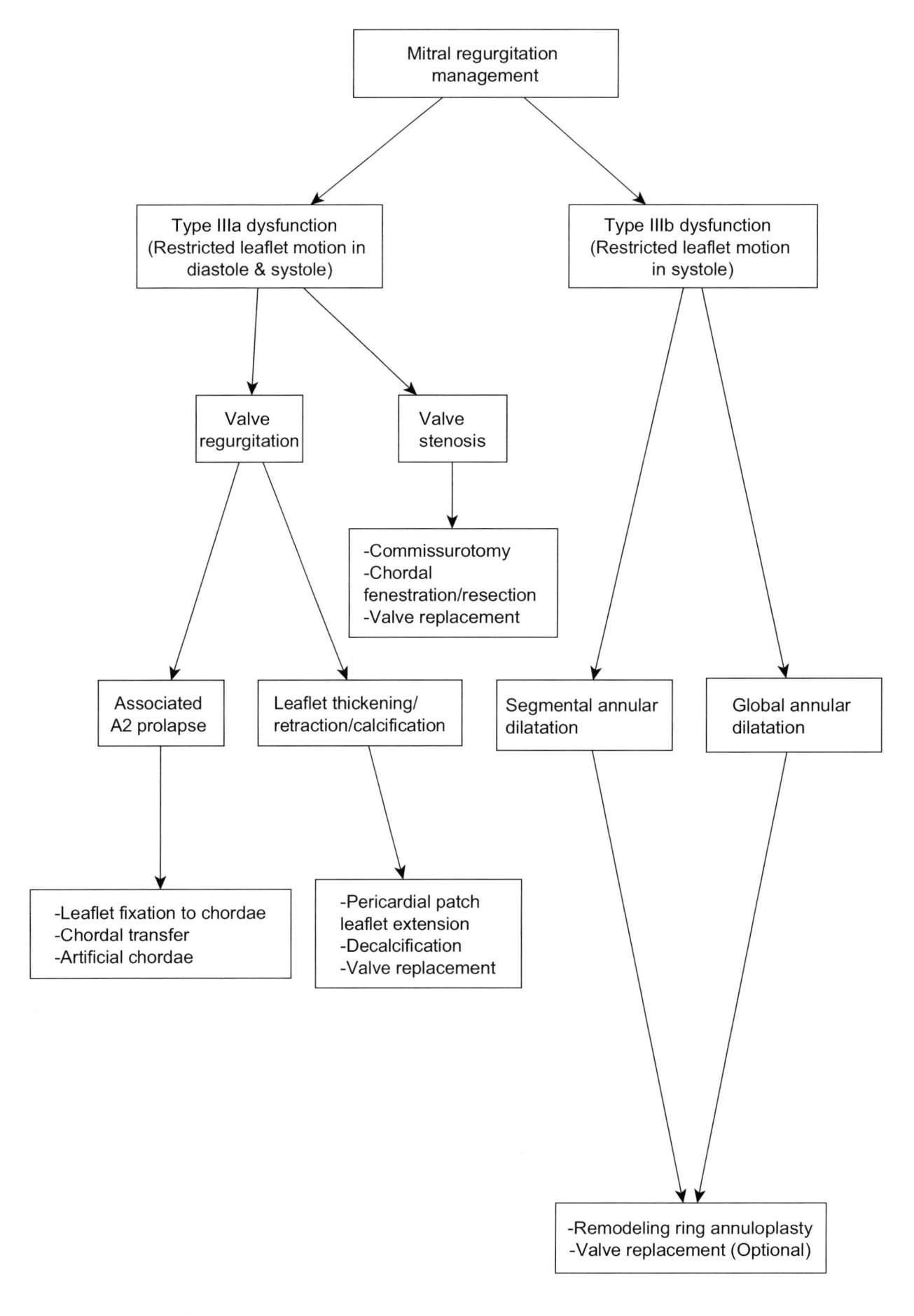

```
                    ┌─────────────────────┐
                    │ Mitral regurgitation│
                    │    management       │
                    └─────────────────────┘
                      ↙               ↘
    ┌──────────────────────┐      ┌──────────────────────┐
    │ Type IIIa dysfunction│      │ Type IIIb dysfunction│
    │(Restricted leaflet   │      │(Restricted leaflet   │
    │ motion in            │      │ motion in systole)   │
    │ diastole & systole)  │      │                      │
    └──────────────────────┘      └──────────────────────┘
         ↙         ↘                    ↙         ↘
   ┌────────┐   ┌────────┐
   │ Valve  │   │ Valve  │
   │regurgi-│   │stenosis│
   │tation  │   │        │
   └────────┘   └────────┘
```

Type IIIa – Valve stenosis:
- Commissurotomy
- Chordal fenestration/resection
- Valve replacement

Type IIIa – Valve regurgitation:

Associated A2 prolapse:
- Leaflet fixation to chordae
- Chordal transfer
- Artificial chordae

Leaflet thickening/retraction/calcification:
- Pericardial patch leaflet extension
- Decalcification
- Valve replacement

Type IIIb – Segmental annular dilatation / Global annular dilatation:
- Remodeling ring annuloplasty
- Valve replacement (Optional)

Mitral regurgitation - Indications for Surgery
Sudhan Nagarajan, Percy Boateng

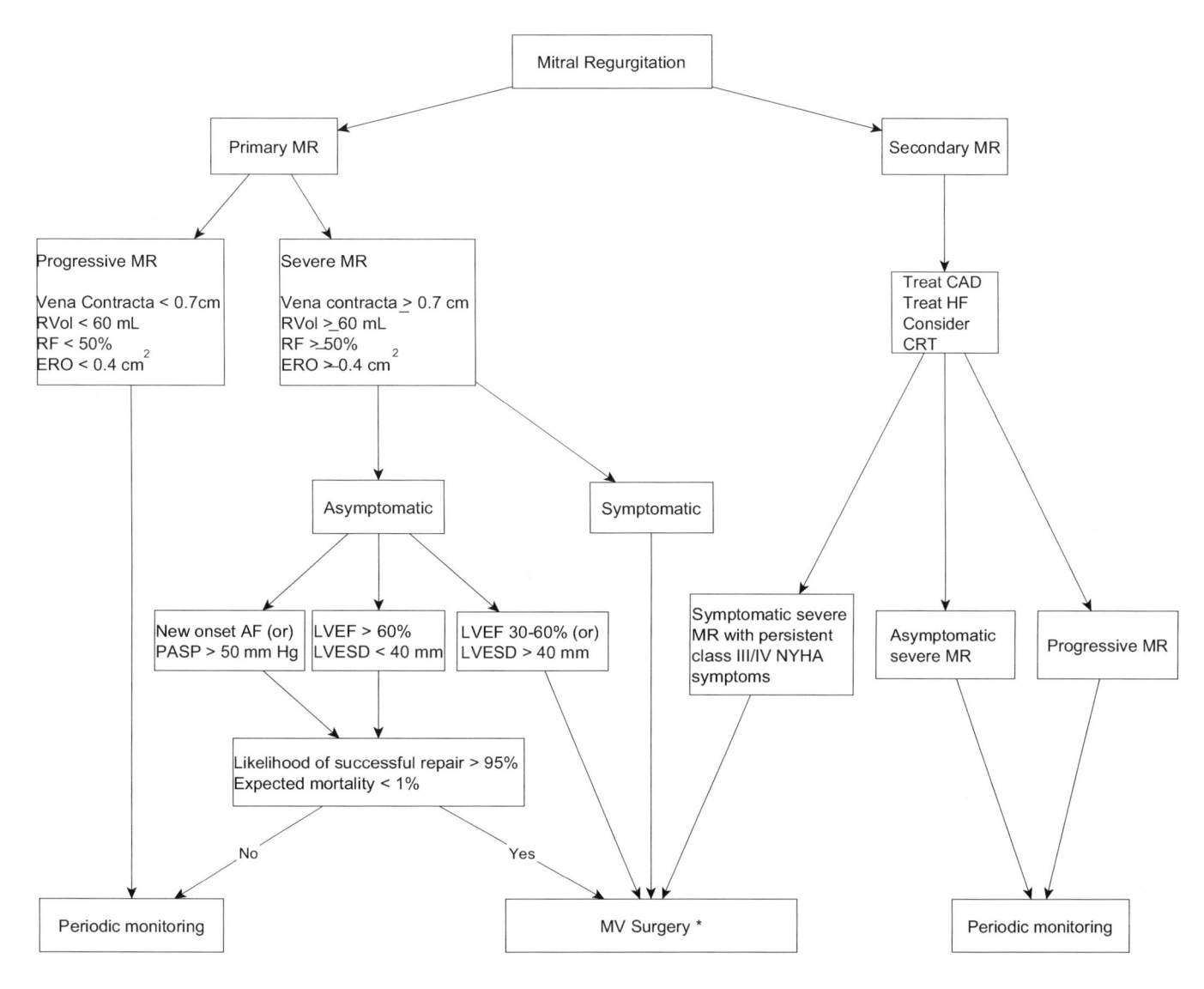

```
                          ┌─────────────────────┐
                          │ Mitral Regurgitation│
                          └──────────┬──────────┘
                      ┌──────────────┴──────────────┐
                ┌─────▼─────┐                 ┌─────▼──────┐
                │ Primary MR│                 │Secondary MR│
                └─────┬─────┘                 └─────┬──────┘
          ┌───────────┴──────────┐                  │
   ┌──────▼─────────┐   ┌────────▼────────┐   ┌─────▼──────┐
   │Progressive MR  │   │ Severe MR       │   │ Treat CAD  │
   │                │   │                 │   │ Treat HF   │
   │VC < 0.7cm      │   │VC ≥ 0.7 cm      │   │ Consider   │
   │RVol < 60 mL    │   │RVol ≥ 60 mL     │   │ CRT        │
   │RF < 50%        │   │RF ≥ 50%         │   └────────────┘
   │ERO < 0.4 cm²   │   │ERO ≥ 0.4 cm²    │
   └────────────────┘   └─────────────────┘
```

Mitral valve repair recommended over replacement, always in severe asymptomatic MR and whenever possible in other situations.

MR, mitral regurgitation; RVol, regurgitant volume; RF, regurgitant fraction; ERO, effective regurgitant orifice; LV, left ventricle; CAD, coronary artery disease; HF, heart failure; CRT, cardiac resynchronization therapy; AF, atrial fibrillation; PASP, pulmonary artery systolic pressure; LVEF, left ventricular ejection fraction; LVESD, left ventricular end-systolic dimension; NYHA, New York Heart Association

Mitral Stenosis
Clauden Louis, Sunil Prasad

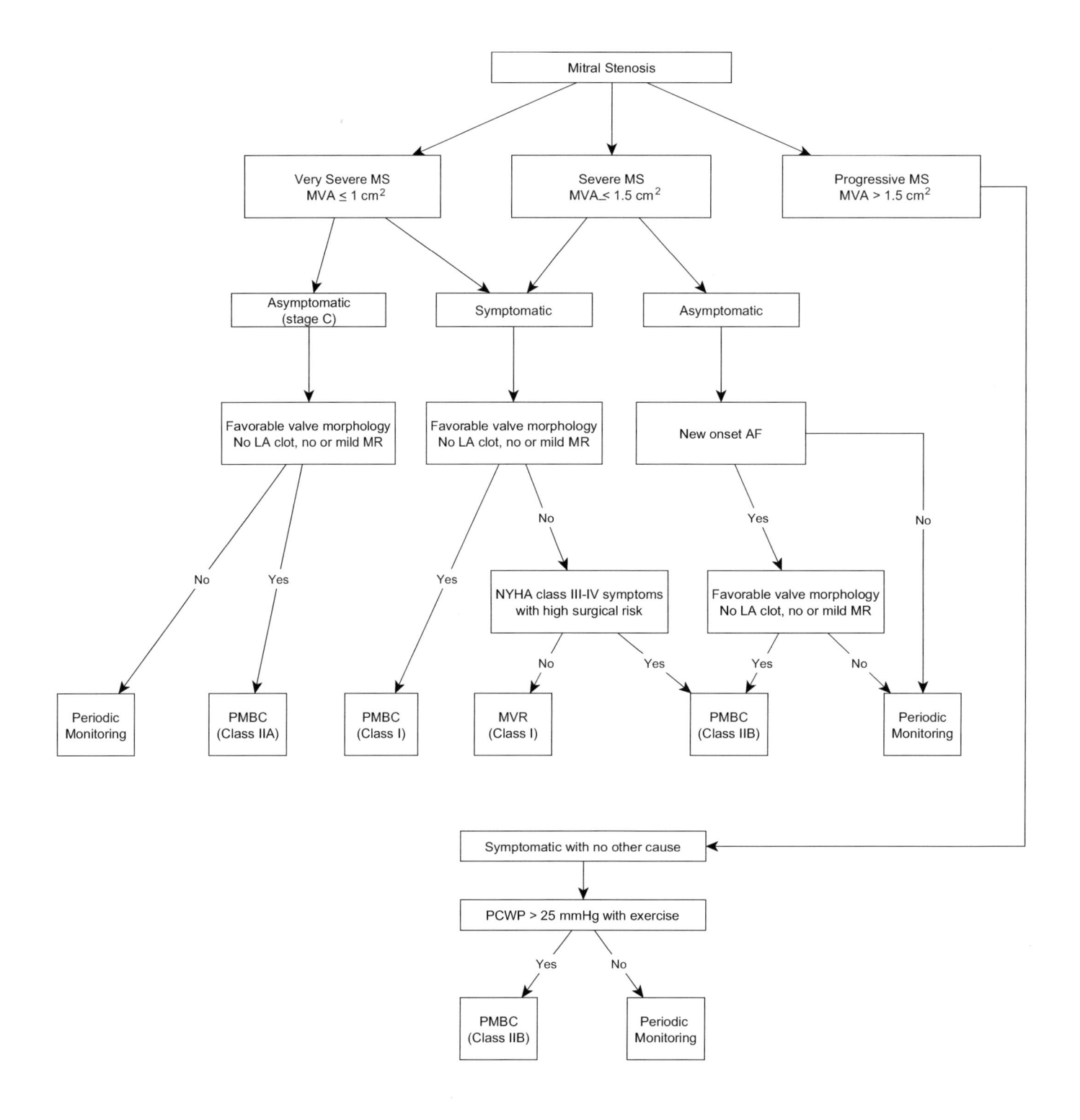

```
                              ┌─────────────────┐
                              │ Mitral Stenosis │
                              └─────────────────┘
            ┌──────────────────────┼──────────────────────┐
            ▼                      ▼                      ▼
   ┌─────────────────┐    ┌─────────────────┐    ┌─────────────────┐
   │ Very Severe MS  │    │   Severe MS     │    │ Progressive MS  │
   │  MVA ≤ 1 cm²    │    │  MVA ≤ 1.5 cm²  │    │  MVA > 1.5 cm²  │
   └─────────────────┘    └─────────────────┘    └─────────────────┘
            │               │            │                │
            ▼               ▼            ▼                │
      ┌───────────┐   ┌───────────┐  ┌───────────┐        │
      │Asymptomatic│  │Symptomatic│  │Asymptomatic│       │
      │ (stage C) │   └───────────┘  └───────────┘        │
      └───────────┘         │             │               │
            │               ▼             ▼               │
            ▼     ┌──────────────────┐  ┌──────────────┐  │
   ┌──────────────┐│Favorable valve  │  │ New onset AF │  │
   │Favorable valve││morphology       │  └──────────────┘  │
   │morphology    ││No LA clot, no    │     Yes │  │ No    │
   │No LA clot,   ││or mild MR        │         │  │       │
   │no or mild MR ││                  │         ▼  │       │
   └──────────────┘└──────────────────┘  ┌──────────────┐  │
      No │  Yes       Yes │    │ No      │Favorable valve│ │
         │              │  │            │morphology      │ │
         ▼              ▼  ▼            │No LA clot, no  │ │
                 ┌─────────────────┐   │or mild MR      │ │
                 │NYHA class III-IV│   └────────────────┘ │
                 │symptoms with     │    Yes │    │ No    │
                 │high surgical risk│        │    │       │
                 └─────────────────┘        ▼    ▼       │
                   No │      │ Yes                        │
   ┌────────┐ ┌────┐ ┌────┐ ┌────┐ ┌────┐  ┌────┐ ┌────────┐
   │Periodic│ │PMBC│ │PMBC│ │MVR │ │PMBC│  │PMBC│ │Periodic│
   │Monitor.│ │(IIA)│ │(I) │ │(I) │ │    │  │(IIB)│ │Monitor.│
   └────────┘ └────┘ └────┘ └────┘ └────┘  └────┘ └────────┘

                     ┌──────────────────────────┐◄─────────┘
                     │Symptomatic with no other │
                     │cause                     │
                     └──────────────────────────┘
                                │
                                ▼
                     ┌──────────────────────────┐
                     │PCWP > 25 mmHg with       │
                     │exercise                  │
                     └──────────────────────────┘
                         Yes │      │ No
                             ▼      ▼
                         ┌──────┐ ┌──────────┐
                         │PMBC  │ │Periodic  │
                         │(IIB) │ │Monitoring│
                         └──────┘ └──────────┘
```

```
                        ┌─────────────────┐
                        │ Mitral Stenosis │
                        └─────────────────┘
              ┌────────────────┼─────────────────────────┐
              ▼                ▼                         ▼
    ┌──────────────────┐ ┌──────────────────┐  ┌──────────────────┐  ☆
    │ Very Severe MS   │ │   Severe MS      │  │  Progressive MS  │──┐
    │ MVA ≤ 1 cm²      │ │ MVA ≤ 1.5 cm²    │  │ MVA > 1.5 cm²    │  │
    └──────────────────┘ └──────────────────┘  └──────────────────┘  │
           │              │           │                  │            │
           ▼              ▼           ▼                  ▼            │
  ┌──────────────┐  ┌────────────┐  ┌──────────────┐                  │
  │ Asymptomatic │  │ Symptomatic│  │ Asymptomatic │                  │
  │  (stage C)   │  │            │  │              │                  │
  └──────────────┘  └────────────┘  └──────────────┘                  │
         │                │                │                          │
         ▼                ▼                ▼                          ▼
  ┌──────────────┐  ┌──────────────┐  ┌──────────────┐         
  │  Favorable   │  │  Favorable   │  │ New onset AF │         
  │valve morph.  │  │valve morph.  │  │              │         
  │No LA clot,   │  │No LA clot,   │  │              │         
  │no or mild MR │  │no or mild MR │  │              │         
  └──────────────┘  └──────────────┘  └──────────────┘         
         │                │                │                          │
         ▼                ▼                ▼                          ▼
      ┌─────┐          ┌─────┐          ┌─────┐                    ┌─────┐
      │Next │          │Next │          │Next │                    │Next │
      │Page │          │Page │          │Page │                    │Page │
      └─────┘          └─────┘          └─────┘                    └─────┘
```

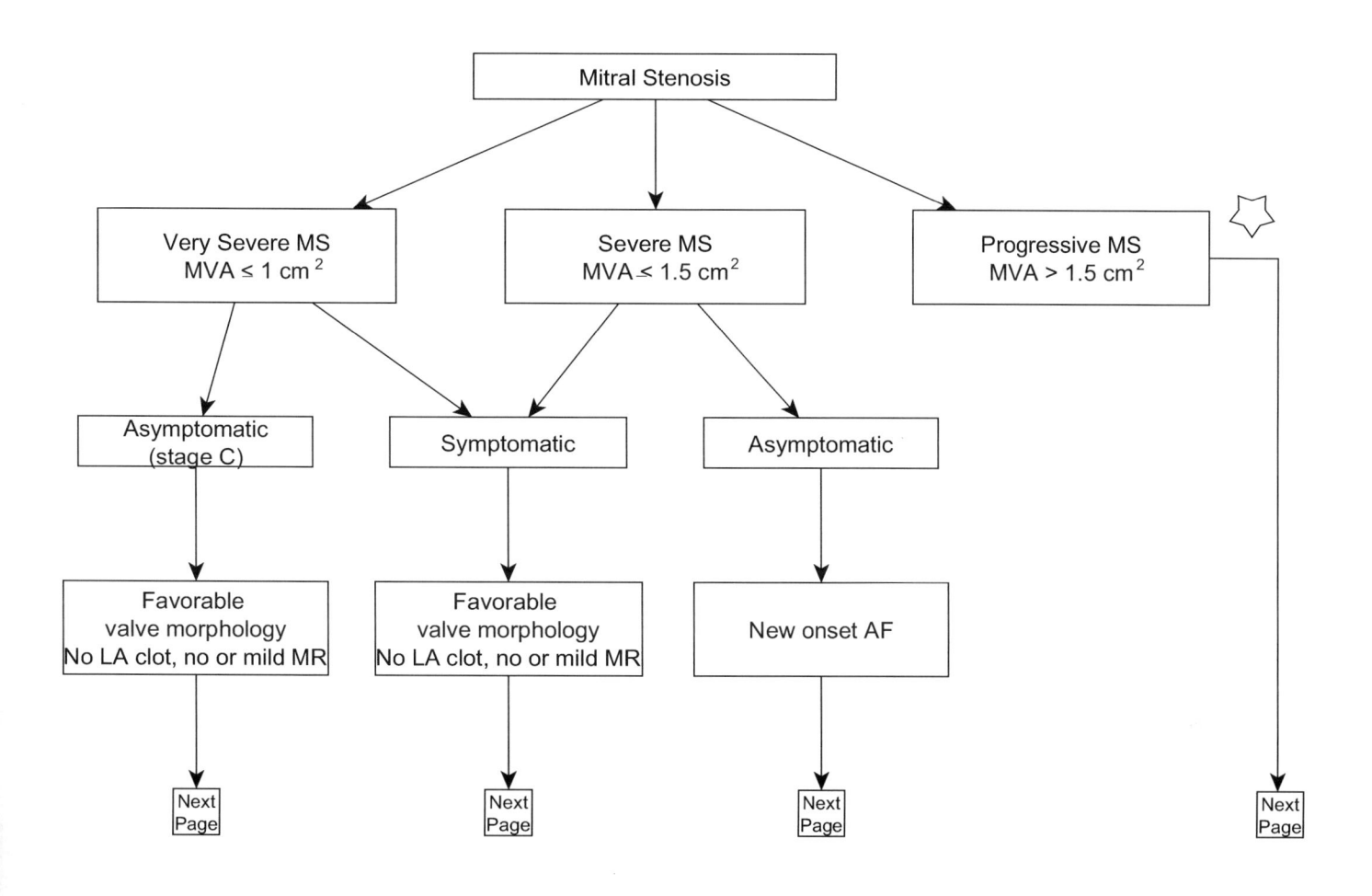

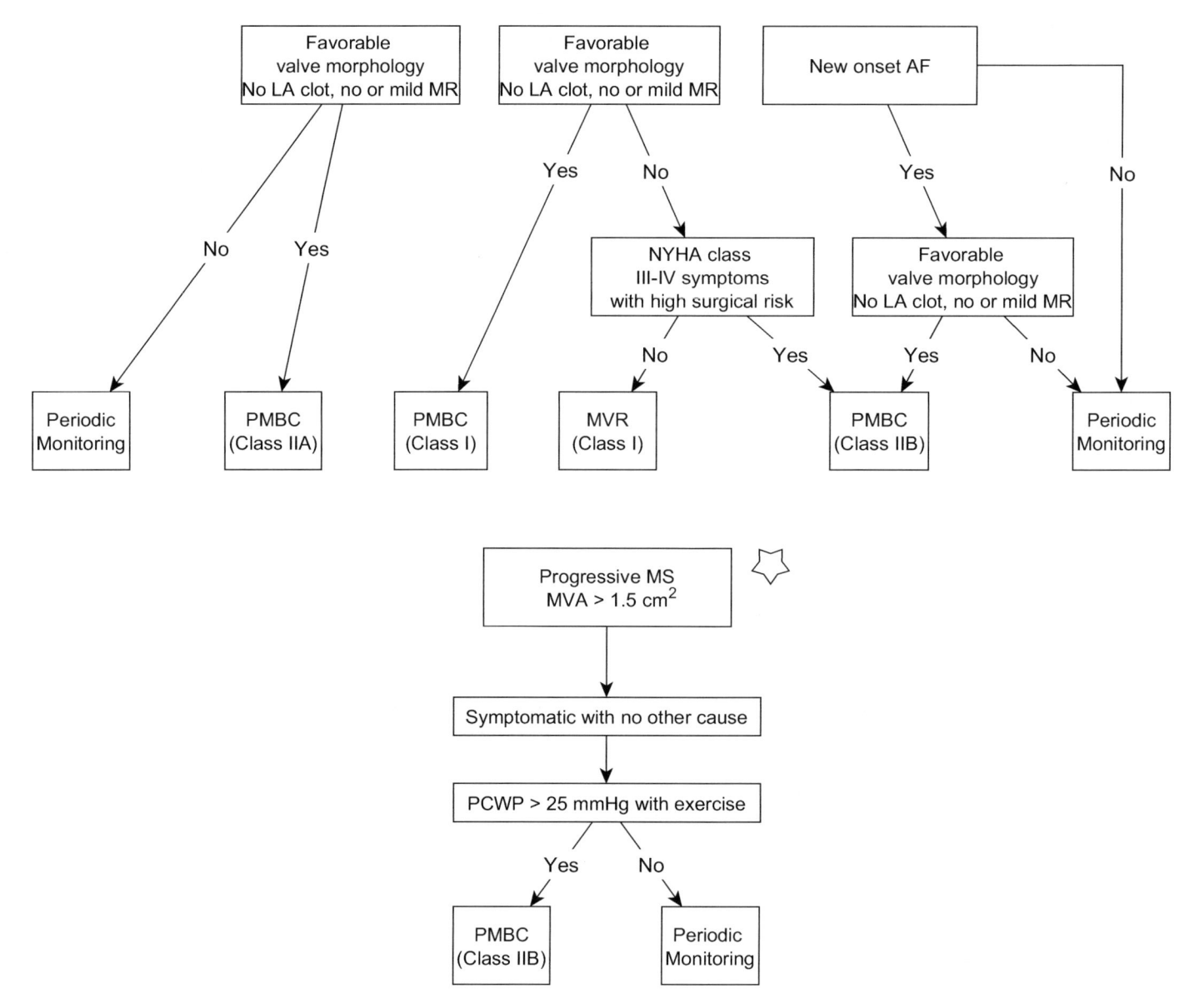

AF, atrial fibrillation; LA, left atrial; MR, mitral regurgitation; MS, mitral stenosis; MVA, mitral valve area; MVR, mitral valve surgery (repair or replacement); NYHA, New York Heart Association; PCWP, pulmonary capillary wedge pressure; PMBC, percutaneous mitral balloon commissurotomy.

Management of Type A Aortic Dissection
Awais Ashfaq, Howard Song

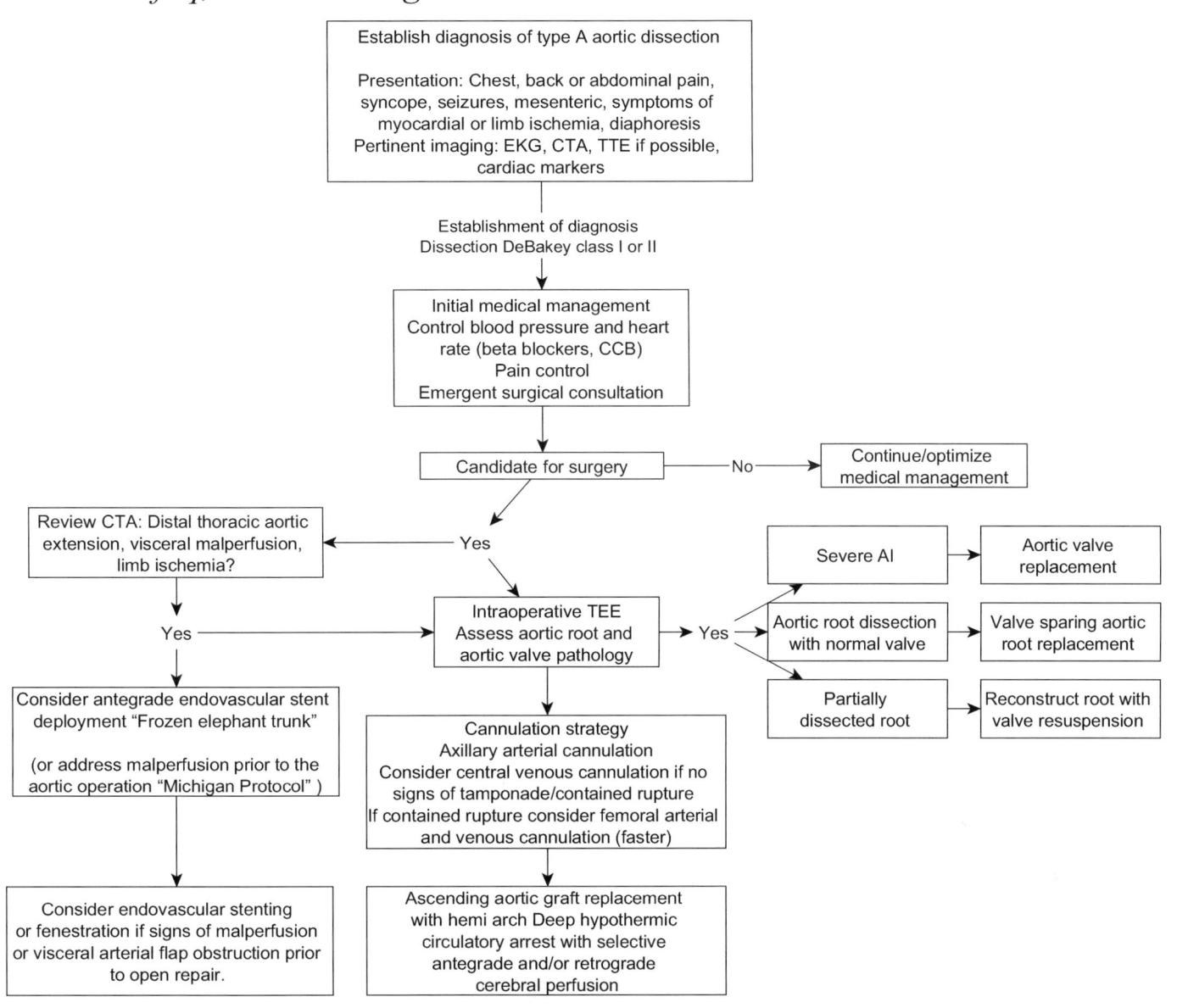

```
┌─────────────────────────────────────────┐
│ Establish diagnosis of type A aortic dissection │
│                                         │
│ Presentation: Chest, back or abdominal pain, │
│ syncope, seizures, mesenteric, symptoms of │
│ myocardial or limb ischemia, diaphoresis │
│ Pertinent imaging: EKG, CTA, TTE if possible, │
│ cardiac markers                         │
└─────────────────────────────────────────┘
                    │
         Establishment of diagnosis
         Dissection DeBakey class I or II
                    ↓
┌─────────────────────────────────────┐
│ Initial medical management          │
│ Control blood pressure and heart    │
│ rate (beta blockers, CCB)           │
│ Pain control                        │
│ Emergent surgical consultation      │
└─────────────────────────────────────┘
                    ↓
         ┌──────────────────────┐      ┌──────────────────────┐
         │ Candidate for surgery │──No→│ Continue/optimize    │
         └──────────────────────┘      │ medical management   │
                    │ Yes              └──────────────────────┘
                    ↓

┌────────────────────────────┐      ┌──────────────────────────┐      ┌──────────────────┐   ┌──────────────────┐
│ Review CTA: Distal thoracic │←─Yes─│ Intraoperative TEE       │─Yes→│ Severe AI        │──→│ Aortic valve     │
│ aortic extension, visceral  │      │ Assess aortic root and   │     └──────────────────┘   │ replacement      │
│ malperfusion, limb ischemia?│      │ aortic valve pathology   │                             └──────────────────┘
└────────────────────────────┘      └──────────────────────────┘     ┌──────────────────┐   ┌──────────────────────┐
            │ Yes                              │                     │ Aortic root      │──→│ Valve sparing aortic │
            ↓                                  ↓                     │ dissection with  │   │ root replacement     │
┌────────────────────────────┐      ┌──────────────────────────┐     │ normal valve     │   └──────────────────────┘
│ Consider antegrade endo-   │      │ Cannulation strategy     │     └──────────────────┘
│ vascular stent deployment  │      │ Axillary arterial        │     ┌──────────────────┐   ┌──────────────────────┐
│ "Frozen elephant trunk"    │      │ cannulation              │     │ Partially        │──→│ Reconstruct root with│
│                            │      │ Consider central venous  │     │ dissected root   │   │ valve resuspension   │
│ (or address malperfusion   │      │ cannulation if no signs  │     └──────────────────┘   └──────────────────────┘
│ prior to the aortic opera- │      │ of tamponade/contained   │
│ tion "Michigan Protocol")  │      │ rupture                  │
└────────────────────────────┘      │ If contained rupture     │
            │                       │ consider femoral arterial│
            ↓                       │ and venous cannulation   │
┌────────────────────────────┐      │ (faster)                 │
│ Consider endovascular      │      └──────────────────────────┘
│ stenting or fenestration   │                  ↓
│ if signs of malperfusion   │      ┌──────────────────────────┐
│ or visceral arterial flap  │      │ Ascending aortic graft   │
│ obstruction prior to open  │      │ replacement with hemi    │
│ repair.                    │      │ arch Deep hypothermic    │
└────────────────────────────┘      │ circulatory arrest with  │
                                    │ selective antegrade      │
                                    │ and/or retrograde        │
                                    │ cerebral perfusion       │
                                    └──────────────────────────┘
```

EKG, Electrocardiogram; CTA, Computed Tomography Angiogram; TTE, Transthoracic Echocardiogram; CCB, Calcium Channel Blocker; TEE, Transesophageal Echocardiogram; AI, Aortic Insufficiency

Management of Type B Aortic Dissection
Laura Seese, Christopher Sciortino

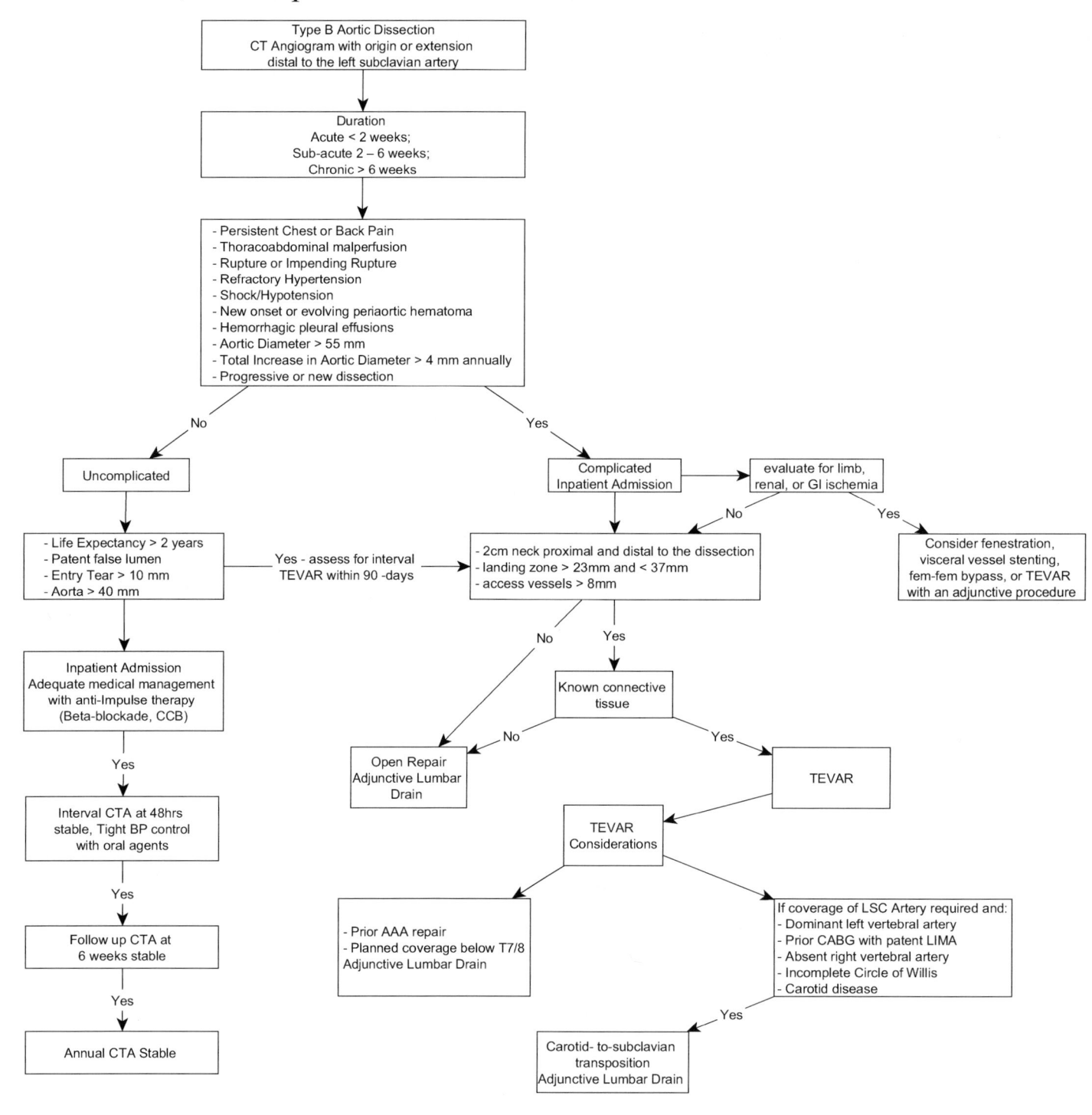

```
┌─────────────────────────────────────┐
│     Type B Aortic Dissection        │
│ CT Angiogram with origin or extension│
│   distal to the left subclavian artery│
└─────────────────────────────────────┘
                 ↓
┌─────────────────────────────────────┐
│            Duration                 │
│        Acute < 2 weeks;             │
│       Sub-acute 2 – 6 weeks;        │
│         Chronic > 6 weeks           │
└─────────────────────────────────────┘
                 ↓
┌─────────────────────────────────────┐
│ - Persistent Chest or Back Pain     │
│ - Thoracoabdominal malperfusion     │
│ - Rupture or Impending Rupture      │
│ - Refractory Hypertension           │
│ - Shock/Hypotension                 │
│ - New onset or evolving periaortic hematoma│
│ - Hemorrhagic pleural effusions     │
│ - Aortic Diameter > 55 mm           │
│ - Total Increase in Aortic Diameter > 4 mm annually│
│ - Progressive or new dissection     │
└─────────────────────────────────────┘
       No ↙              ↘ Yes
```

No (Uncomplicated) branch:
- Life Expectancy > 2 years
- Patent false lumen
- Entry Tear > 10 mm
- Aorta > 40 mm

→ Yes - assess for interval TEVAR within 90 -days

Otherwise:
- Inpatient Admission, Adequate medical management with anti-Impulse therapy (Beta-blockade, CCB)
- Yes → Interval CTA at 48hrs stable, Tight BP control with oral agents
- Yes → Follow up CTA at 6 weeks stable
- Yes → Annual CTA Stable

Yes (Complicated) branch:
Complicated Inpatient Admission → evaluate for limb, renal, or GI ischemia
- Yes → Consider fenestration, visceral vessel stenting, fem-fem bypass, or TEVAR with an adjunctive procedure
- No →
  - 2cm neck proximal and distal to the dissection
  - landing zone > 23mm and < 37mm
  - access vessels > 8mm

  - No → Open Repair, Adjunctive Lumbar Drain
  - Yes → Known connective tissue
    - Yes → TEVAR
    - No → Open Repair, Adjunctive Lumbar Drain

TEVAR Considerations:
- Prior AAA repair
- Planned coverage below T7/8
  Adjunctive Lumbar Drain

If coverage of LSC Artery required and:
- Dominant left vertebral artery
- Prior CABG with patent LIMA
- Absent right vertebral artery
- Incomplete Circle of Willis
- Carotid disease

Yes → Carotid- to-subclavian transposition, Adjunctive Lumbar Drain

```
┌─────────────────────────────────────────┐
│       Type B Aortic Dissection          │
│ CT Angiogram with origin or extension   │
│   distal to the left subclavian artery  │
└─────────────────────────────────────────┘
                    │
                    ▼
┌─────────────────────────────────────────┐
│               Duration                  │
│          Acute < 2 weeks;               │
│         Sub-acute 2 – 6 weeks;          │
│           Chronic > 6 weeks             │
└─────────────────────────────────────────┘
                    │
                    ▼
┌─────────────────────────────────────────┐
│ - Persistent Chest or Back Pain         │
│ - Thoracoabdominal malperfusion         │
│ - Rupture or Impending Rupture          │
│ - Refractory Hypertension               │
│ - Shock/Hypotension                     │
│ - New onset or evolving periaortic      │
│   hematoma                              │
│ - Hemorrhagic pleural effusions         │
│ - Aortic Diameter > 55 mm               │
│ - Total Increase in Aortic Diameter     │
│   > 4 mm annually                       │
│ - Progressive or new dissection         │
└─────────────────────────────────────────┘
         │                        │
        No                       Yes
         ▼                        ▼
┌─────────────────┐      ┌─────────────────────┐
│  Uncomplicated  │      │     Complicated     │
│                 │      │ Inpatient Admission │
└─────────────────┘      └─────────────────────┘
```

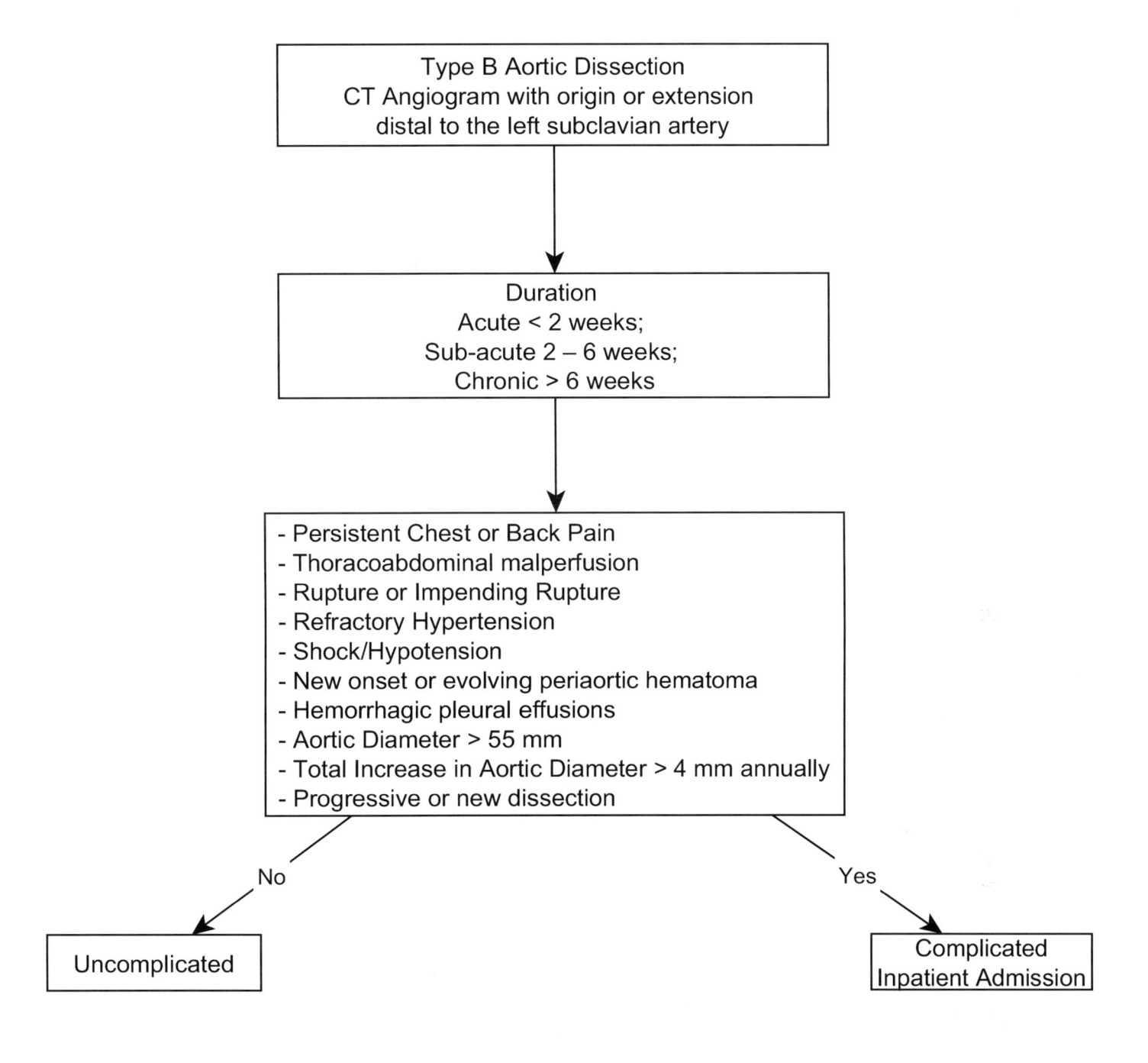

Uncomplicated

- Life Expectancy > 2 years
- Patent false lumen
- Entry Tear > 10 mm
- Aorta > 40 mm

→ Yes - assess for interval TEVAR within 90-days

↓

Inpatient Admission
Adequate medical management with anti-Impulse therapy (Beta-blockade, CCB)

↓ Yes

Interval CTA at 48hrs stable, Tight BP control with oral agents

↓ Yes

Follow up CTA at 6 weeks stable

↓ Yes

Annual CTA Stable

Complicated Inpatient Admission

→ evaluate for limb, renal, or GI ischemia
- No → continue
- Yes → Consider fenestration, visceral vessel stenting, fem-fem bypass, or TEVAR with an adjunctive procedure

- 2cm neck proximal and distal to the dissection
- landing zone > 23mm and < 37mm
- access vessels > 8mm

- No → Open Repair / Adjunctive Lumbar Drain
- Yes → Known connective tissue
  - No → Open Repair / Adjunctive Lumbar Drain
  - Yes → TEVAR

→ TEVAR Considerations

- Prior AAA repair
- Planned coverage below T7/8
  Adjunctive Lumbar Drain

If coverage of LSC Artery required and:
- Dominant left vertebral artery
- Prior CABG with patent LIMA
- Absent right vertebral artery
- Incomplete Circle of Willis
- Carotid disease

↓ Yes

Carotid- to-subclavian transposition
Adjunctive Lumbar Drain

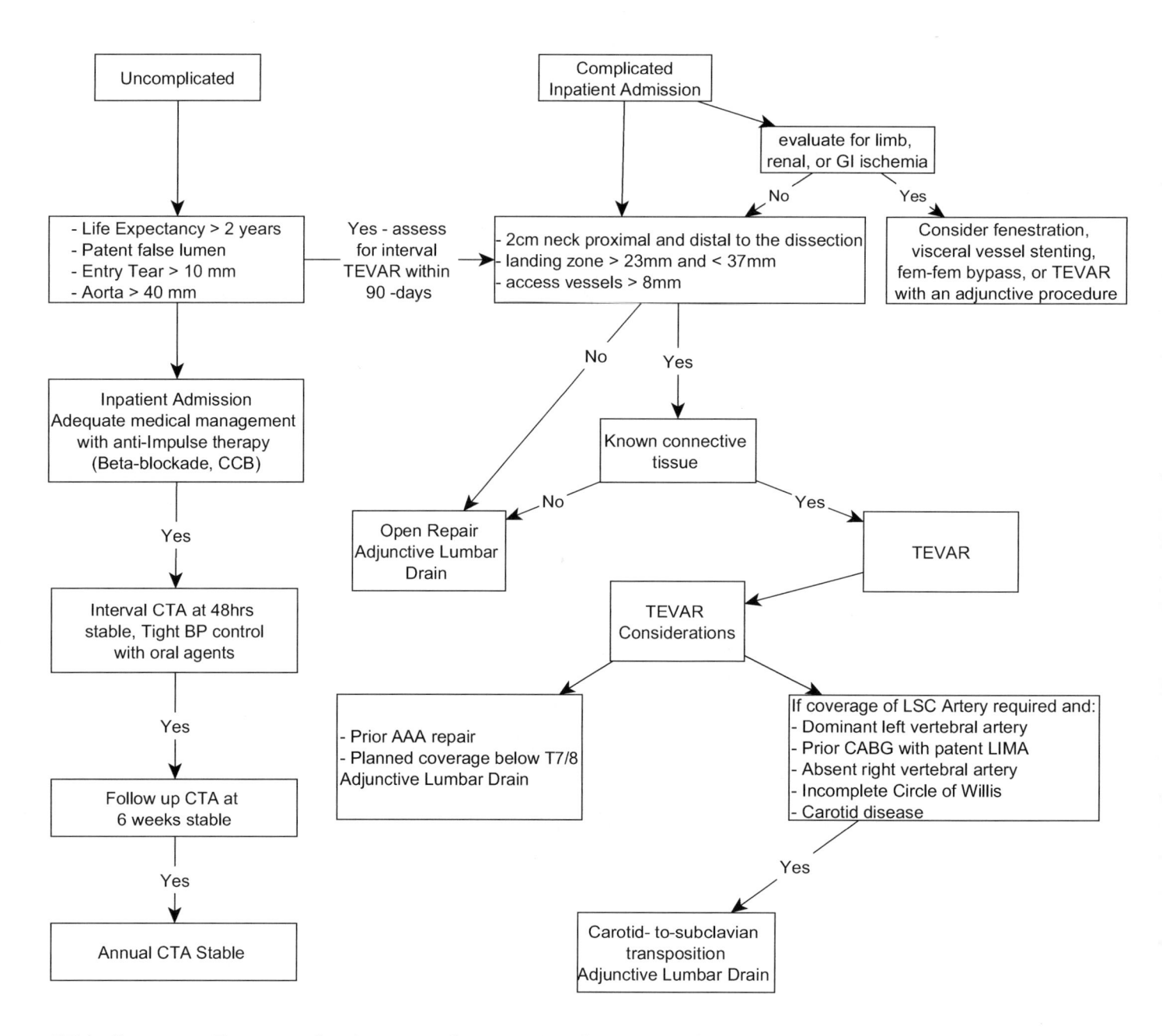

CTA, Computer Tomography Angiography; TEVAR, thoracic endovascular aortic repair; SBP, systolic blood pressure; CCB, calcium channel blocker; ACEi, angiotensin converting enzyme inhibitor; LIMA left internal mammary artery; CABG coronary artery bypass grafting

Ascending Aortic Aneurysm
Tedi Vlahu, Jeffrey Schwartz

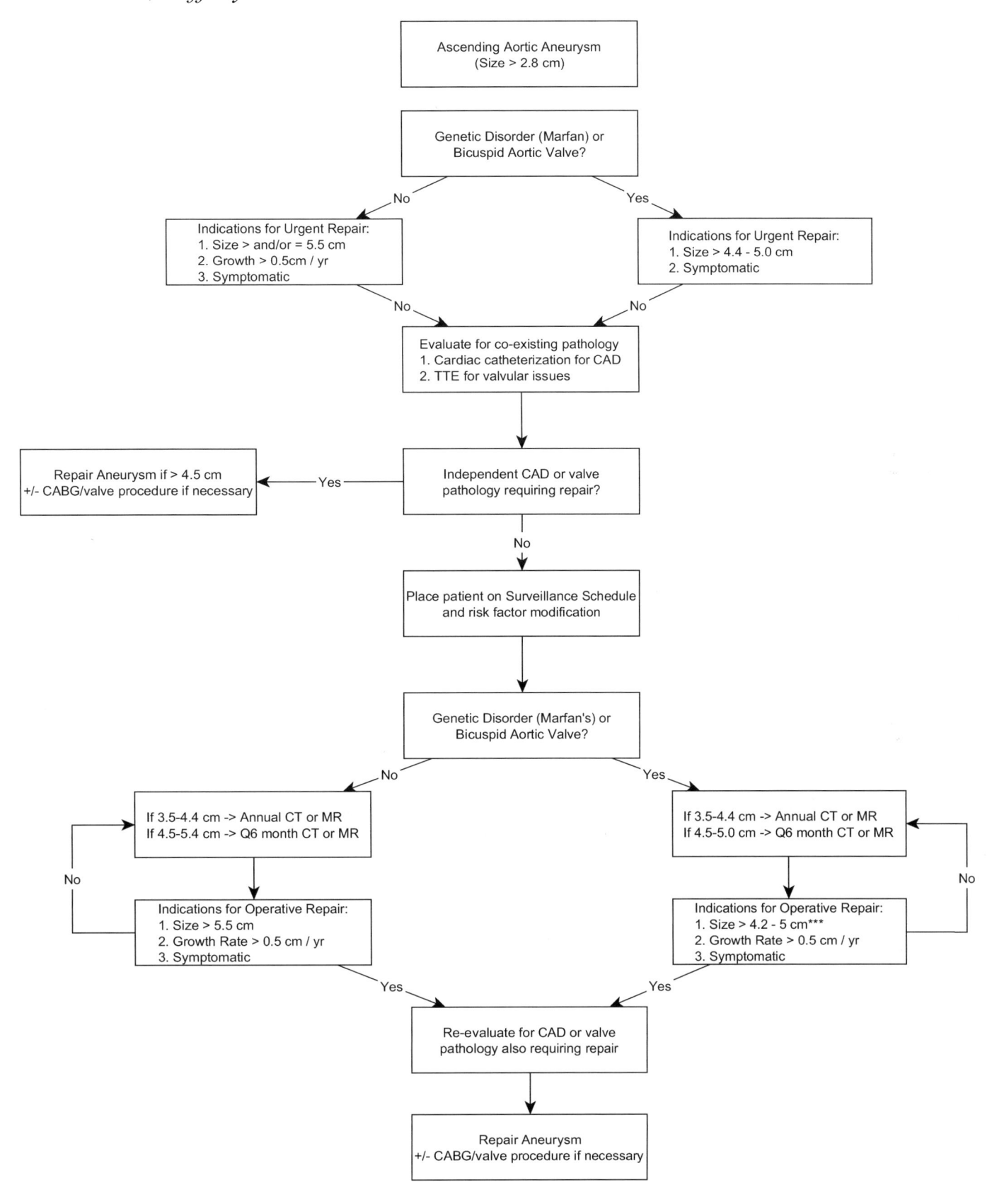

```
                    ┌─────────────────────────────┐
                    │  Ascending Aortic Aneurysm  │
                    │       (Size > 2.8 cm)       │
                    └──────────────┬──────────────┘
                                   │
                    ┌──────────────▼──────────────┐
                    │  Genetic Disorder (Marfan) or│
                    │   Bicuspid Aortic Valve?    │
                    └──────┬───────────────┬──────┘
                       No  │               │  Yes
          ┌────────────────▼──┐         ┌──▼──────────────────┐
          │ Indications for   │         │ Indications for     │
          │ Urgent Repair:    │         │ Urgent Repair:      │
          │ 1. Size > and/or  │         │ 1. Size > 4.4-5.0 cm│
          │    = 5.5 cm       │         │ 2. Symptomatic      │
          │ 2. Growth>0.5cm/yr│         │                     │
          │ 3. Symptomatic    │         │                     │
          └─────────┬─────────┘         └─────────┬───────────┘
                 No │                          No │
                    ▼                             ▼
                ┌──────────────────────────────────┐
                │ Evaluate for co-existing pathology│
                │ 1. Cardiac catheterization for CAD│
                │ 2. TTE for valvular issues       │
                └──────────────┬───────────────────┘
                               ▼
                ┌──────────────────────────┐
   ┌──Yes───────│ Independent CAD or valve │
   │            │ pathology requiring repair?│
   │            └──────────────┬───────────┘
   ▼                           │ No
┌──────────────────────────┐   ▼
│ Repair Aneurysm if >4.5cm│  ┌──────────────────────────────┐
│ +/- CABG/valve procedure │  │ Place patient on Surveillance│
│ if necessary             │  │ Schedule and risk factor     │
└──────────────────────────┘  │ modification                 │
                              └──────────────┬───────────────┘
                                             ▼
                              ┌─────────────────────────────┐
                              │ Genetic Disorder (Marfan's) │
                              │  or Bicuspid Aortic Valve?  │
                              └──────┬──────────────┬───────┘
                                 No  │              │  Yes
             ┌───────────────────────▼──┐      ┌────▼─────────────────────┐
        ┌───►│ If 3.5-4.4 cm -> Annual  │      │ If 3.5-4.4 cm -> Annual  │◄───┐
        │    │    CT or MR              │      │    CT or MR              │    │
        │    │ If 4.5-5.4 cm -> Q6 month│      │ If 4.5-5.0 cm -> Q6 month│    │
        │    │    CT or MR              │      │    CT or MR              │    │
        │    └───────────┬──────────────┘      └────────────┬─────────────┘    │
     No │                ▼                                  ▼                  │ No
        │    ┌──────────────────────────┐      ┌──────────────────────────┐    │
        └────│ Indications for Operative│      │ Indications for Operative│────┘
             │ Repair:                  │      │ Repair:                  │
             │ 1. Size > 5.5 cm         │      │ 1. Size > 4.2 - 5 cm***  │
             │ 2. Growth Rate>0.5 cm/yr │      │ 2. Growth Rate>0.5 cm/yr │
             │ 3. Symptomatic           │      │ 3. Symptomatic           │
             └──────────────┬───────────┘      └───────────┬──────────────┘
                         Yes│                              │Yes
                            ▼                              ▼
                       ┌──────────────────────────────────────┐
                       │ Re-evaluate for CAD or valve         │
                       │ pathology also requiring repair      │
                       └──────────────────┬───────────────────┘
                                          ▼
                       ┌──────────────────────────────────────┐
                       │ Repair Aneurysm                      │
                       │ +/- CABG/valve procedure if necessary│
                       └──────────────────────────────────────┘
```

```
                    ┌─────────────────────────┐
                    │ Ascending Aortic Aneurysm│
                    │    (Size > 2.8 cm)      │
                    └─────────────────────────┘
                                │
                                ▼
                    ┌─────────────────────────┐
                    │ Genetic Disorder (Marfan) or │
                    │   Bicuspid Aortic Valve? │
                    └─────────────────────────┘
                       No │            │ Yes
                          ▼            ▼
        ┌──────────────────────────┐   ┌──────────────────────────┐
        │ Indications for Urgent Repair:│   │ Indications for Urgent Repair:│
        │ 1. Size > and/or = 5.5 cm │   │ 1. Size > 4.4 - 5.0 cm   │
        │ 2. Growth > 0.5cm / yr   │   │ 2. Symptomatic           │
        │ 3. Symptomatic           │   └──────────────────────────┘
        └──────────────────────────┘
                       No │            │ No
                          ▼            ▼
                    ┌─────────────────────────────┐
                    │ Evaluate for co-existing pathology│
                    │ 1. Cardiac catheterization for CAD│
                    │ 2. TTE for valvular issues  │
                    └─────────────────────────────┘
                                │
                                ▼
┌────────────────────┐    ┌─────────────────────────┐
│ Repair Aneurysm    │    │ Independent CAD or valve│
│   if > 4.5 cm      │◄Yes│ pathology requiring repair?│
│ +/- CABG/valve     │    └─────────────────────────┘
│ procedure if necessary│              │ No
└────────────────────┘              ▼
                    ┌─────────────────────────────────┐
                    │ Place patient on Surveillance Schedule│
                    │    and risk factor modification │
                    └─────────────────────────────────┘
```

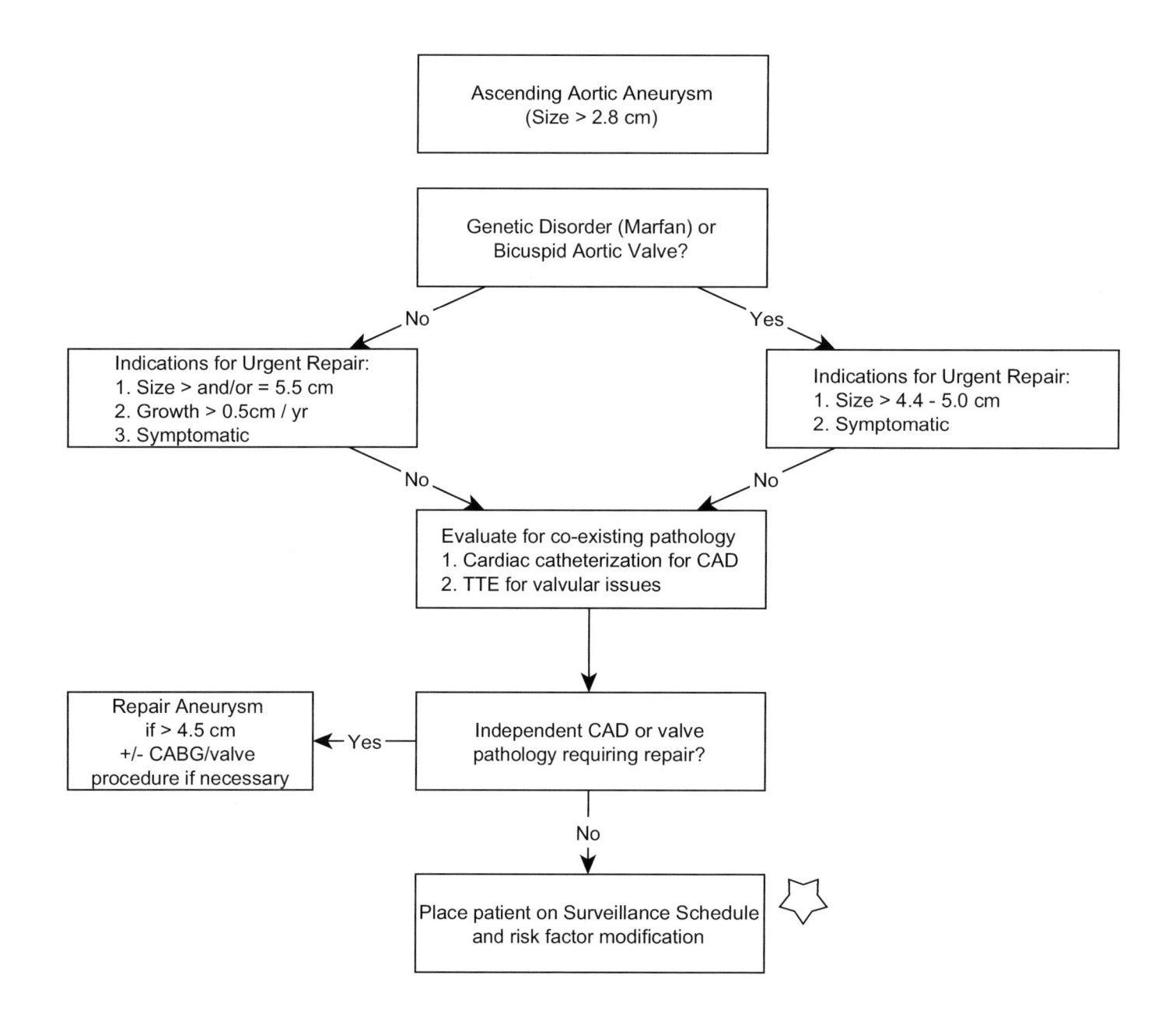

```
┌─────────────────────────────────┐
│ Place patient on Surveillance   │ ☆
│ Schedule and risk factor        │
│ modification                    │
└─────────────────────────────────┘
                │
                ▼
┌─────────────────────────────────┐
│ Genetic Disorder (Marfan's) or  │
│ Bicuspid Aortic Valve?          │
└─────────────────────────────────┘
         No  /        \  Yes
```

Left branch (No):
- If 3.5-4.4 cm -> Annual CT or MR
- If 4.5-5.4 cm -> Q6 month CT or MR

Indications for Operative Repair:
1. Size > 5.5 cm
2. Growth Rate > 0.5 cm / yr
3. Symptomatic

Right branch (Yes):
- If 3.5-4.4 cm -> Annual CT or MR
- If 4.5-5.0 cm -> Q6 month CT or MR

Indications for Operative Repair:
1. Size > 4.2 - 5 cm***
2. Growth Rate > 0.5 cm / yr
3. Symptomatic

Both Yes →

Re-evaluate for CAD or valve pathology also requiring repair

↓

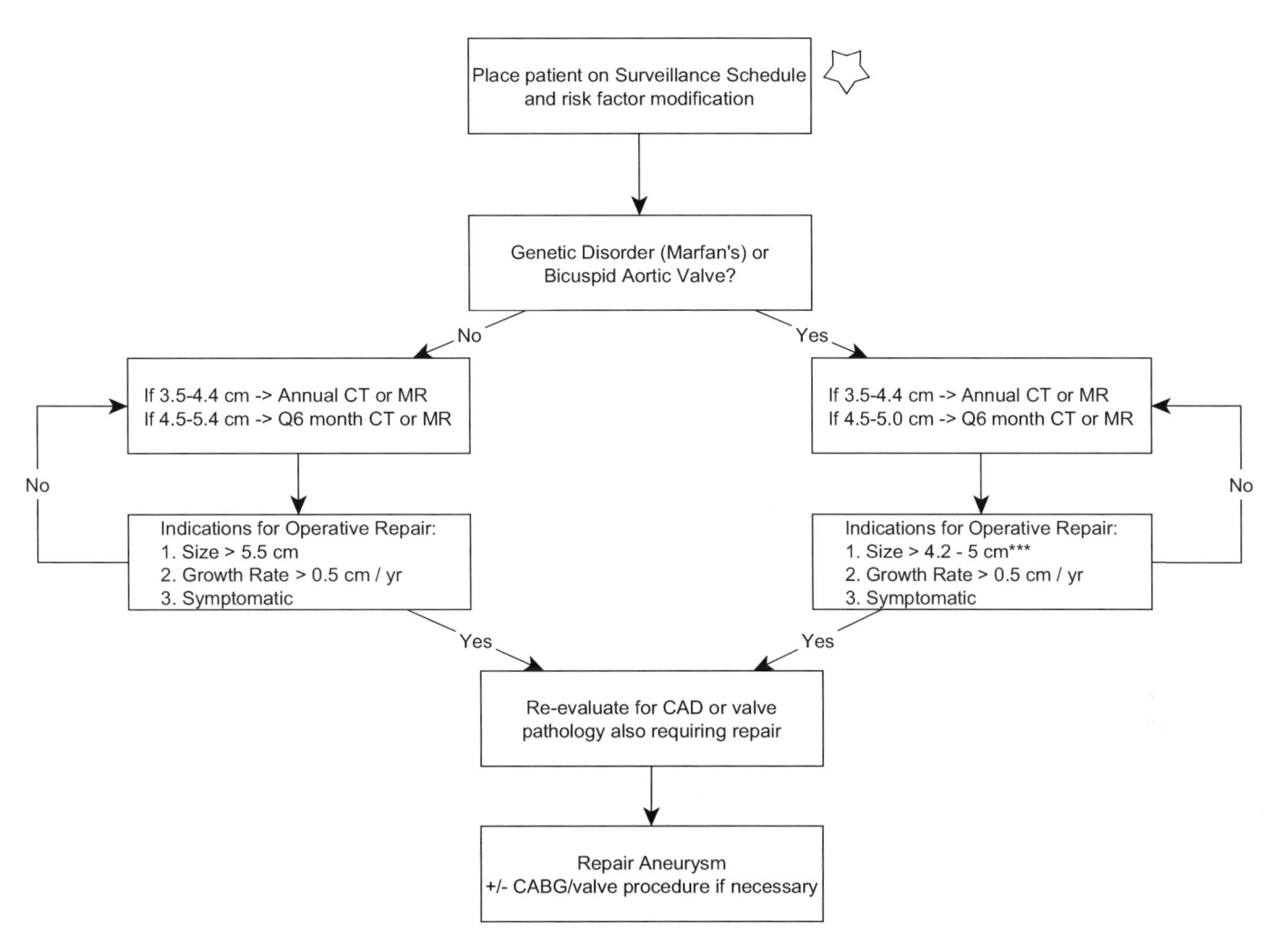

Repair Aneurysm +/- CABG/valve procedure if necessary

***Repair at following sizes:

1. >4.0 cm if woman with Marfan Syndrome and contemplating pregnancy (also need to replace root)
2. >4.2 cm by TEE or 4.4-4.6 by CT if patient with Loeys-Dietz syndrome or TGFBR1/TGFBR2 mutation
3. >4.5 cm if family history of aortic dissection
4. Ratio of maximum ascending aortic root area $(3.14 \times r^2)$ in cm2 divided pt. height in meters > 10 in Marfan Syndrome, BAV and other genetic disorders.

BAV, Bicuspid Aortic Valve; CAD, Coronary Artery Disease; TEE, Transesophageal Echocardiogram; TTE, Transthoracic Echocardiogram

Aortic Root Aneurysms
Kevin Graham, Joel Corvera

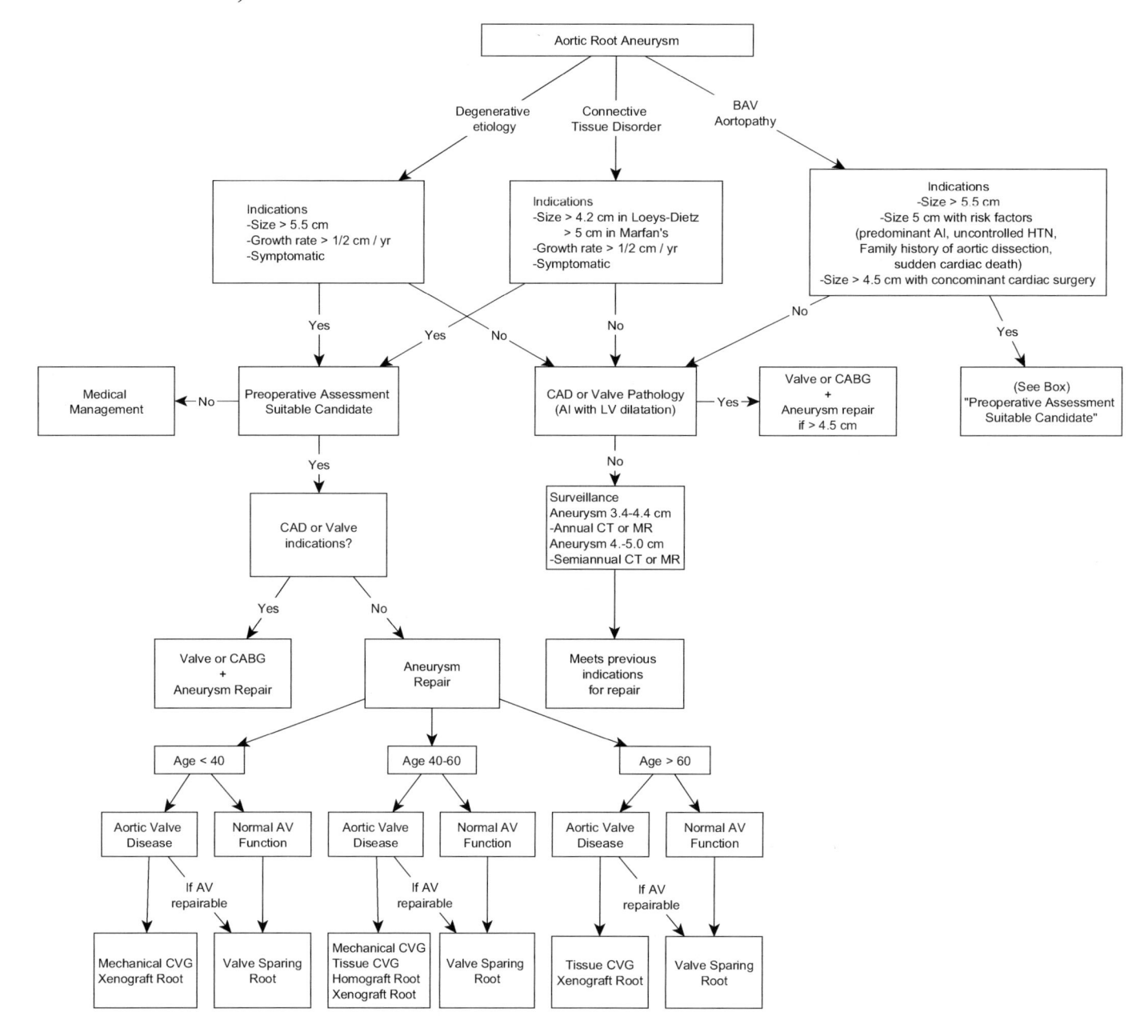

```
                              ┌─────────────────────────┐
                              │  Aortic Root Aneurysm   │
                              └─────────────────────────┘
                    Degenerative    Connective        BAV
                     etiology     Tissue Disorder   Aortopathy
                        │              │                │
                        ▼              ▼                ▼
            ┌──────────────────┐  ┌──────────────────┐  ┌─────────────────────────────────┐
            │ Indications      │  │ Indications      │  │ Indications                     │
            │ -Size > 5.5 cm   │  │ -Size > 4.2 cm   │  │ -Size > 5.5 cm                  │
            │ -Growth rate     │  │  in Loeys-Dietz  │  │ -Size 5 cm with risk factors    │
            │  > 1/2 cm / yr   │  │  > 5 cm in       │  │  (predominant AI, uncontrolled  │
            │ -Symptomatic     │  │   Marfan's       │  │  HTN, Family history of aortic  │
            │                  │  │ -Growth rate     │  │  dissection, sudden cardiac     │
            │                  │  │  > 1/2 cm / yr   │  │  death)                         │
            │                  │  │ -Symptomatic     │  │ -Size > 4.5 cm with concominant │
            │                  │  │                  │  │  cardiac surgery                │
            └──────────────────┘  └──────────────────┘  └─────────────────────────────────┘
                  │Yes    Yes│  No       │No                    │No          │Yes
                  ▼          ▼           ▼                      ▼            ▼
    ┌─────────┐  ┌──────────────────┐  ┌──────────────────┐  ┌──────────┐  ┌──────────────────┐
    │Medical  │◄─│Preoperative      │  │CAD or Valve      │─►│Valve or  │  │(See Box)         │
    │Manage-  │No│Assessment        │  │Pathology         │Yes│CABG +   │  │"Preoperative     │
    │ment     │  │Suitable Candidate│  │(AI with LV dila- │  │Aneurysm  │  │Assessment        │
    └─────────┘  └──────────────────┘  │tation)           │  │repair    │  │Suitable          │
                         │Yes          └──────────────────┘  │if > 4.5cm│  │Candidate"        │
                         ▼                      │No          └──────────┘  └──────────────────┘
                  ┌──────────────┐              ▼
                  │CAD or Valve  │     ┌──────────────────┐
                  │indications?  │     │Surveillance      │
                  └──────────────┘     │Aneurysm 3.4-4.4cm│
                     Yes│  │No         │-Annual CT or MR  │
                        │  │           │Aneurysm 4.-5.0cm │
                        ▼  ▼           │-Semiannual CT/MR │
              ┌──────────┐ ┌────────┐  └──────────────────┘
              │Valve or  │ │Aneurysm│           │
              │CABG +    │ │Repair  │           ▼
              │Aneurysm  │ │        │  ┌──────────────┐
              │Repair    │ │        │  │Meets previous│
              └──────────┘ └────────┘  │indications   │
                              │        │for repair    │
               ┌──────────────┼──────────────┐
               ▼              ▼              ▼
          ┌────────┐      ┌────────┐      ┌────────┐
          │Age < 40│      │Age40-60│      │Age > 60│
          └────────┘      └────────┘      └────────┘
           │     │         │     │         │     │
           ▼     ▼         ▼     ▼         ▼     ▼
        ┌────┐ ┌────┐   ┌────┐ ┌────┐   ┌────┐ ┌────┐
        │Aor.│ │Norm│   │Aor.│ │Norm│   │Aor.│ │Norm│
        │Valve│ │AV  │   │Valve│ │AV  │   │Valve│ │AV  │
        │Dis.│ │Func│   │Dis.│ │Func│   │Dis.│ │Func│
        └────┘ └────┘   └────┘ └────┘   └────┘ └────┘
         │If AV  │        │If AV │        │If AV │
         │repair-│        │repair│        │repair│
         │able   │        │able  │        │able  │
         ▼       ▼        ▼      ▼        ▼      ▼
       ┌──────┐┌──────┐ ┌──────┐┌──────┐ ┌──────┐┌──────┐
       │Mech. ││Valve │ │Mech. ││Valve │ │Tissue││Valve │
       │CVG   ││Spar- │ │CVG   ││Spar- │ │CVG   ││Spar- │
       │Xeno- ││ing   │ │Tissue││ing   │ │Xeno- ││ing   │
       │graft ││Root  │ │CVG   ││Root  │ │graft ││Root  │
       │Root  ││      │ │Homo- ││      │ │Root  ││      │
       │      ││      │ │graft ││      │ │      ││      │
       │      ││      │ │Root  ││      │ │      ││      │
       │      ││      │ │Xeno- ││      │ │      ││      │
       │      ││      │ │graft ││      │ │      ││      │
       │      ││      │ │Root  ││      │ │      ││      │
       └──────┘└──────┘ └──────┘└──────┘ └──────┘└──────┘
```

```
                        Aortic Root Aneurysm
                       /        |         \
          Degenerative     Connective     BAV
          etiology         Tissue Disorder Aortopathy
               |                |              |
        Indications        Indications      Indications
        -Size > 5.5 cm     -Size > 4.2 cm    -Size > 5.5 cm
        -Growth rate       in Loeys-Dietz    -Size 5 cm with risk factors
         > 1/2 cm / yr     > 5 cm in Marfan's (predominant AI, uncontrolled HTN,
        -Symptomatic       -Growth rate      Family history of aortic dissection,
                            > 1/2 cm / yr    sudden cardiac death)
                           -Symptomatic      -Size > 4.5 cm with concominant cardiac surgery
```

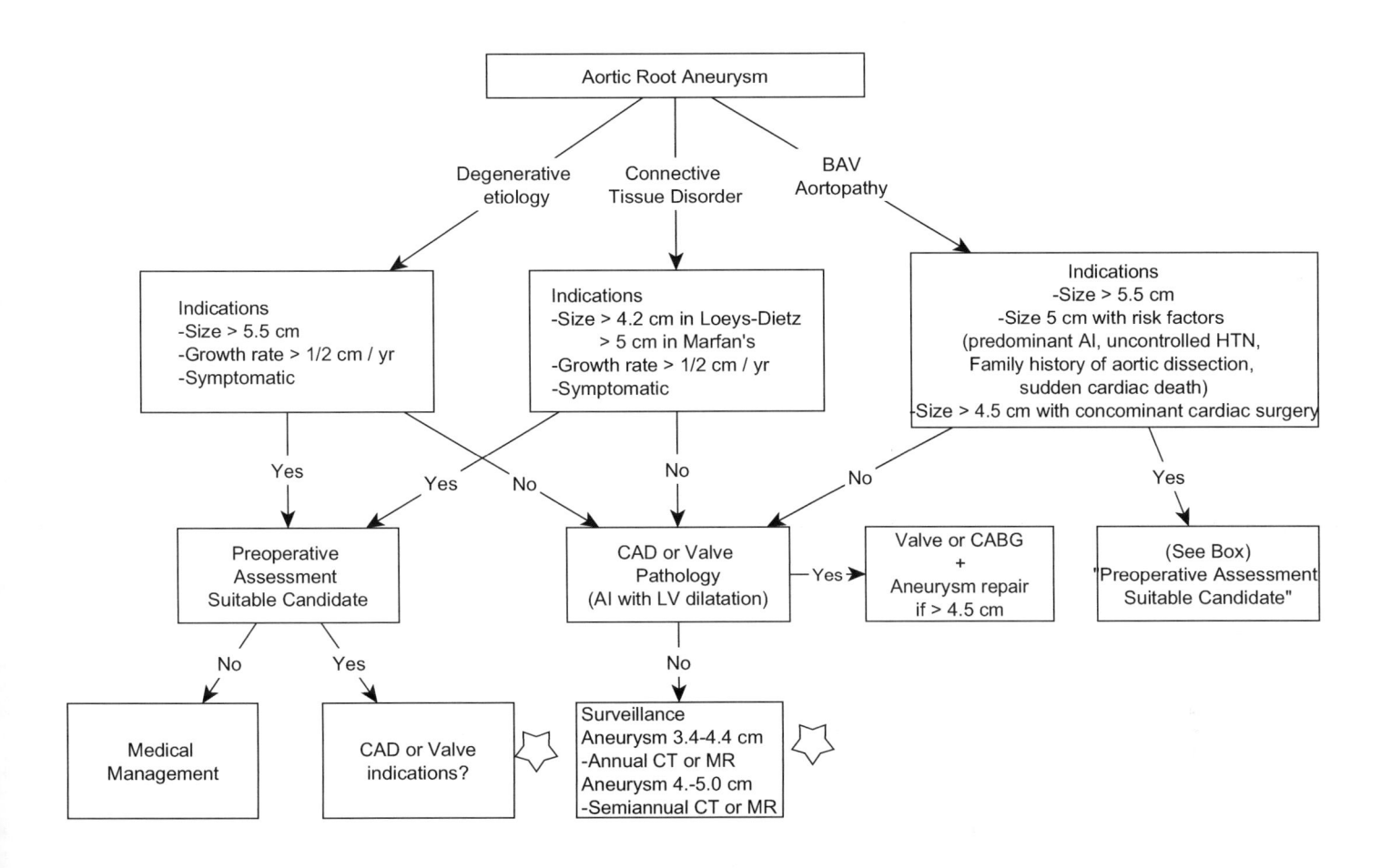

Yes / No branches lead to:

- Preoperative Assessment Suitable Candidate
  - No → Medical Management
  - Yes → CAD or Valve indications?
- CAD or Valve Pathology (AI with LV dilatation)
  - Yes → Valve or CABG + Aneurysm repair if > 4.5 cm
  - No → Surveillance
    - Aneurysm 3.4-4.4 cm - Annual CT or MR
    - Aneurysm 4.-5.0 cm - Semiannual CT or MR
- BAV Yes → (See Box) "Preoperative Assessment Suitable Candidate"

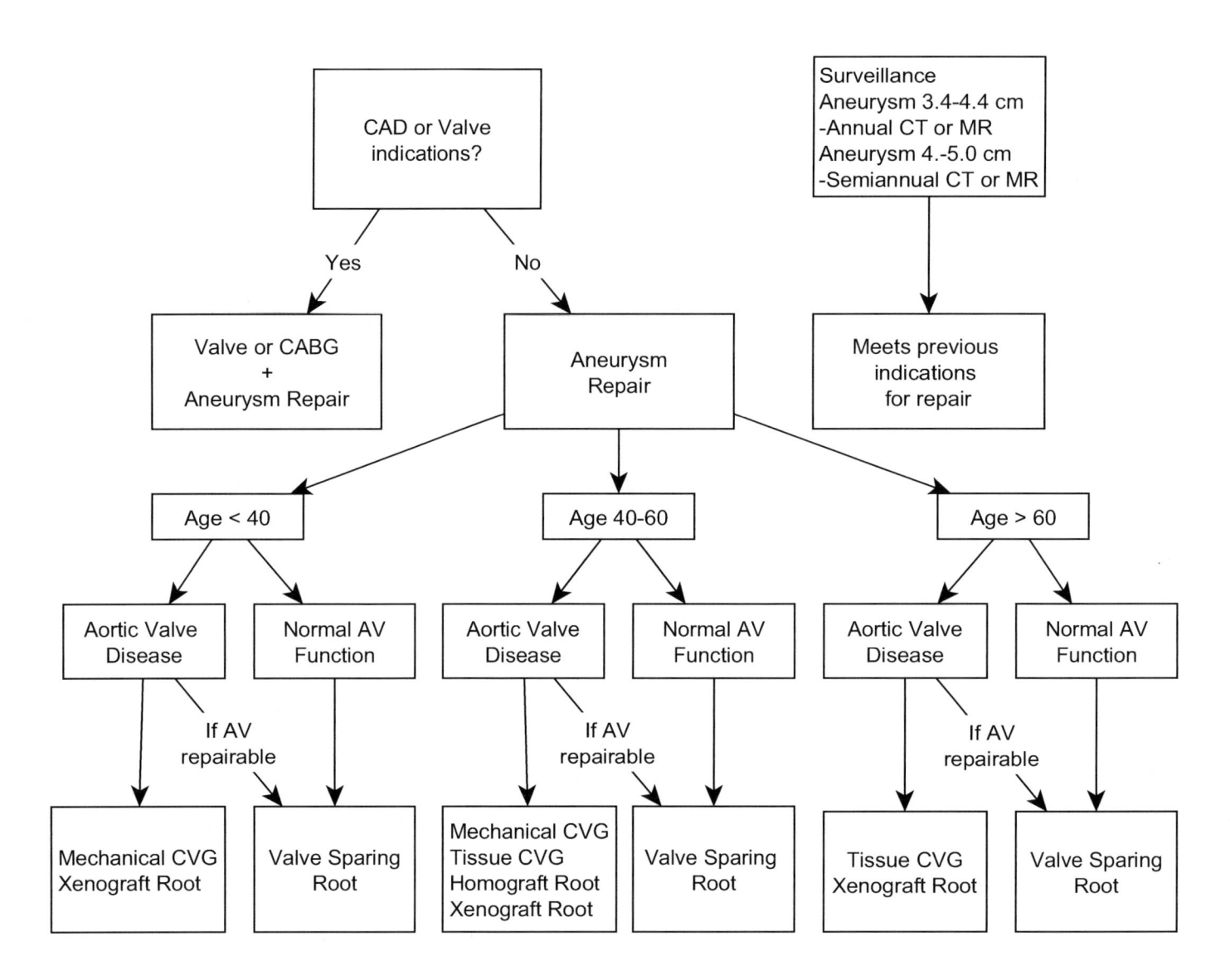

```
                    ┌─────────────────┐                      ┌──────────────────────┐
                    │  CAD or Valve   │                      │ Surveillance         │
                    │  indications?   │                      │ Aneurysm 3.4-4.4 cm  │
                    └─────────────────┘                      │ -Annual CT or MR     │
                      Yes        No                          │ Aneurysm 4.-5.0 cm   │
                     ↓            ↓                          │ -Semiannual CT or MR │
          ┌──────────────────┐  ┌──────────┐                 └──────────────────────┘
          │  Valve or CABG   │  │ Aneurysm │                            ↓
          │        +         │  │  Repair  │                 ┌──────────────────────┐
          │ Aneurysm Repair  │  └──────────┘                 │   Meets previous     │
          └──────────────────┘                               │   indications        │
                                                             │   for repair         │
                                                             └──────────────────────┘
```

Aneurysm Repair branches:

- **Age < 40**
  - Aortic Valve Disease → Mechanical CVG / Xenograft Root
  - If AV repairable → Valve Sparing Root
  - Normal AV Function → Valve Sparing Root

- **Age 40-60**
  - Aortic Valve Disease → Mechanical CVG / Tissue CVG / Homograft Root / Xenograft Root
  - If AV repairable → Valve Sparing Root
  - Normal AV Function → Valve Sparing Root

- **Age > 60**
  - Aortic Valve Disease → Tissue CVG / Xenograft Root
  - If AV repairable → Valve Sparing Root
  - Normal AV Function → Valve Sparing Root

BAV, Bicuspid Aortic Valve; CAD, Coronary Artery Disease; CT, Computed Tomography; MR, Magnetic Resonance; CABG, Coronary Artery Bypass Grafting; AV, Aortic Valve; CVG, Composite Valve Graft; AI, Aortic Insufficiency; HTN, Hypertension

Descending Thoracic Aortic Aneurysms
Carlo Maria Rosati, Leonard Girardi

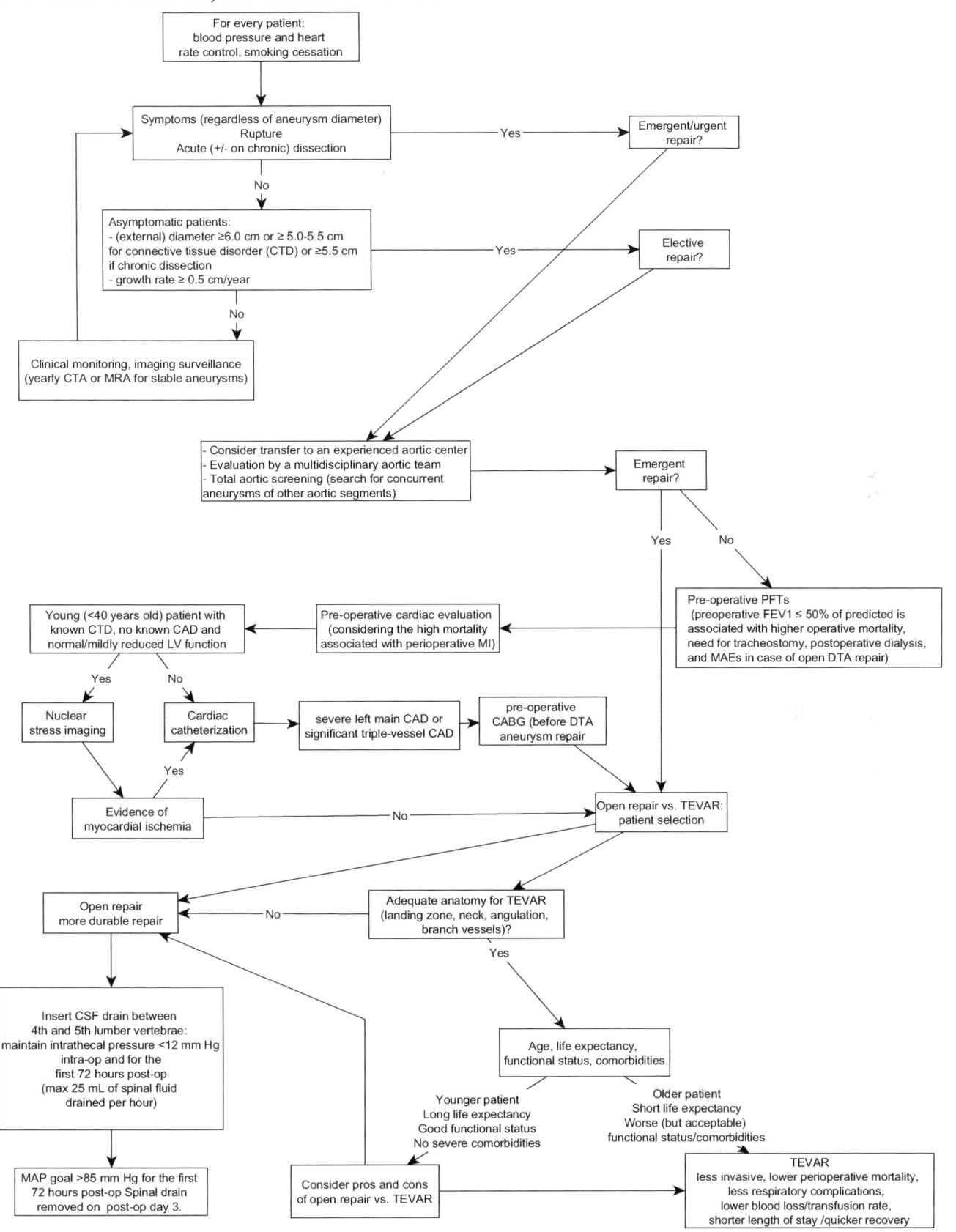

```
┌─────────────────────────────┐
│ For every patient:          │
│ blood pressure and heart    │
│ rate control, smoking       │
│ cessation                   │
└──────────────┬──────────────┘
               ▼
┌─────────────────────────────┐              ┌──────────────┐
│ Symptoms (regardless of     │── Yes ──────▶│ Emergent/    │
│ aneurysm diameter)          │              │ urgent       │
│ Rupture                     │              │ repair?      │
│ Acute (+/- on chronic)      │              └──────────────┘
│ dissection                  │
└──────────────┬──────────────┘
               │ No
               ▼
┌─────────────────────────────┐              ┌──────────────┐
│ Asymptomatic patients:      │              │ Elective     │
│ - (external) diameter ≥6.0  │── Yes ──────▶│ repair?      │
│   cm or ≥ 5.0-5.5 cm for    │              └──────────────┘
│   connective tissue         │
│   disorder (CTD) or ≥5.5 cm │
│   if chronic dissection     │
│ - growth rate ≥ 0.5 cm/year │
└──────────────┬──────────────┘
               │ No
               ▼
┌─────────────────────────────┐
│ Clinical monitoring,        │
│ imaging surveillance        │
│ (yearly CTA or MRA for      │
│ stable aneurysms)           │
└─────────────────────────────┘

┌─────────────────────────────────────────────┐          ┌──────────────┐
│ - Consider transfer to an experienced       │          │ Emergent     │
│   aortic center                             │─────────▶│ repair?      │
│ - Evaluation by a multidisciplinary         │          └──────┬───────┘
│   aortic team                               │            Yes / \ No
│ - Total aortic screening (search for        │                /   \
│   concurrent aneurysms of other aortic      │               /     \
│   segments)                                 │              /       ▼
└─────────────────────────────────────────────┘             /   ┌─────────────────────────────┐
                                                           /    │ Pre-operative PFTs           │
                                                          /     │ (preoperative FEV1 ≤ 50% of  │
                                                         /      │ predicted is associated with │
                                                        /       │ higher operative mortality,  │
                                                       /        │ need for tracheostomy,       │
                                                      /         │ postoperative dialysis, and  │
                                                     /          │ MAEs in case of open DTA     │
                                                    /           │ repair)                      │
                                                   /            └─────────────────────────────┘
```

Young (<40 years old) patient with known CTD, no known CAD and normal/mildly reduced LV function

Pre-operative cardiac evaluation (considering the high mortality associated with perioperative MI)

- Yes → Nuclear stress imaging
- No → Cardiac catheterization

→ severe left main CAD or significant triple-vessel CAD → pre-operative CABG (before DTA aneurysm repair)

Evidence of myocardial ischemia — No → Open repair vs. TEVAR: patient selection

Open repair — more durable repair ← No — Adequate anatomy for TEVAR (landing zone, neck, angulation, branch vessels)?
→ Yes → Age, life expectancy, functional status, comorbidities

Insert CSF drain between 4th and 5th lumber vertebrae: maintain intrathecal pressure <12 mm Hg intra-op and for the first 72 hours post-op (max 25 mL of spinal fluid drained per hour)

MAP goal >85 mm Hg for the first 72 hours post-op Spinal drain removed on post-op day 3.

Younger patient — Long life expectancy, Good functional status, No severe comorbidities → Consider pros and cons of open repair vs. TEVAR

Older patient — Short life expectancy, Worse (but acceptable) functional status/comorbidities

TEVAR — less invasive, lower perioperative mortality, less respiratory complications, lower blood loss/transfusion rate, shorter length of stay /quicker recovery

85

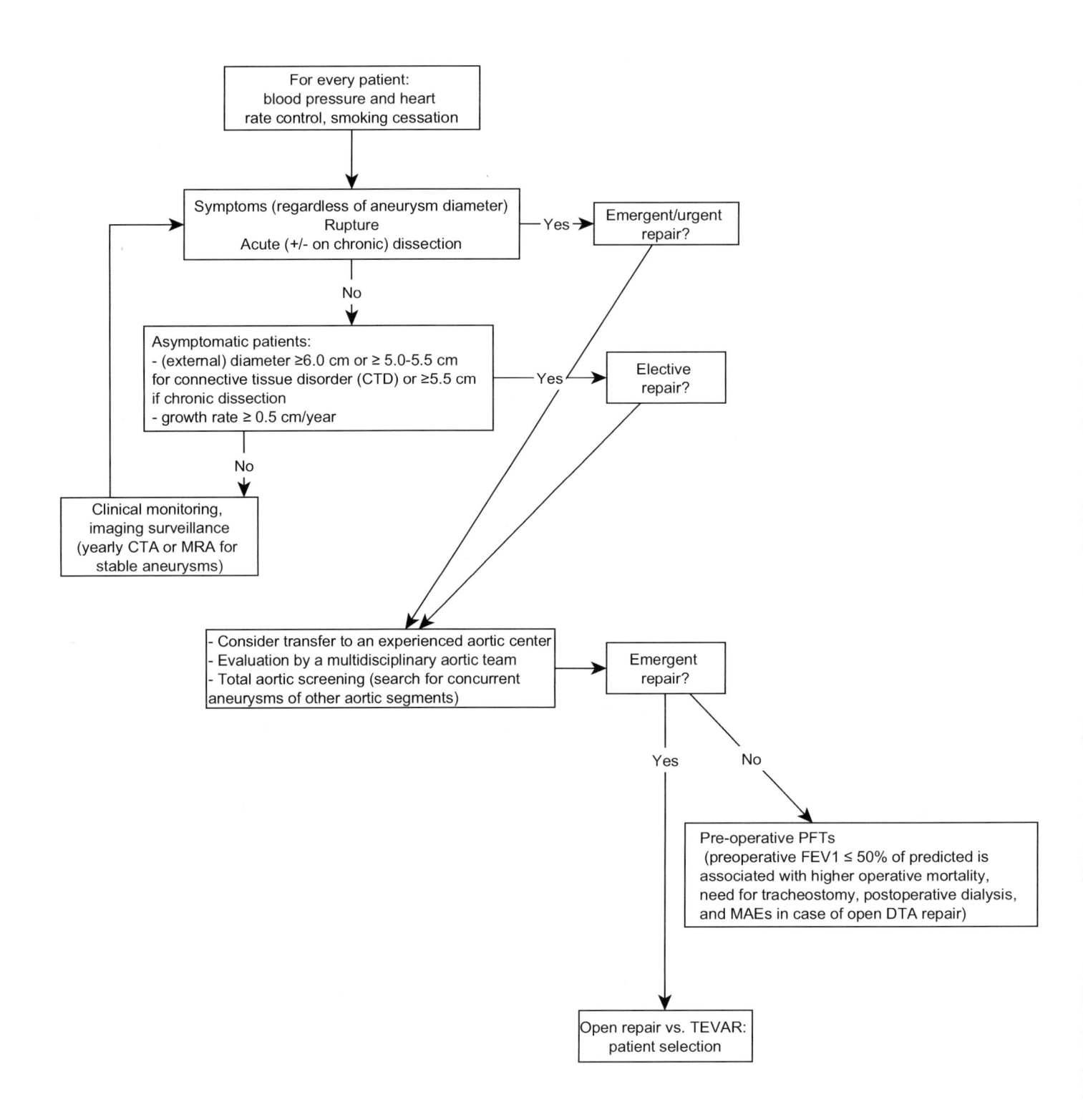

```
┌─────────────────────────────┐
│ For every patient:          │
│ blood pressure and heart    │
│ rate control, smoking cessation │
└──────────────┬──────────────┘
               │
               ▼
┌─────────────────────────────────────┐
│ Symptoms (regardless of aneurysm diameter) │──Yes──▶ Emergent/urgent repair?
│ Rupture                                    │
│ Acute (+/- on chronic) dissection          │
└──────────────┬──────────────────────┘
               │ No
               ▼
┌─────────────────────────────────────────────┐
│ Asymptomatic patients:                      │
│ - (external) diameter ≥6.0 cm or ≥ 5.0-5.5 cm│──Yes──▶ Elective repair?
│ for connective tissue disorder (CTD) or ≥5.5 cm│
│ if chronic dissection                       │
│ - growth rate ≥ 0.5 cm/year                 │
└──────────────┬──────────────────────────────┘
               │ No
               ▼
┌─────────────────────────────┐
│ Clinical monitoring,        │
│ imaging surveillance        │
│ (yearly CTA or MRA for      │
│ stable aneurysms)           │
└─────────────────────────────┘

┌─────────────────────────────────────────────┐
│ - Consider transfer to an experienced aortic center │
│ - Evaluation by a multidisciplinary aortic team     │──▶ Emergent repair?
│ - Total aortic screening (search for concurrent     │      │        │
│   aneurysms of other aortic segments)               │     Yes      No
└─────────────────────────────────────────────┘                      │
                                                                     ▼
                                              ┌────────────────────────────────────────┐
                                              │ Pre-operative PFTs                     │
                                              │ (preoperative FEV1 ≤ 50% of predicted is│
                                              │ associated with higher operative mortality,│
                                              │ need for tracheostomy, postoperative dialysis,│
                                              │ and MAEs in case of open DTA repair)   │
                                              └────────────────────────────────────────┘

                            ┌─────────────────────────────┐
                            │ Open repair vs. TEVAR:      │
                            │ patient selection           │
                            └─────────────────────────────┘
```

```
                                                    ┌──────────────┐
                                                    │  Emergent    │
                                                    │  repair?     │
                                                    └──────┬───────┘
                                                    Yes  ／  ＼  No
```

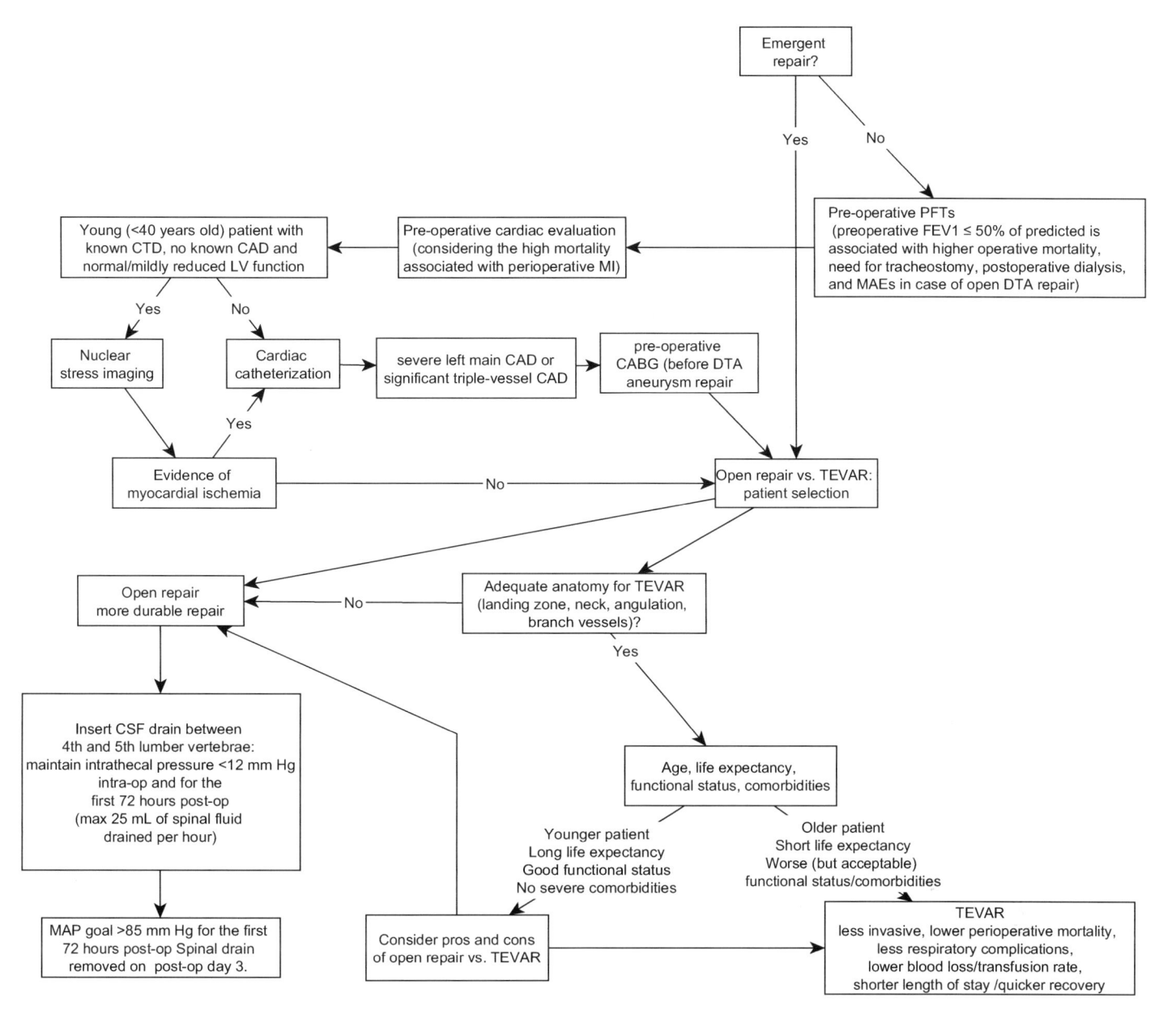

```
┌─────────────────────────┐   ┌──────────────────────────┐   ┌──────────────────────────────────┐
│ Young (<40 years old)   │   │ Pre-operative cardiac    │   │ Pre-operative PFTs               │
│ patient with known CTD, │◄──│ evaluation (considering  │◄──│ (preoperative FEV1 ≤ 50% of      │
│ no known CAD and        │   │ the high mortality       │   │ predicted is associated with     │
│ normal/mildly reduced   │   │ associated with          │   │ higher operative mortality,      │
│ LV function             │   │ perioperative MI)        │   │ need for tracheostomy,           │
└──────┬──────────┬───────┘   └──────────────────────────┘   │ postoperative dialysis, and      │
    Yes│       No │                                          │ MAEs in case of open DTA repair) │
       ▼          ▼                                          └──────────────────────────────────┘
┌──────────┐  ┌──────────────┐   ┌────────────────────┐   ┌──────────────────┐
│ Nuclear  │  │ Cardiac      │──▶│ severe left main   │──▶│ pre-operative    │
│ stress   │  │catheterization│   │ CAD or significant │   │ CABG (before DTA │
│ imaging  │  │              │   │ triple-vessel CAD  │   │ aneurysm repair  │
└────┬─────┘  └──────┬───────┘   └────────────────────┘   └────────┬─────────┘
     │            Yes│                                              │
     ▼               ▼                                              ▼
┌─────────────────────┐                                   ┌──────────────────────┐
│ Evidence of         │────────── No ────────────────────▶│ Open repair vs. TEVAR│
│ myocardial ischemia │                                   │ patient selection    │
└─────────────────────┘                                   └──────────┬───────────┘
                                                                     │
┌─────────────────┐        ┌──────────────────────┐                 │
│ Open repair     │◄── No ─│ Adequate anatomy for │◄────────────────┘
│ more durable    │        │ TEVAR (landing zone, │
│ repair          │        │ neck, angulation,    │
└────────┬────────┘        │ branch vessels)?     │
         │                 └──────────┬───────────┘
         ▼                          Yes│
┌─────────────────────────┐            ▼
│ Insert CSF drain between│    ┌────────────────────────┐
│ 4th and 5th lumber      │    │ Age, life expectancy,  │
│ vertebrae: maintain     │    │ functional status,     │
│ intrathecal pressure    │    │ comorbidities          │
│ <12 mm Hg intra-op and  │    └────┬──────────────┬────┘
│ for the first 72 hours  │  Younger patient   Older patient
│ post-op (max 25 mL of   │  Long life exp.    Short life exp.
│ spinal fluid drained    │  Good functional   Worse (but acceptable)
│ per hour)               │  status            functional status/
└──────────┬──────────────┘  No severe         comorbidities
           │                 comorbidities
           ▼                      │                  ▼
┌─────────────────────────┐       ▼         ┌─────────────────────────────┐
│ MAP goal >85 mm Hg for  │  ┌──────────────┐│ TEVAR                       │
│ the first 72 hours      │  │ Consider pros││ less invasive, lower        │
│ post-op Spinal drain    │  │ and cons of  ││ perioperative mortality,    │
│ removed on post-op      │  │ open repair  ││ less respiratory            │
│ day 3.                  │  │ vs. TEVAR    ││ complications, lower blood  │
└─────────────────────────┘  └──────────────┘│ loss/transfusion rate,      │
                                             │ shorter length of stay /    │
                                             │ quicker recovery            │
                                             └─────────────────────────────┘
```

CABG, coronary artery bypass grafting; CAD, coronary artery disease; CSF, cerebrospinal fluid; CTA, computed tomography angiography; CTD, connective tissue disorder; DTA, descending thoracic aorta; FEV1, forced expiratory volume in 1 second; LV, left ventricle; MAP, mean arterial pressure; MI, myocardial infarction; MRA, magnetic resonance angiography; PFTs, pulmonary function tests; TEVAR, thoracic endovascular aortic repair

Extracorporeal Membrane Oxygenation
Saikus CE, Piercecchi CW, Blum JM

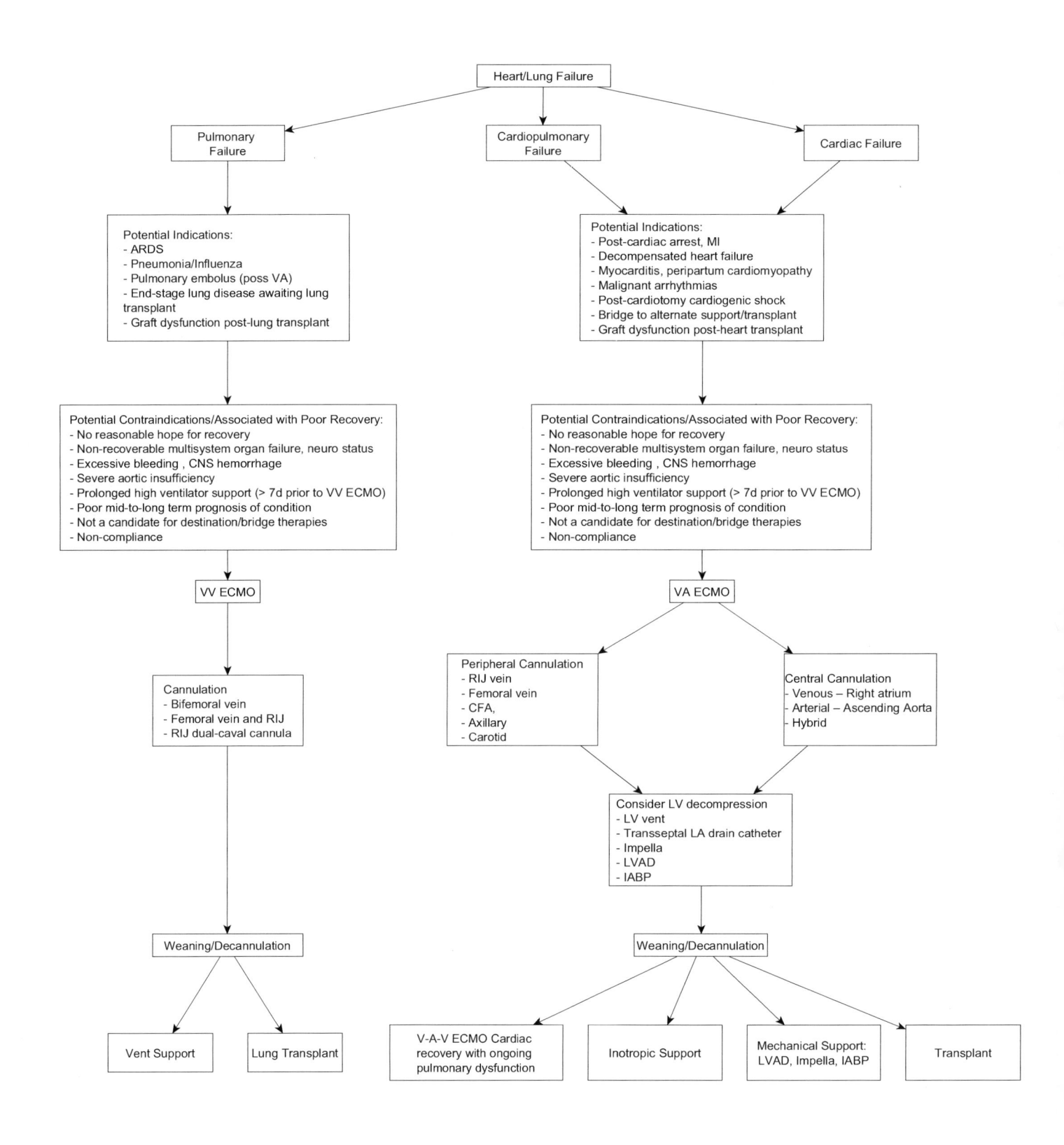

```
                          Heart/Lung Failure
              ┌──────────────────┼──────────────────┐
     Pulmonary Failure   Cardiopulmonary      Cardiac Failure
                             Failure
```

Potential Indications (Pulmonary):
- ARDS
- Pneumonia/Influenza
- Pulmonary embolus (poss VA)
- End-stage lung disease awaiting lung transplant
- Graft dysfunction post-lung transplant

Potential Indications (Cardiac/Cardiopulmonary):
- Post-cardiac arrest, MI
- Decompensated heart failure
- Myocarditis, peripartum cardiomyopathy
- Malignant arrhythmias
- Post-cardiotomy cardiogenic shock
- Bridge to alternate support/transplant
- Graft dysfunction post-heart transplant

Potential Contraindications/Associated with Poor Recovery:
- No reasonable hope for recovery
- Non-recoverable multisystem organ failure, neuro status
- Excessive bleeding, CNS hemorrhage
- Severe aortic insufficiency
- Prolonged high ventilator support (> 7d prior to VV ECMO)
- Poor mid-to-long term prognosis of condition
- Not a candidate for destination/bridge therapies
- Non-compliance

Potential Contraindications/Associated with Poor Recovery:
- No reasonable hope for recovery
- Non-recoverable multisystem organ failure, neuro status
- Excessive bleeding, CNS hemorrhage
- Severe aortic insufficiency
- Prolonged high ventilator support (> 7d prior to VV ECMO)
- Poor mid-to-long term prognosis of condition
- Not a candidate for destination/bridge therapies
- Non-compliance

VV ECMO

Cannulation
- Bifemoral vein
- Femoral vein and RIJ
- RIJ dual-caval cannula

VA ECMO

Peripheral Cannulation
- RIJ vein
- Femoral vein
- CFA
- Axillary
- Carotid

Central Cannulation
- Venous – Right atrium
- Arterial – Ascending Aorta
- Hybrid

Consider LV decompression
- LV vent
- Transseptal LA drain catheter
- Impella
- LVAD
- IABP

Weaning/Decannulation (VV ECMO):
- Vent Support
- Lung Transplant

Weaning/Decannulation (VA ECMO):
- V-A-V ECMO Cardiac recovery with ongoing pulmonary dysfunction
- Inotropic Support
- Mechanical Support: LVAD, Impella, IABP
- Transplant

```
┌─────────────────┐
│ Heart/Lung Failure │
└─────────────────┘
         │
   ┌─────┼─────┐
   ▼     ▼     ▼
```

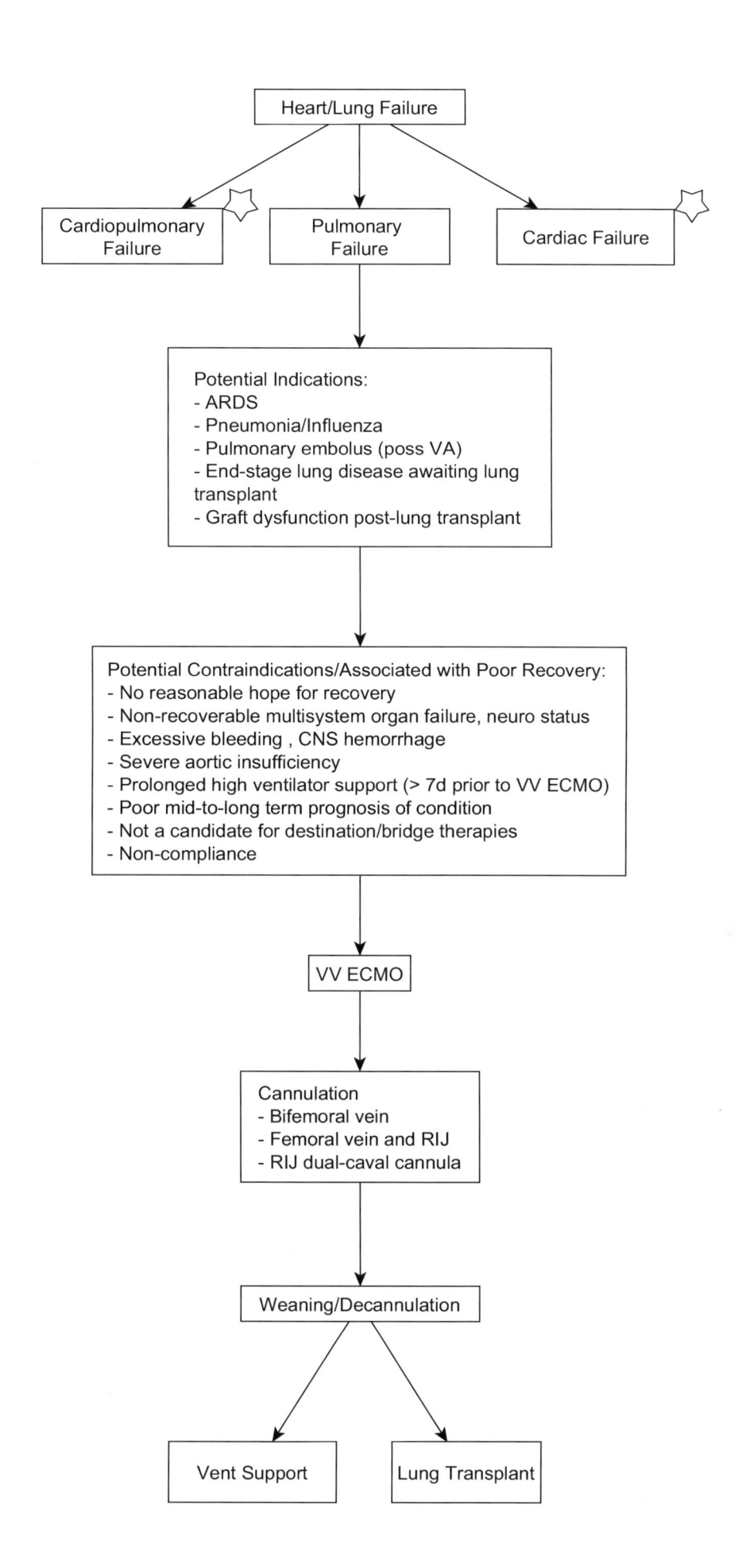

- **Cardiopulmonary Failure**
- **Pulmonary Failure**
- **Cardiac Failure**

Potential Indications:
- ARDS
- Pneumonia/Influenza
- Pulmonary embolus (poss VA)
- End-stage lung disease awaiting lung transplant
- Graft dysfunction post-lung transplant

Potential Contraindications/Associated with Poor Recovery:
- No reasonable hope for recovery
- Non-recoverable multisystem organ failure, neuro status
- Excessive bleeding, CNS hemorrhage
- Severe aortic insufficiency
- Prolonged high ventilator support (> 7d prior to VV ECMO)
- Poor mid-to-long term prognosis of condition
- Not a candidate for destination/bridge therapies
- Non-compliance

VV ECMO

Cannulation
- Bifemoral vein
- Femoral vein and RIJ
- RIJ dual-caval cannula

Weaning/Decannulation

- Vent Support
- Lung Transplant

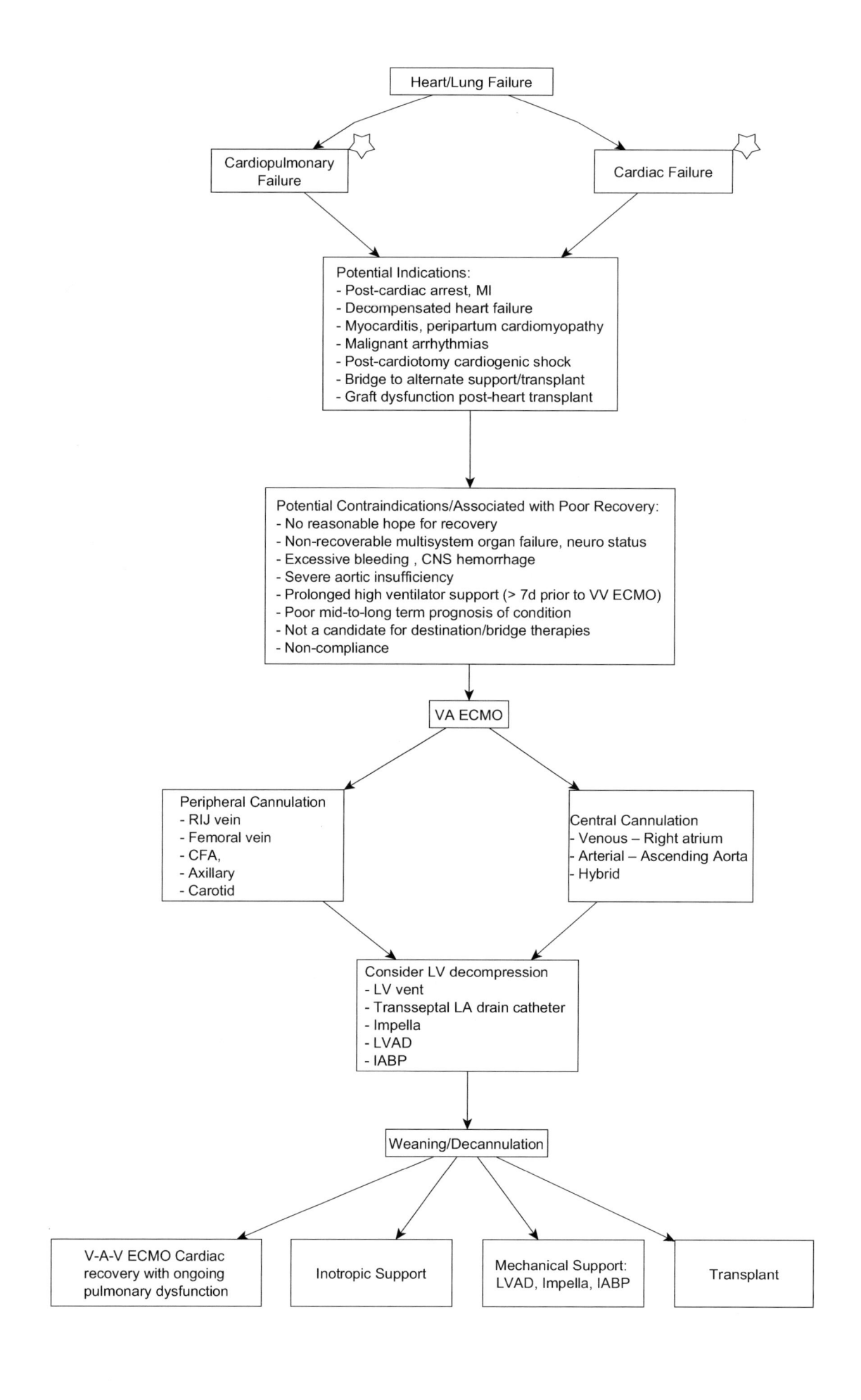

```
┌─────────────────┐
│ Heart/Lung Failure │
└─────────────────┘
        │
   ┌────┴────┐
   ▼         ▼
┌──────────────┐   ┌──────────────┐
│Cardiopulmonary│   │Cardiac Failure│
│   Failure    │   │              │
└──────────────┘   └──────────────┘
        │         │
        └────┬────┘
             ▼
┌─────────────────────────────────────────┐
│ Potential Indications:                  │
│  - Post-cardiac arrest, MI              │
│  - Decompensated heart failure          │
│  - Myocarditis, peripartum cardiomyopathy│
│  - Malignant arrhythmias                │
│  - Post-cardiotomy cardiogenic shock    │
│  - Bridge to alternate support/transplant│
│  - Graft dysfunction post-heart transplant│
└─────────────────────────────────────────┘
             │
             ▼
┌─────────────────────────────────────────────────────┐
│ Potential Contraindications/Associated with Poor Recovery: │
│  - No reasonable hope for recovery                  │
│  - Non-recoverable multisystem organ failure, neuro status │
│  - Excessive bleeding, CNS hemorrhage               │
│  - Severe aortic insufficiency                      │
│  - Prolonged high ventilator support (> 7d prior to VV ECMO)│
│  - Poor mid-to-long term prognosis of condition     │
│  - Not a candidate for destination/bridge therapies │
│  - Non-compliance                                   │
└─────────────────────────────────────────────────────┘
             │
             ▼
        ┌─────────┐
        │ VA ECMO │
        └─────────┘
          │     │
     ┌────┘     └────┐
     ▼               ▼
┌──────────────┐  ┌──────────────────┐
│Peripheral    │  │Central Cannulation│
│Cannulation   │  │ - Venous – Right atrium│
│ - RIJ vein   │  │ - Arterial – Ascending Aorta│
│ - Femoral vein│  │ - Hybrid         │
│ - CFA,       │  │                  │
│ - Axillary   │  │                  │
│ - Carotid    │  │                  │
└──────────────┘  └──────────────────┘
          │     │
          └──┬──┘
             ▼
┌──────────────────────────────┐
│ Consider LV decompression    │
│  - LV vent                   │
│  - Transseptal LA drain catheter│
│  - Impella                   │
│  - LVAD                      │
│  - IABP                      │
└──────────────────────────────┘
             │
             ▼
    ┌──────────────────┐
    │Weaning/Decannulation│
    └──────────────────┘
     │      │      │      │
     ▼      ▼      ▼      ▼
┌─────────┐ ┌────────┐ ┌──────────┐ ┌──────────┐
│V-A-V ECMO│ │Inotropic│ │Mechanical│ │Transplant│
│Cardiac   │ │Support  │ │Support:  │ │          │
│recovery  │ │         │ │LVAD,     │ │          │
│with ongoing│ │         │ │Impella,  │ │          │
│pulmonary │ │         │ │IABP      │ │          │
│dysfunction│ │         │ │          │ │          │
└─────────┘ └────────┘ └──────────┘ └──────────┘
```

ECMO, extracorporeal membrane oxygenation; VV, Veno-venous; VA, Veno-arterial; V-A-V, Veno-arterial-venous; IABP, Intra-aortic balloon pump; LVAD, Left ventricular assist device; BiVAD, Bi-ventricular assist device; TAH, Total artificial heart; MI, Myocardial infarction; LV, Left ventricle; LA, Left atrium; CFA, Common femoral artery; ARDS, Acute respiratory distress syndrome; RIJ, Right internal jugular; SvO2, Mixed venous oxygen saturation; CNS, Central nervous system; ICH, Intracranial hemorrhage; PEDS, Pediatrics

Left Ventricular Assist Devices
Marvin Atkins, Pavin Atluri

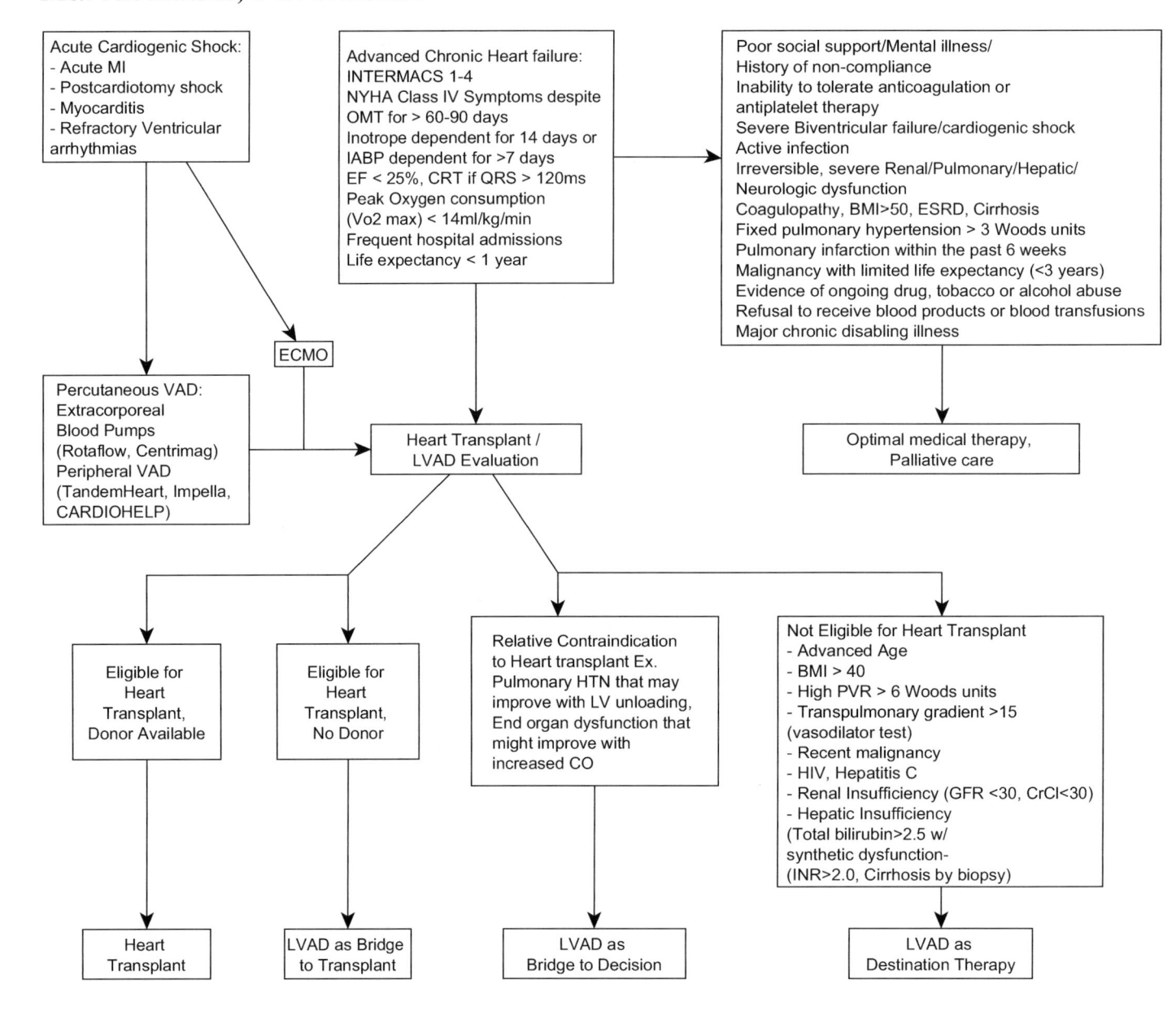

```
┌─────────────────────────┐  ┌──────────────────────────────┐  ┌────────────────────────────────────────────┐
│ Acute Cardiogenic Shock:│  │ Advanced Chronic Heart       │  │ Poor social support/Mental illness/        │
│ - Acute MI              │  │ failure:                     │  │ History of non-compliance                  │
│ - Postcardiotomy shock  │  │ INTERMACS 1-4                │  │ Inability to tolerate anticoagulation or   │
│ - Myocarditis           │  │ NYHA Class IV Symptoms       │  │ antiplatelet therapy                       │
│ - Refractory Ventricular│  │ despite OMT for > 60-90 days │  │ Severe Biventricular failure/cardiogenic   │
│ arrhythmias             │  │ Inotrope dependent for 14    │  │ shock                                      │
│                         │  │ days or IABP dependent for   │  │ Active infection                           │
│                         │  │ >7 days                      │  │ Irreversible, severe Renal/Pulmonary/      │
│                         │  │ EF < 25%, CRT if QRS > 120ms │  │ Hepatic/Neurologic dysfunction             │
│                         │  │ Peak Oxygen consumption      │  │ Coagulopathy, BMI>50, ESRD, Cirrhosis      │
│                         │  │ (Vo2 max) < 14ml/kg/min      │  │ Fixed pulmonary hypertension > 3 Woods units│
│                         │  │ Frequent hospital admissions │  │ Pulmonary infarction within the past 6 weeks│
│                         │  │ Life expectancy < 1 year     │  │ Malignancy with limited life expectancy (<3 years)│
│                         │  │                              │  │ Evidence of ongoing drug, tobacco or alcohol abuse│
│                         │  │                              │  │ Refusal to receive blood products or blood transfusions│
│                         │  │                              │  │ Major chronic disabling illness            │
└─────────────────────────┘  └──────────────────────────────┘  └────────────────────────────────────────────┘
                  │   ┌──────┐           │                                       │
                  │   │ ECMO │           │                                       ▼
                  ▼   └──────┘           ▼                          ┌────────────────────────┐
┌──────────────────────┐         ┌──────────────────┐               │ Optimal medical therapy│
│ Percutaneous VAD:    │         │ Heart Transplant │               │ Palliative care        │
│ Extracorporeal       │         │ / LVAD Evaluation│               └────────────────────────┘
│ Blood Pumps          │         └──────────────────┘
│ (Rotaflow, Centrimag)│
│ Peripheral VAD       │
│ (TandemHeart,Impella,│
│ CARDIOHELP)          │
└──────────────────────┘
```

Branches from Heart Transplant / LVAD Evaluation:

- **Eligible for Heart Transplant, Donor Available** → Heart Transplant
- **Eligible for Heart Transplant, No Donor** → LVAD as Bridge to Transplant
- **Relative Contraindication to Heart transplant Ex. Pulmonary HTN that may improve with LV unloading, End organ dysfunction that might improve with increased CO** → LVAD as Bridge to Decision
- **Not Eligible for Heart Transplant**
  - Advanced Age
  - BMI > 40
  - High PVR > 6 Woods units
  - Transpulmonary gradient >15 (vasodilator test)
  - Recent malignancy
  - HIV, Hepatitis C
  - Renal Insufficiency (GFR <30, CrCl<30)
  - Hepatic Insufficiency (Total bilirubin>2.5 w/ synthetic dysfunction- (INR>2.0, Cirrhosis by biopsy))

  → LVAD as Destination Therapy

INTERMACS, Interagency Registry for Mechanically Assisted Circulatory Support; OMT, Optimal medical therapy; CRT, Cardiac Resynchronization Therapy; ESRD, End Stage Renal Disease; ECMO, Extra Corporeal Membrane Oxygenation; PVR, Peripheral Vascular Resistance; GFR, Glomerular filtration rate; Cr Cl, Creatinine clearance; BMI, Body Mass Index

Right Ventricular Assist Device
Awais Ashfaq, Fred Tibayan

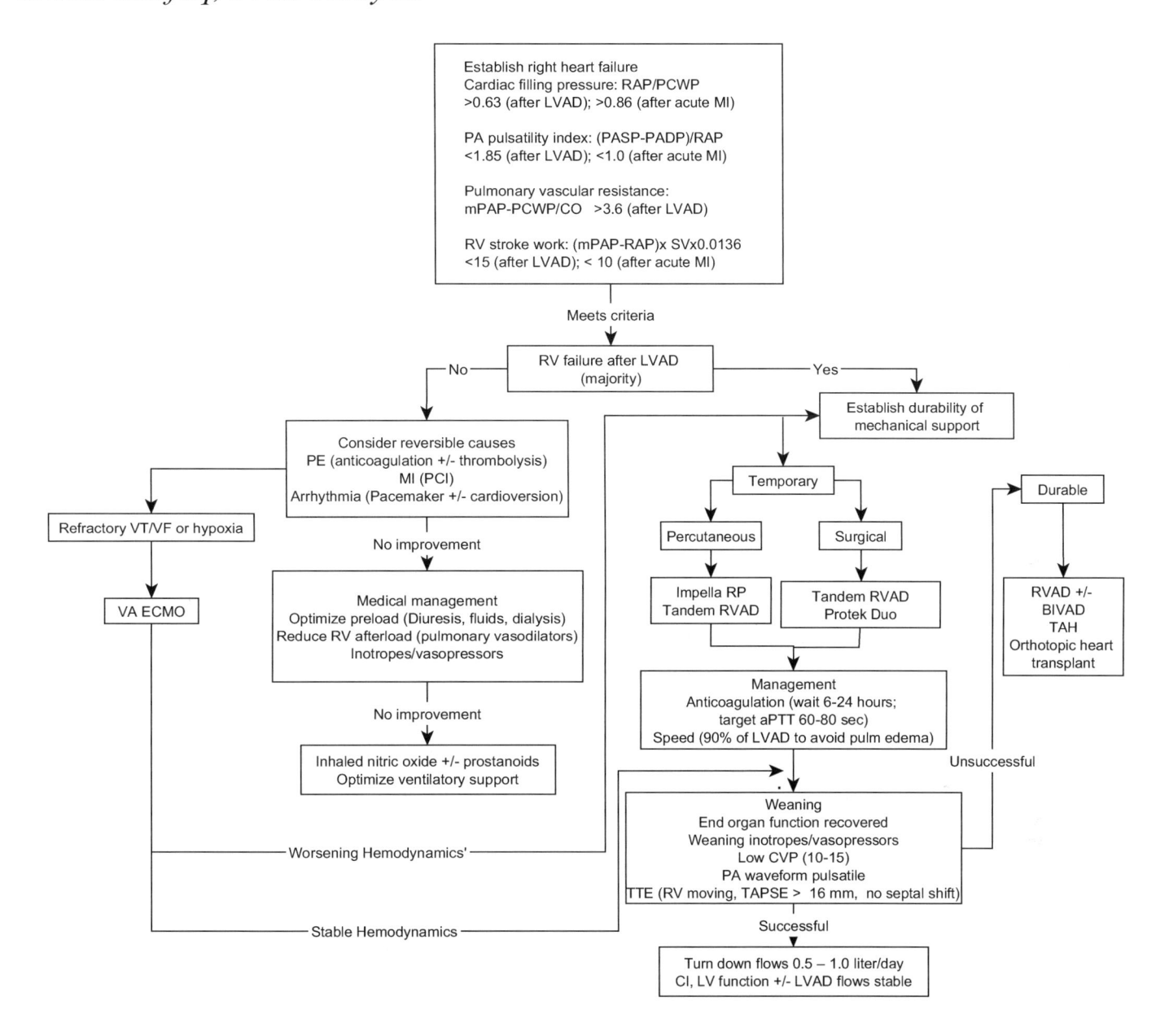

```
┌─────────────────────────────────────────┐
│ Establish right heart failure            │
│ Cardiac filling pressure: RAP/PCWP       │
│ >0.63 (after LVAD); >0.86 (after acute MI)│
│                                          │
│ PA pulsatility index: (PASP-PADP)/RAP    │
│ <1.85 (after LVAD); <1.0 (after acute MI)│
│                                          │
│ Pulmonary vascular resistance:           │
│ mPAP-PCWP/CO  >3.6 (after LVAD)          │
│                                          │
│ RV stroke work: (mPAP-RAP)x SVx0.0136    │
│ <15 (after LVAD); < 10 (after acute MI)  │
└─────────────────────────────────────────┘
                   │ Meets criteria
                   ▼
        ┌──────────────────────┐
   No ──│ RV failure after LVAD │── Yes
   │    │     (majority)        │    │
   │    └──────────────────────┘    │
   ▼                                 ▼
                              Establish durability of
                               mechanical support
                              ┌──────┴──────┐
                           Temporary     Durable
                          ┌────┴────┐       │
                    Percutaneous  Surgical  │
                    Impella RP  Tandem RVAD RVAD +/-
                    Tandem RVAD Protek Duo  BIVAD
                                            TAH
                                            Orthotopic heart
                                            transplant
```

Consider reversible causes
PE (anticoagulation +/- thrombolysis)
MI (PCI)
Arrhythmia (Pacemaker +/- cardioversion)

Refractory VT/VF or hypoxia → VA ECMO

Medical management
Optimize preload (Diuresis, fluids, dialysis)
Reduce RV afterload (pulmonary vasodilators)
Inotropes/vasopressors

Inhaled nitric oxide +/- prostanoids
Optimize ventilatory support

Management
Anticoagulation (wait 6-24 hours;
target aPTT 60-80 sec)
Speed (90% of LVAD to avoid pulm edema)

Weaning
End organ function recovered
Weaning inotropes/vasopressors
Low CVP (10-15)
PA waveform pulsatile
TTE (RV moving, TAPSE > 16 mm, no septal shift)

Turn down flows 0.5 – 1.0 liter/day
CI, LV function +/- LVAD flows stable

RVAD, Right ventricular assist device; RAP, Right atrial pressure; PCWP, Pulmonary capillary wedge pressure; PA, Pulmonary artery; PASP, Pulmonary artery systolic pressure; PADP, Pulmonary artery diastolic pressure; LVAD, Left ventricular assist device; PE, Pulmonary embolism; MI, Myocardial infarction; PCI, Percutaneous coronary intervention; VT/VF, Ventricular tachycardia, ventricular fibrillation; VA ECMO, Veno-arterial extracorporeal membrane oxygenation; CVP, Central venous pressure; TTE, transthoracic echocardiogram; TAPSE, Tricuspid annular plane systolic excursion; CI, Cardiac index; BIVAD, Biventricular assist device; TAH, Total artificial heart.

Pump Thrombosis
J Hunter Mehaffey, Leora Yarboro

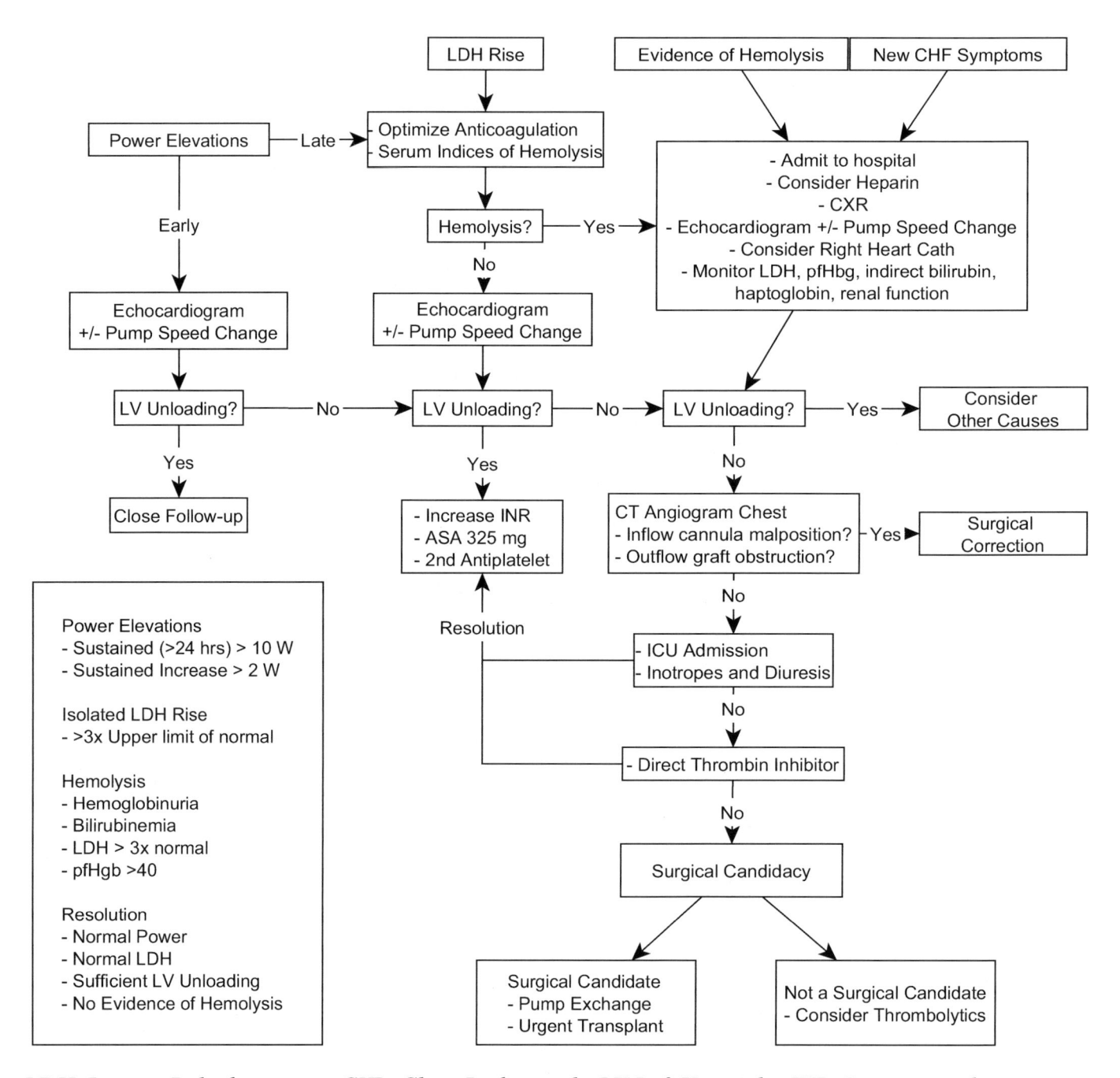

```
                                    LDH Rise          Evidence of Hemolysis    New CHF Symptoms
                                        │                      │                      │
                                        ▼                      └──────────┬───────────┘
  Power Elevations  ──Late──▶  - Optimize Anticoagulation                  │
                               - Serum Indices of Hemolysis                ▼
         │                              │                      - Admit to hospital
       Early                            ▼                      - Consider Heparin
         │                          Hemolysis? ──Yes──▶        - CXR
         ▼                              │                      - Echocardiogram +/- Pump Speed Change
  Echocardiogram                       No                      - Consider Right Heart Cath
  +/- Pump Speed Change                 ▼                      - Monitor LDH, pfHbg, indirect bilirubin,
         │                        Echocardiogram                 haptoglobin, renal function
         ▼                        +/- Pump Speed Change                    │
   LV Unloading? ──No──▶           │                                       ▼
         │                         ▼                                 LV Unloading? ──Yes──▶ Consider
        Yes                   LV Unloading? ──No──────────────────▶        │                Other Causes
         ▼                         │                                      No
   Close Follow-up                Yes                                      ▼
                                   ▼                               CT Angiogram Chest
                              - Increase INR                       - Inflow cannula malposition? ──Yes──▶ Surgical
                              - ASA 325 mg                         - Outflow graft obstruction?            Correction
                              - 2nd Antiplatelet                           │
                                   ▲                                      No
                              Resolution                                   ▼
                                                                   - ICU Admission
                                                                   - Inotropes and Diuresis
                                                                           │
                                                                          No
                                                                           ▼
                                                                   - Direct Thrombin Inhibitor
                                                                           │
                                                                          No
                                                                           ▼
                                                                   Surgical Candidacy
                                                                   ┌───────┴────────┐
                                                                   ▼                ▼
                                                          Surgical Candidate   Not a Surgical Candidate
                                                          - Pump Exchange      - Consider Thrombolytics
                                                          - Urgent Transplant
```

Power Elevations
- Sustained (>24 hrs) > 10 W
- Sustained Increase > 2 W

Isolated LDH Rise
- >3x Upper limit of normal

Hemolysis
- Hemoglobinuria
- Bilirubinemia
- LDH > 3x normal
- pfHgb >40

Resolution
- Normal Power
- Normal LDH
- Sufficient LV Unloading
- No Evidence of Hemolysis

LDH, Lactate Dehydrogenase; CXR, Chest Radiograph; LV Left Ventricle; INR, International Normalized Ratio; ASA, Aspirin; CT, Computed Tomography; ICU, Intensive Care Unit; pfHgb, plasma free hemoglobin

Orthotopic Heart Transplantation
Brittany A. Zwischenberger, Carmelo A. Milano

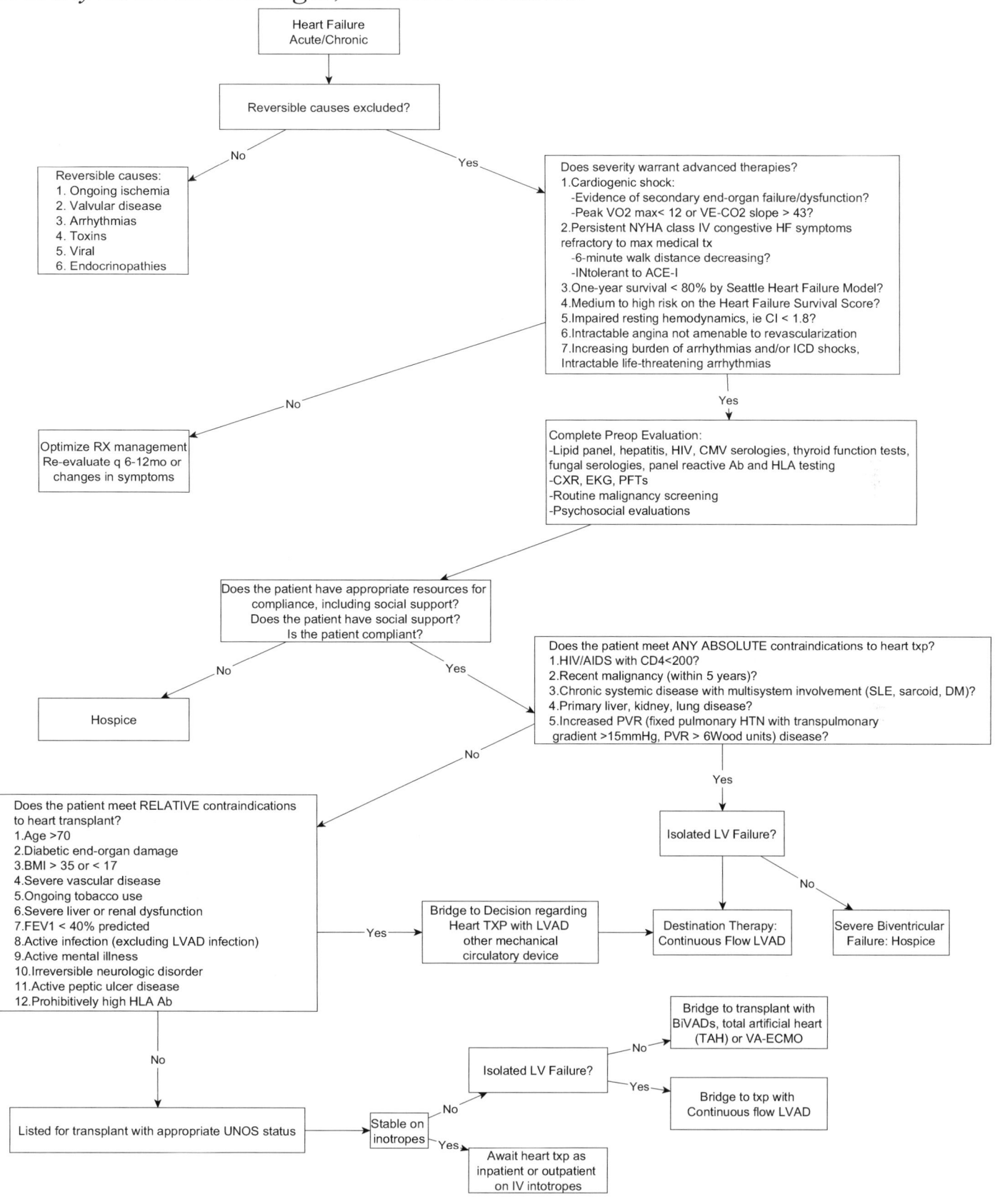

```
                    ┌─────────────────┐
                    │  Heart Failure  │
                    │  Acute/Chronic  │
                    └────────┬────────┘
                             │
                    ┌────────▼──────────────┐
                    │ Reversible causes     │
                    │ excluded?             │
                    └───┬───────────────┬───┘
                     No │               │ Yes
```

Reversible causes:
1. Ongoing ischemia
2. Valvular disease
3. Arrhythmias
4. Toxins
5. Viral
6. Endocrinopathies

Does severity warrant advanced therapies?
1. Cardiogenic shock:
   - Evidence of secondary end-organ failure/dysfunction?
   - Peak VO2 max< 12 or VE-CO2 slope > 43?
2. Persistent NYHA class IV congestive HF symptoms refractory to max medical tx
   - 6-minute walk distance decreasing?
   - INtolerant to ACE-I
3. One-year survival < 80% by Seattle Heart Failure Model?
4. Medium to high risk on the Heart Failure Survival Score?
5. Impaired resting hemodynamics, ie CI < 1.8?
6. Intractable angina not amenable to revascularization
7. Increasing burden of arrhythmias and/or ICD shocks, Intractable life-threatening arrhythmias

Optimize RX management Re-evaluate q 6-12mo or changes in symptoms

Complete Preop Evaluation:
- Lipid panel, hepatitis, HIV, CMV serologies, thyroid function tests, fungal serologies, panel reactive Ab and HLA testing
- CXR, EKG, PFTs
- Routine malignancy screening
- Psychosocial evaluations

Does the patient have appropriate resources for compliance, including social support?
Does the patient have social support?
Is the patient compliant?

No → **Hospice**

Yes → **Does the patient meet ANY ABSOLUTE contraindications to heart txp?**
1. HIV/AIDS with CD4<200?
2. Recent malignancy (within 5 years)?
3. Chronic systemic disease with multisystem involvement (SLE, sarcoid, DM)?
4. Primary liver, kidney, lung disease?
5. Increased PVR (fixed pulmonary HTN with transpulmonary gradient >15mmHg, PVR > 6Wood units) disease?

Yes → **Isolated LV Failure?**
- Yes → **Destination Therapy: Continuous Flow LVAD**
- No → **Severe Biventricular Failure: Hospice**

No → **Does the patient meet RELATIVE contraindications to heart transplant?**
1. Age >70
2. Diabetic end-organ damage
3. BMI > 35 or < 17
4. Severe vascular disease
5. Ongoing tobacco use
6. Severe liver or renal dysfunction
7. FEV1 < 40% predicted
8. Active infection (excluding LVAD infection)
9. Active mental illness
10. Irreversible neurologic disorder
11. Active peptic ulcer disease
12. Prohibitively high HLA Ab

Yes → **Bridge to Decision regarding Heart TXP with LVAD other mechanical circulatory device**

No → **Listed for transplant with appropriate UNOS status** → **Stable on inotropes**
- Yes → **Await heart txp as inpatient or outpatient on IV intotropes**
- No → **Isolated LV Failure?**
  - Yes → **Bridge to txp with Continuous flow LVAD**
  - No → **Bridge to transplant with BiVADs, total artificial heart (TAH) or VA-ECMO**

95

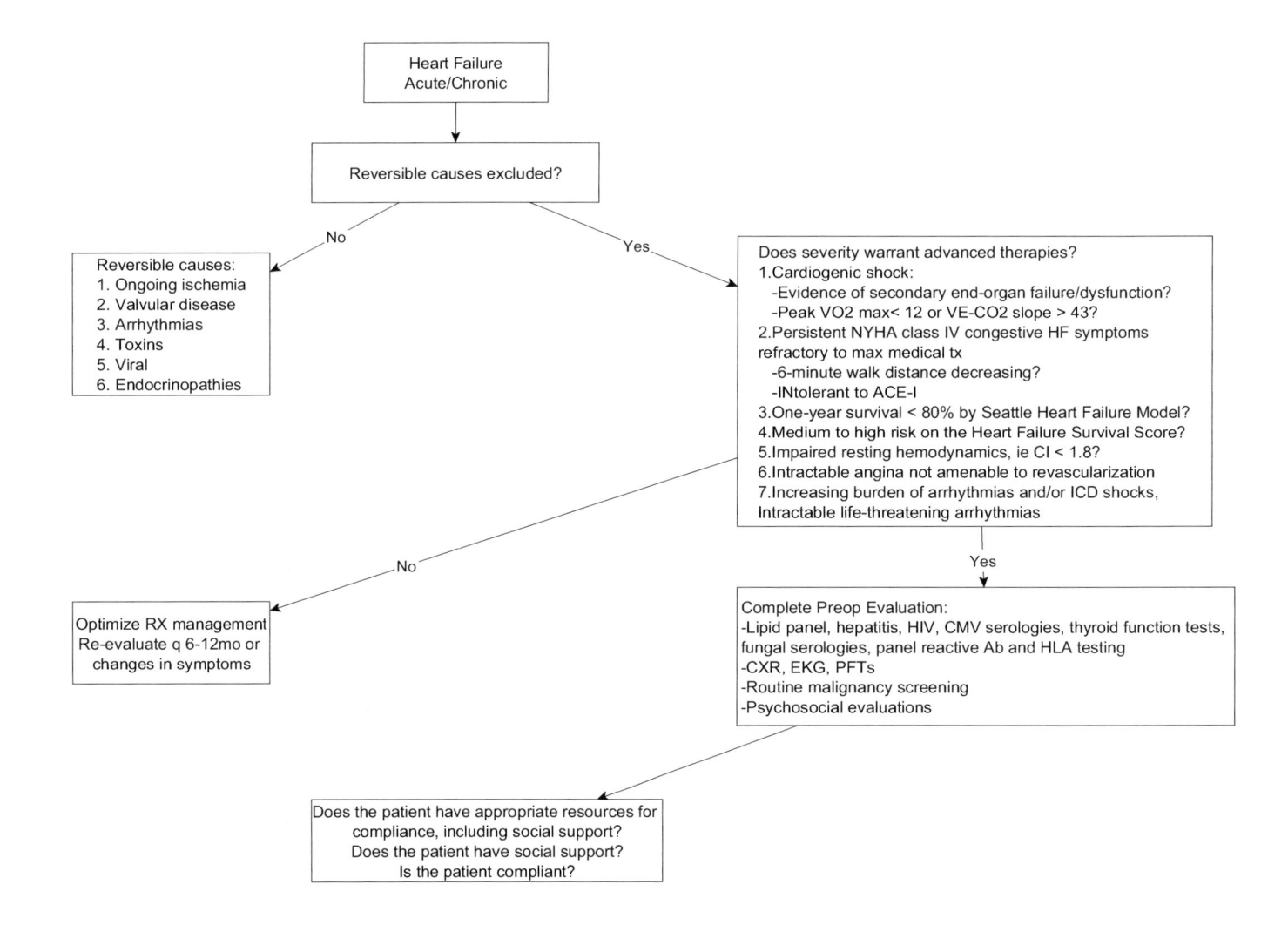

```
                    ┌─────────────────┐
                    │  Heart Failure  │
                    │  Acute/Chronic  │
                    └────────┬────────┘
                             ▼
                    ┌─────────────────────────┐
                    │ Reversible causes excluded? │
                    └──┬───────────────────┬──┘
                  No  /                     \  Yes
                     ▼                       ▼
```

Reversible causes:
1. Ongoing ischemia
2. Valvular disease
3. Arrhythmias
4. Toxins
5. Viral
6. Endocrinopathies

Does severity warrant advanced therapies?
1. Cardiogenic shock:
   - Evidence of secondary end-organ failure/dysfunction?
   - Peak VO2 max< 12 or VE-CO2 slope > 43?
2. Persistent NYHA class IV congestive HF symptoms refractory to max medical tx
   - 6-minute walk distance decreasing?
   - INtolerant to ACE-I
3. One-year survival < 80% by Seattle Heart Failure Model?
4. Medium to high risk on the Heart Failure Survival Score?
5. Impaired resting hemodynamics, ie CI < 1.8?
6. Intractable angina not amenable to revascularization
7. Increasing burden of arrhythmias and/or ICD shocks, Intractable life-threatening arrhythmias

No → **Optimize RX management Re-evaluate q 6-12mo or changes in symptoms**

Yes ↓

Complete Preop Evaluation:
- Lipid panel, hepatitis, HIV, CMV serologies, thyroid function tests, fungal serologies, panel reactive Ab and HLA testing
- CXR, EKG, PFTs
- Routine malignancy screening
- Psychosocial evaluations

Does the patient have appropriate resources for compliance, including social support?
Does the patient have social support?
Is the patient compliant?

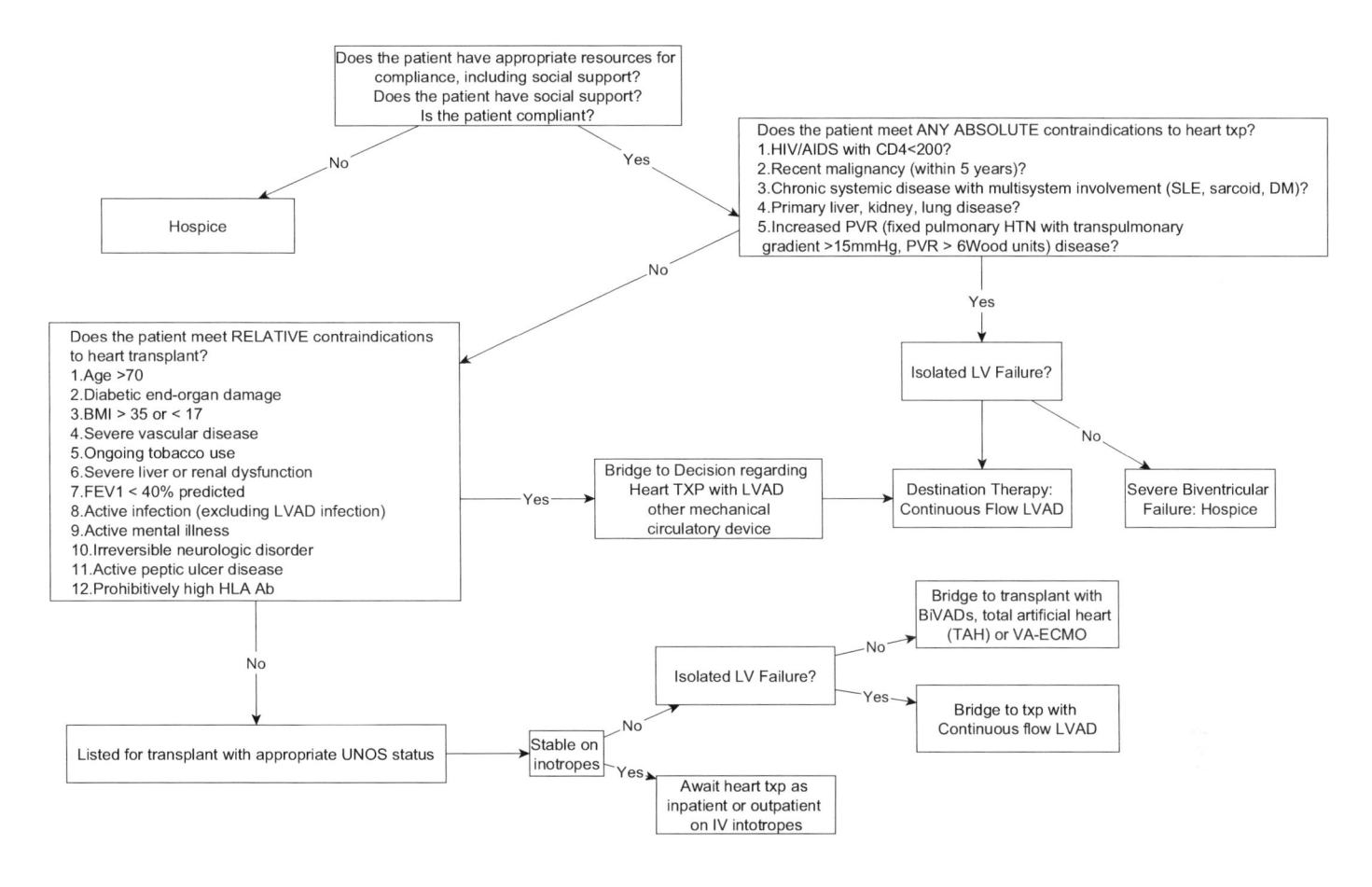

VO₂ max, maximum oxygen uptake; *VE-CO2*, minute ventilation-to-carbon dioxide output; *HF*, heart failure; *RX*, medication; *CI*, cardiac index; *PFT*, pulmonary function testing; *LV*, left ventricle; *RV*, right ventricle; *LVAD*, left ventricular assist device; *RVAD*, right ventricular assist device; *BiVAD*, biventricular assist device; *PVR*, pulmonary vascular resistance; *FEV1*, forced expiratory volume during first second of exhale; *ECMO*, extracorporeal membrane oxygenation; *ICD*, implantable cardioverter defibrillator; *HTN*, hypertension; *UNOS*, United Network for Organ Sharing

Hypertrophic Cardiomyopathy
Yuriy Dudiy, Howard Song

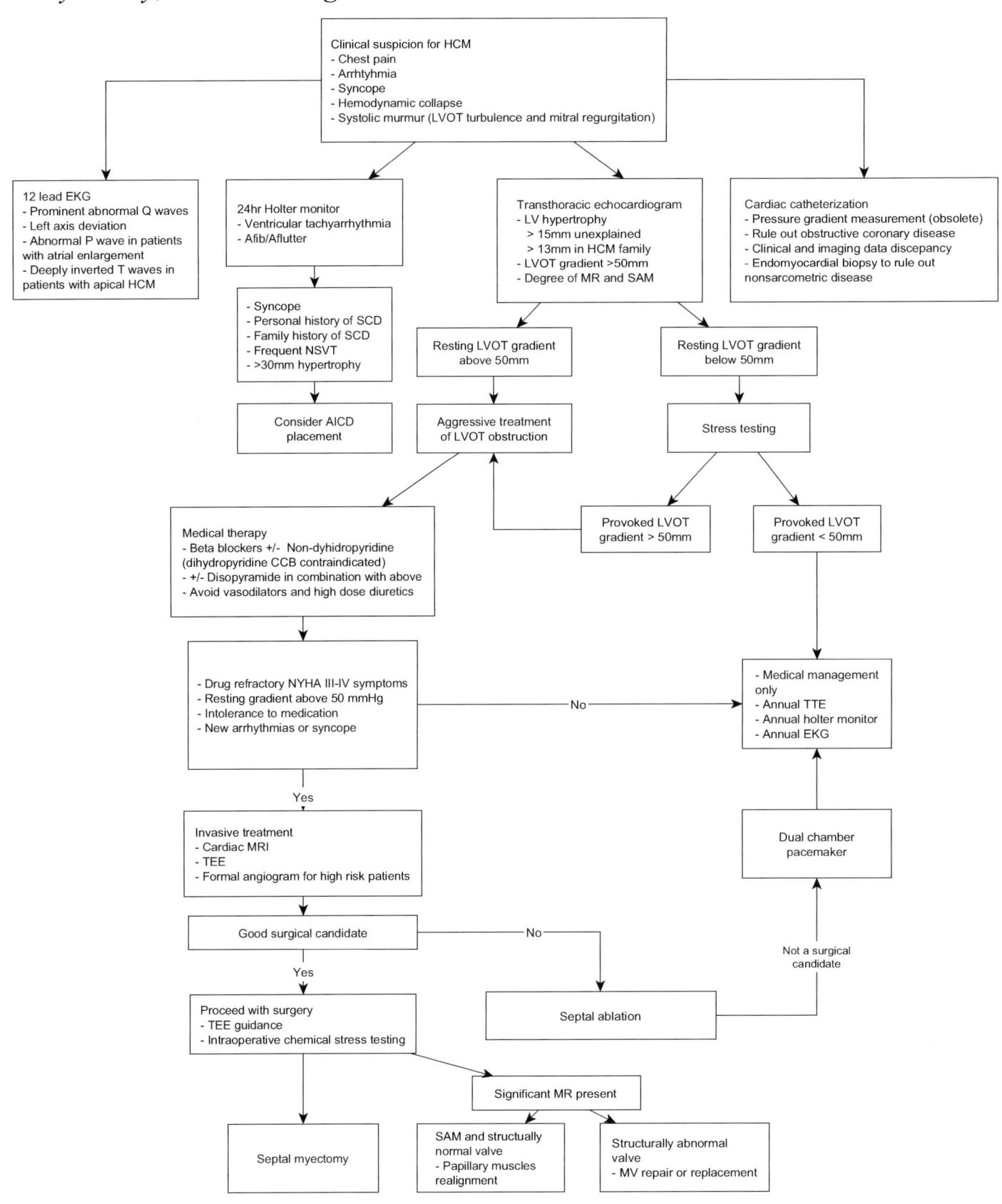

```
┌─────────────────────────────────────────────┐
│ Clinical suspicion for HCM                  │
│   - Chest pain                              │
│   - Arrhtyhmia                              │
│   - Syncope                                 │
│   - Hemodynamic collapse                    │
│   - Systolic murmur (LVOT turbulence and    │
│     mitral regurgitation)                   │
└─────────────────────────────────────────────┘
```

12 lead EKG
- Prominent abnormal Q waves
- Left axis deviation
- Abnormal P wave in patients with atrial enlargement
- Deeply inverted T waves in patients with apical HCM

24hr Holter monitor
- Ventricular tachyarrhythmia
- Afib/Aflutter

Transthoracic echocardiogram
- LV hypertrophy
  - > 15mm unexplained
  - > 13mm in HCM family
- LVOT gradient >50mm
- Degree of MR and SAM

Cardiac catheterization
- Pressure gradient measurement (obsolete)
- Rule out obstructive coronary disease
- Clinical and imaging data discepancy
- Endomyocardial biopsy to rule out nonsarcometric disease

- Syncope
- Personal history of SCD
- Family history of SCD
- Frequent NSVT
- >30mm hypertrophy

→ **Consider AICD placement**

Resting LVOT gradient above 50mm → **Aggressive treatment of LVOT obstruction**

Resting LVOT gradient below 50mm → **Stress testing**

Provoked LVOT gradient > 50mm

Provoked LVOT gradient < 50mm

Medical therapy
- Beta blockers +/- Non-dyhidropyridine (dihydropyridine CCB contraindicated)
- +/- Disopyramide in combination with above
- Avoid vasodilators and high dose diuretics

- Drug refractory NYHA III-IV symptoms
- Resting gradient above 50 mmHg
- Intolerance to medication
- New arrhythmias or syncope

→ No → **Medical management only**
- Annual TTE
- Annual holter monitor
- Annual EKG

Yes ↓

Invasive treatment
- Cardiac MRI
- TEE
- Formal angiogram for high risk patients

Good surgical candidate
- No → **Septal ablation** → Not a surgical candidate → **Dual chamber pacemaker**

Yes ↓

Proceed with surgery
- TEE guidance
- Intraoperative chemical stress testing

→ **Septal myectomy**

Significant MR present
- **SAM and structurally normal valve** – Papillary muscles realignment
- **Structurally abnormal valve** – MV repair or replacement

98

HCM, hypertrophic cardiomyopathy, LVOT, left ventricular outflow tract; SCD, sudden cardiac death; AICD, automated implantable cardioverter-defibrillator; CCB, calcium channels blockers; MR, mitral regurgitation; SAM, systolic anterior motion.

Cardiac Tumors
Michael Kasten, Mark Turrentine

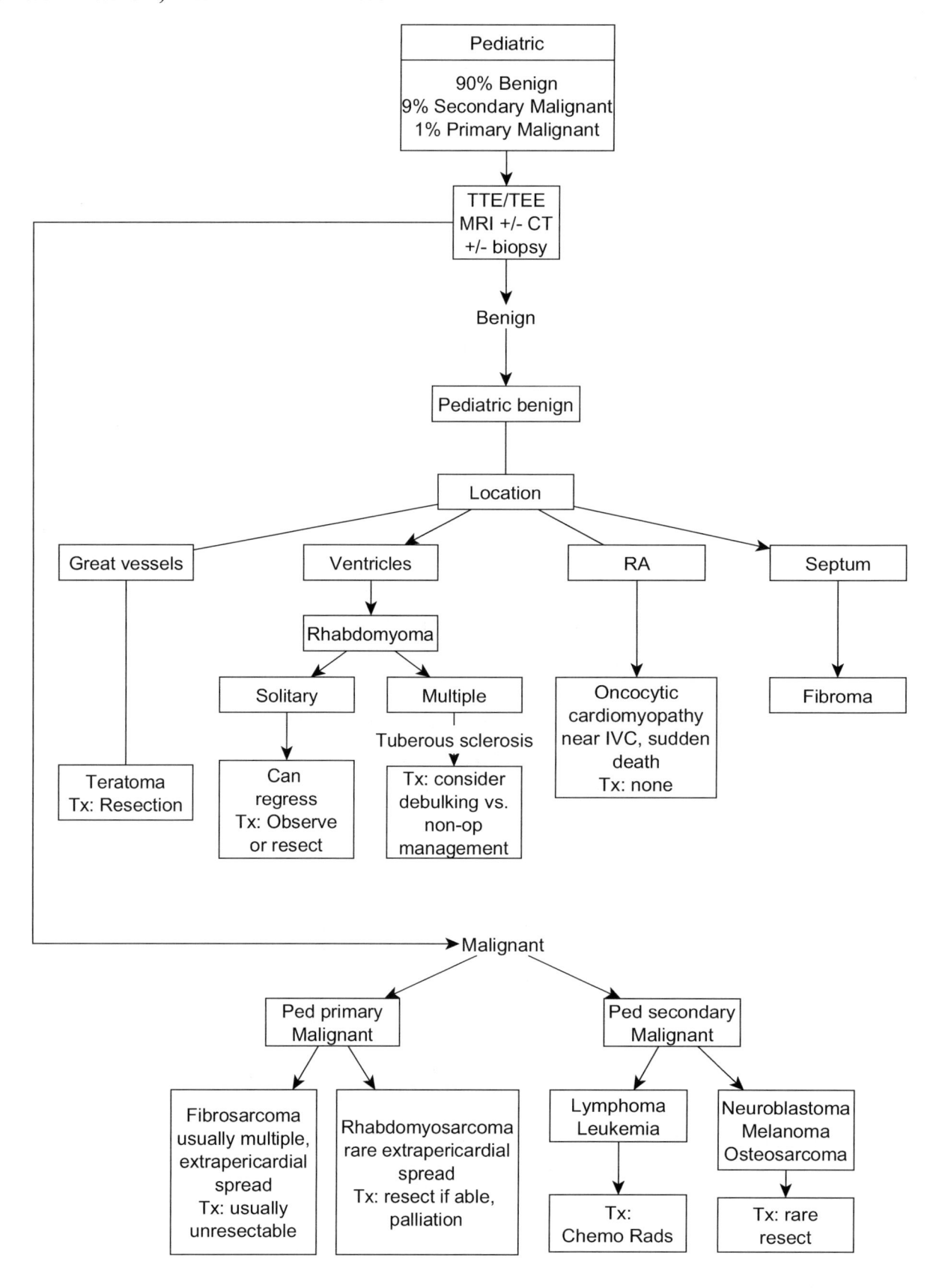

```
                    ┌─────────────────────┐
                    │     Pediatric       │
                    │   90% Benign        │
                    │ 9% Secondary Malignant │
                    │  1% Primary Malignant │
                    └──────────┬──────────┘
                               ↓
                    ┌─────────────────┐
                    │    TTE/TEE      │
                    │   MRI +/- CT    │
                    │   +/- biopsy    │
                    └─────────────────┘
                               │ Benign
                               ↓
                    ┌─────────────────┐
                    │ Pediatric benign│
                    └─────────────────┘
                               ↓
                    ┌─────────────────┐
                    │    Location     │
                    └─────────────────┘
```

Branches from Location:

- **Great vessels** → **Teratoma** — Tx: Resection
- **Ventricles** → **Rhabdomyoma**
  - Solitary → Can regress — Tx: Observe or resect
  - Multiple → Tuberous sclerosis — Tx: consider debulking vs. non-op management
- **RA** → Oncocytic cardiomyopathy near IVC, sudden death — Tx: none
- **Septum** → Fibroma

Malignant

- **Ped primary Malignant**
  - Fibrosarcoma usually multiple, extrapericardial spread — Tx: usually unresectable
  - Rhabdomyosarcoma rare extrapericardial spread — Tx: resect if able, palliation
- **Ped secondary Malignant**
  - Lymphoma, Leukemia — Tx: Chemo Rads
  - Neuroblastoma, Melanoma, Osteosarcoma — Tx: rare resect

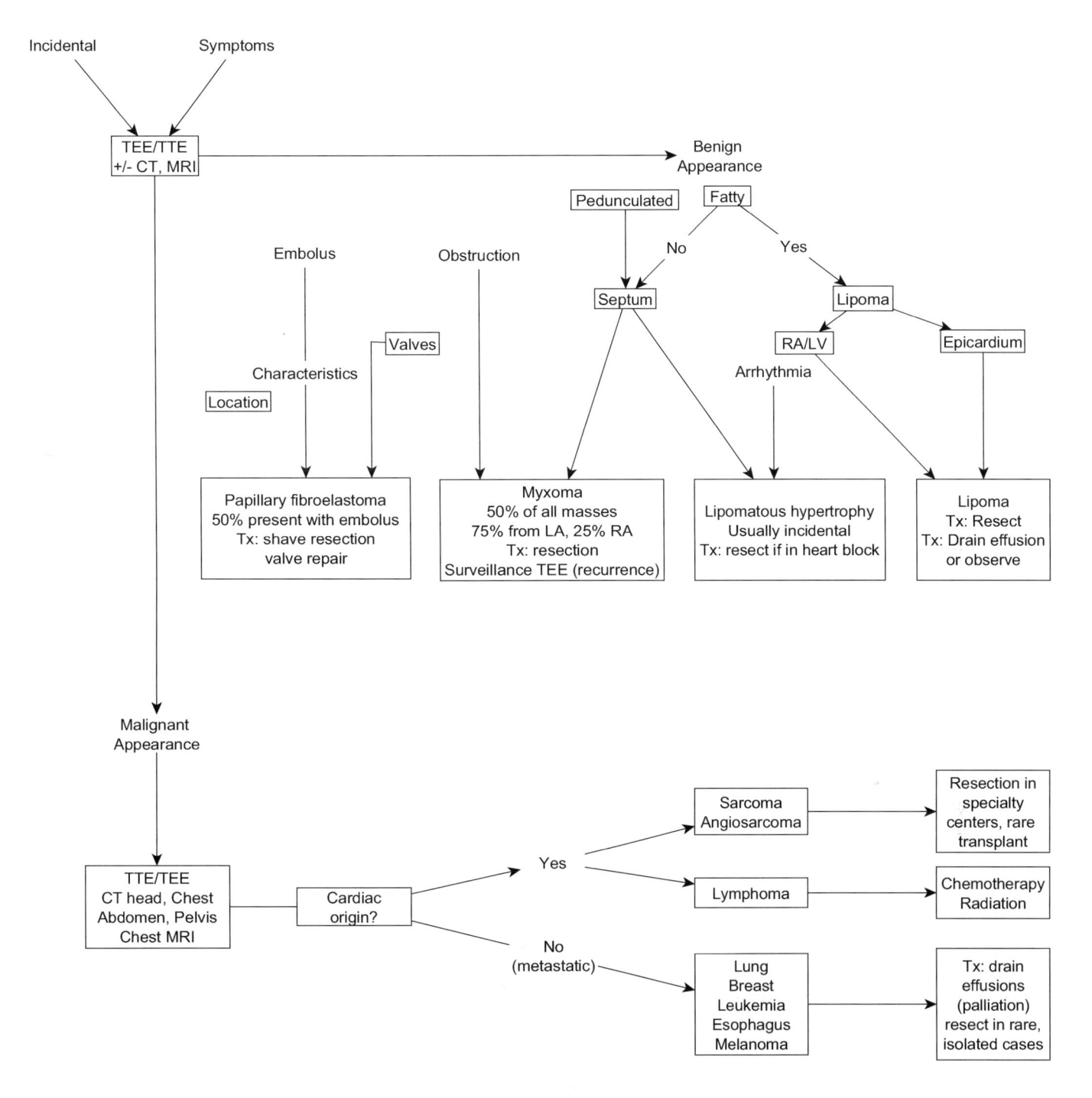

```
Incidental      Symptoms
     \          /
      ↓        ↓
    ┌─────────────┐                                    Benign
    │  TEE/TTE    │─────────────────────────────────→ Appearance
    │  +/- CT, MRI│
    └─────────────┘                          ┌──────────┐  ┌──────┐
         │                                   │Pedunculated│ │Fatty │
         │                                   └──────────┘  └──────┘
         │         Embolus      Obstruction       │ No      │ Yes
         │            │             │             ↓         ↓
         │            │          ┌──────┐      ┌──────┐  ┌──────┐
         │            │  ┌──────┐│      │      │Septum│  │Lipoma│
         │            │  │Valves││      │      └──────┘  └──────┘
         │       Characteristics │      │         │      │      │
         │  ┌────────┐│          │      │         │    RA/LV  Epicardium
         │  │Location││          │      │         │   Arrhythmia  │
         │  └────────┘↓          ↓      ↓         ↓      ↓        ↓
         │  ┌──────────────────┐ ┌─────────────┐ ┌──────────────┐ ┌──────────────┐
         │  │Papillary fibro-  │ │Myxoma       │ │Lipomatous    │ │Lipoma        │
         │  │elastoma          │ │50% of all   │ │hypertrophy   │ │Tx: Resect    │
         │  │50% present with  │ │masses       │ │Usually       │ │Tx: Drain     │
         │  │embolus           │ │75% from LA, │ │incidental    │ │effusion      │
         │  │Tx: shave resection│ │25% RA       │ │Tx: resect if │ │or observe    │
         │  │valve repair      │ │Tx: resection│ │in heart block│ │              │
         │  │                  │ │Surveillance │ │              │ │              │
         │  │                  │ │TEE (recurrence)│              │ │              │
         │  └──────────────────┘ └─────────────┘ └──────────────┘ └──────────────┘
         │
    Malignant
    Appearance
         │
         ↓
    ┌─────────────┐                                        ┌──────────┐   ┌─────────────┐
    │TTE/TEE      │                                    ┌──→│Sarcoma   │──→│Resection in │
    │CT head, Chest│   ┌────────┐       Yes            │   │Angiosarcoma│ │specialty    │
    │Abdomen, Pelvis│→ │Cardiac │──────────────────────┤   └──────────┘   │centers, rare│
    │Chest MRI    │   │origin? │                      │                  │transplant   │
    └─────────────┘   └────────┘                      │   ┌──────────┐   └─────────────┘
                          │                            └──→│Lymphoma  │──→┌─────────────┐
                          │  No                            └──────────┘   │Chemotherapy │
                          │  (metastatic)                                 │Radiation    │
                          ↓                                               └─────────────┘
                       ┌──────────┐                       ┌─────────────┐
                       │Lung      │                       │Tx: drain    │
                       │Breast    │                       │effusions    │
                       │Leukemia  │──────────────────────→│(palliation) │
                       │Esophagus │                       │resect in rare,│
                       │Melanoma  │                       │isolated cases│
                       └──────────┘                       └─────────────┘
```

TTE, transthoracic echocardiography; TEE, transesophageal echocardiography; CT, computed tomography; MRI, magnetic resonance imaging; RA, right atrium; Tx, therapy; IVC, inferior vena cava; LV, left ventricle

Sternal Wound Infection
Stevan Pupovac, Frank Manetta

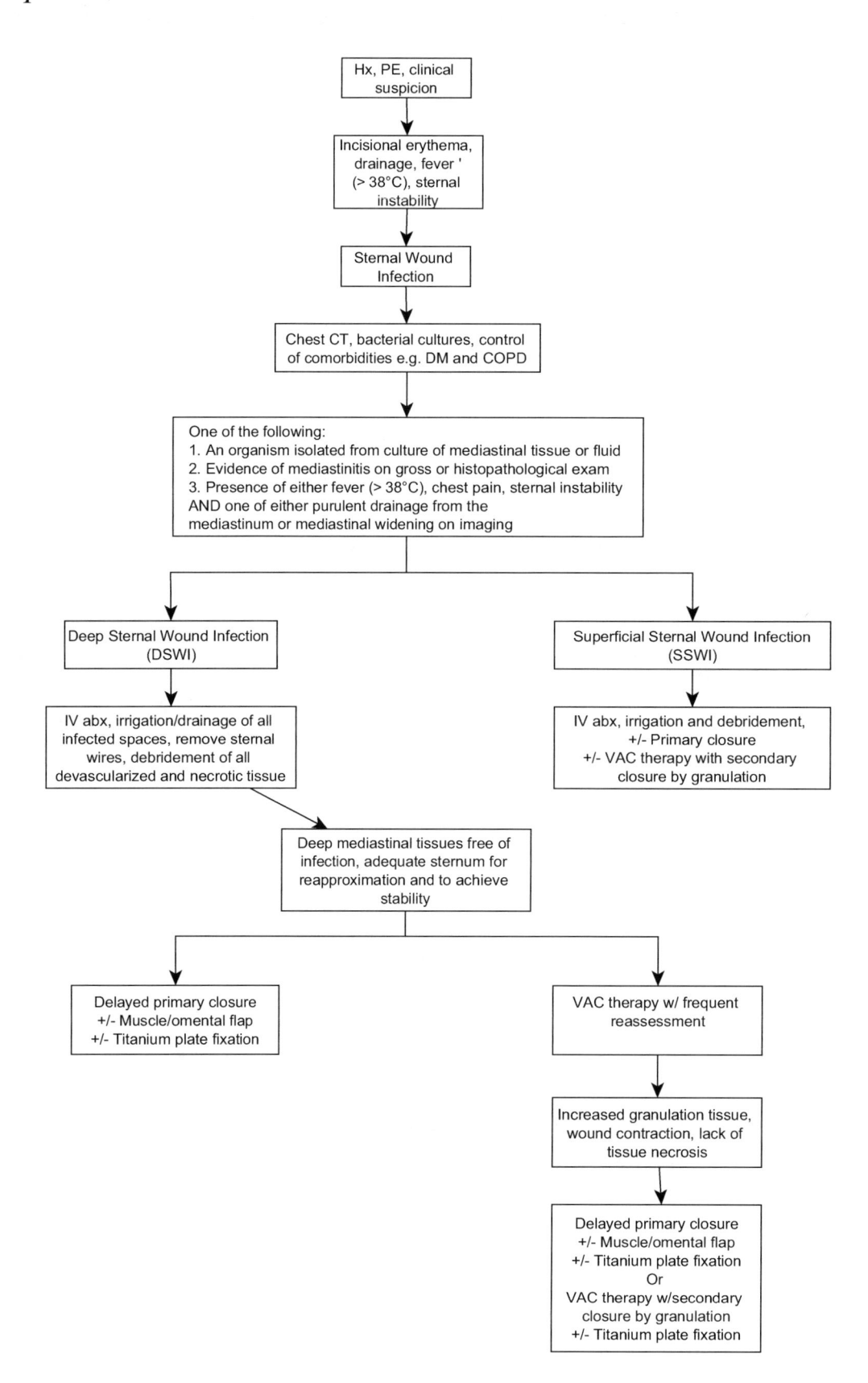

```
┌─────────────────────┐
│ Hx, PE, clinical    │
│ suspicion           │
└──────────┬──────────┘
           ▼
┌─────────────────────┐
│ Incisional erythema,│
│ drainage, fever     │
│ (> 38°C), sternal   │
│ instability         │
└──────────┬──────────┘
           ▼
┌─────────────────────┐
│ Sternal Wound       │
│ Infection           │
└──────────┬──────────┘
           ▼
┌──────────────────────────────┐
│ Chest CT, bacterial cultures,│
│ control of comorbidities     │
│ e.g. DM and COPD             │
└──────────┬───────────────────┘
           ▼
┌──────────────────────────────────────────────────────────┐
│ One of the following:                                    │
│ 1. An organism isolated from culture of mediastinal      │
│    tissue or fluid                                       │
│ 2. Evidence of mediastinitis on gross or                 │
│    histopathological exam                                │
│ 3. Presence of either fever (> 38°C), chest pain,        │
│    sternal instability AND one of either purulent        │
│    drainage from the mediastinum or mediastinal          │
│    widening on imaging                                   │
└────────────┬─────────────────────────────┬───────────────┘
             ▼                             ▼
┌────────────────────────┐    ┌────────────────────────────┐
│ Deep Sternal Wound     │    │ Superficial Sternal Wound  │
│ Infection (DSWI)       │    │ Infection (SSWI)           │
└───────────┬────────────┘    └──────────────┬─────────────┘
            ▼                                ▼
┌─────────────────────────────┐  ┌──────────────────────────┐
│ IV abx, irrigation/drainage │  │ IV abx, irrigation and   │
│ of all infected spaces,     │  │ debridement,             │
│ remove sternal wires,       │  │ +/- Primary closure      │
│ debridement of all          │  │ +/- VAC therapy with     │
│ devascularized and necrotic │  │ secondary closure by     │
│ tissue                      │  │ granulation              │
└──────────────┬──────────────┘  └──────────────────────────┘
               ▼
┌──────────────────────────────┐
│ Deep mediastinal tissues     │
│ free of infection, adequate  │
│ sternum for reapproximation  │
│ and to achieve stability     │
└────────┬──────────────┬──────┘
         ▼              ▼
┌────────────────────┐  ┌────────────────────┐
│ Delayed primary    │  │ VAC therapy w/     │
│ closure            │  │ frequent           │
│ +/- Muscle/omental │  │ reassessment       │
│ flap               │  └──────────┬─────────┘
│ +/- Titanium plate │             ▼
│ fixation           │  ┌────────────────────┐
└────────────────────┘  │ Increased          │
                        │ granulation tissue,│
                        │ wound contraction, │
                        │ lack of tissue     │
                        │ necrosis           │
                        └──────────┬─────────┘
                                   ▼
                        ┌────────────────────────┐
                        │ Delayed primary closure│
                        │ +/- Muscle/omental flap│
                        │ +/- Titanium plate     │
                        │ fixation               │
                        │ Or                     │
                        │ VAC therapy w/secondary│
                        │ closure by granulation │
                        │ +/- Titanium plate     │
                        │ fixation               │
                        └────────────────────────┘
```

Hx, history; PE, physical exam; CXR, chest radiogram; IV abx, intravenous antibiotics; CT, computed tomography; DM, diabetes mellitus; COPD, chronic obstructive pulmonary disorder; VAC, vacuum-assisted closure

Penetrating Chest Trauma
Tedi Vlahu, Jason Frazier

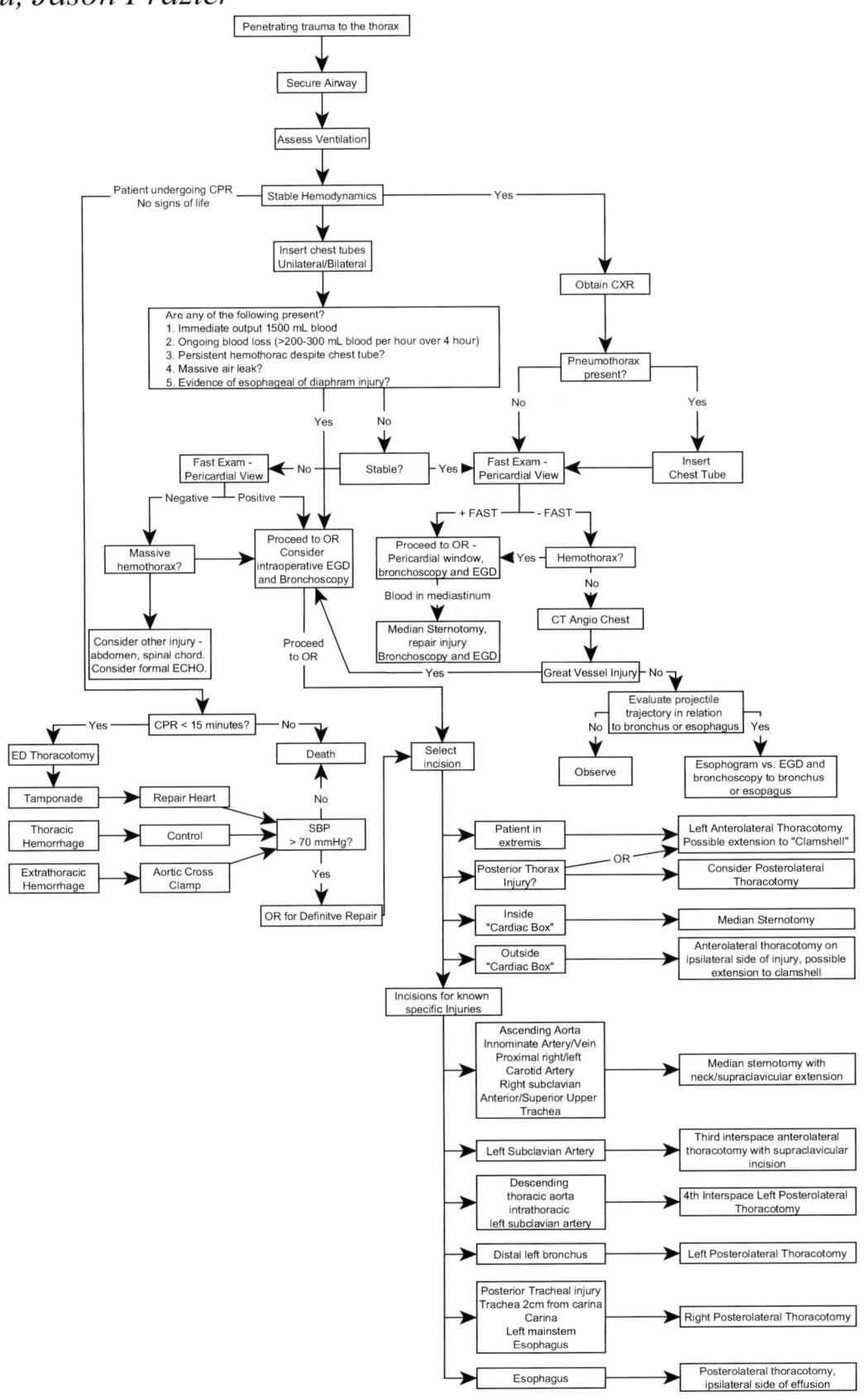

```
                        Penetrating trauma to the thorax
                                    │
                                    ▼
                             Secure Airway
                                    │
                                    ▼
                           Assess Ventilation
                                    │
     Patient undergoing CPR         ▼
     No signs of life  ◄──── Stable Hemodynamics ────Yes──┐
            │                                             │
            │                                             ▼
            │                                    Insert chest tubes
            │                                    Unilateral/Bilateral
            │                                             │
            │                                             ▼                  Obtain CXR
            │          ┌──────────────────────────────────────┐                  │
            │          │ Are any of the following present?     │                  ▼
            │          │ 1. Immediate output 1500 mL blood     │          Pneumothorax present?
            │          │ 2. Ongoing blood loss (>200-300 mL    │            │           │
            │          │    blood per hour over 4 hour)        │           No          Yes
            │          │ 3. Persistent hemothorax despite      │            │           │
            │          │    chest tube?                        │            │           ▼
            │          │ 4. Massive air leak?                  │            │      Insert Chest Tube
            │          │ 5. Evidence of esophageal of          │            │           │
            │          │    diaphram injury?                   │            ▼           ▼
            │          └──────────────────────────────────────┘        Fast Exam -
            │                       │         │                        Pericardial View
            │                      Yes        No                        │        │
            │                       │         ▼                       +FAST    -FAST
            │                       ▼    Stable? ──Yes──┐               │        │
            │            Fast Exam -   ──No─►           │               ▼        ▼
            │            Pericardial View               │        Proceed to OR    Hemothorax?
            │             │         │                   │        Pericardial       │      │
            │          Negative  Positive               │        window,          Yes    No
            │             │         │                   │        bronchoscopy      │      │
            │             ▼         ▼                   │        and EGD           │      ▼
            │       Massive      Proceed to OR          │             │            │  CT Angio Chest
            │     hemothorax?    Consider               │      Blood in            │      │
            │          │         intraoperative EGD     │      mediastinum         │      ▼
            │          ▼         and Bronchoscopy       │             ▼            │  Great Vessel Injury ──No──┐
            │    Consider other                         │      Median Sternotomy,  │      │                      │
            │    injury - abdomen,  Proceed             │      repair injury       │     Yes                     ▼
            │    spinal chord.      to OR               │      Bronchoscopy and EGD│      │             Evaluate projectile
            │    Consider formal ECHO.                  │                          │      │             trajectory in relation
            │                                           │                          └──────┤       No    to bronchus or esophagus  Yes
            ▼                                           │                                 │        │                        │
    ┌─Yes── CPR < 15 minutes? ──No─┐                    │                                 │        ▼                        ▼
    │              │                │                   │                                 │    Observe              Esophogram vs. EGD and
    ▼              │                ▼                   │                                 │                         bronchoscopy to bronchus
ED Thoracotomy                   Death                  │                                 │                         or esopagus
    │                              │                    ▼                                 │
    ▼                              No              Select incision                        │
 Tamponade ──► Repair Heart        │                    │                                 │
    │                              ▼                    ├─► Patient in extremis  ──┐     │
    ▼                        SBP > 70 mmHg?             │                           OR──► Left Anterolateral Thoracotomy
Thoracic Hemorrhage ──► Control    │                    ├─► Posterior Thorax      ──┘     Possible extension to "Clamshell"
    │                             Yes                   │   Injury?                       │
    ▼                              │                    │                          ──────► Consider Posterolateral
Extrathoracic                      ▼                    │                                  Thoracotomy
Hemorrhage ──► Aortic Cross    OR for Definitve Repair  ├─► Inside "Cardiac Box" ────► Median Sternotomy
              Clamp                                     │
                                                        └─► Outside "Cardiac Box" ──► Anterolateral thoracotomy on
                                                                                       ipsilateral side of injury, possible
                                                                                       extension to clamshell
                                         Incisions for known specific Injuries
                                                        │
                                         ├─► Ascending Aorta
                                         │   Innominate Artery/Vein
                                         │   Proximal right/left         ──► Median sternotomy with
                                         │   Carotid Artery                  neck/supraclavicular extension
                                         │   Right subclavian
                                         │   Anterior/Superior Upper Trachea
                                         │
                                         ├─► Left Subclavian Artery    ──► Third interspace anterolateral
                                         │                                  thoracotomy with supraclavicular incision
                                         │
                                         ├─► Descending thoracic aorta ──► 4th Interspace Left Posterolateral
                                         │   intrathoracic                 Thoracotomy
                                         │   left subclavian artery
                                         │
                                         ├─► Distal left bronchus      ──► Left Posterolateral Thoracotomy
                                         │
                                         ├─► Posterior Tracheal injury
                                         │   Trachea 2cm from carina   ──► Right Posterolateral Thoracotomy
                                         │   Carina
                                         │   Left mainstem
                                         │   Esophagus
                                         │
                                         └─► Esophagus                 ──► Posterolateral thoracotomy,
                                                                            ipsilateral side of effusion
```

```
Penetrating trauma to the thorax
          ↓
     Secure Airway
          ↓
   Assess Ventilation
          ↓
Patient undergoing CPR ← Stable Hemodynamics → Yes
No signs of life              ↓
                    Insert chest tubes
                    Unilateral/Bilateral
                              ↓
              Are any of the following present?
              1. Immediate output 1500 mL blood
              2. Ongoing blood loss (>200-300 mL blood per hour over 4 hour)
              3. Persistent hemothorac despite chest tube?
              4. Massive air leak?
              5. Evidence of esophageal of diaphram injury?
                      Yes ↓      No ↓
```

On "Yes" (right) branch:
- Obtain CXR → Pneumothorax present?
  - No → Fast Exam - Pericardial View
  - Yes → Insert Chest Tube → Fast Exam - Pericardial View
- Fast Exam - Pericardial View:
  - + FAST → Proceed to OR - Pericardial window, bronchoscopy and EGD → Blood in mediastinum → Median Sternotomy, repair injury Bronchoscopy and EGD
  - − FAST → Hemothorax?
    - Yes → Proceed to OR - Pericardial window, bronchoscopy and EGD
    - No → CT Angio Chest → Great Vessel Injury?
      - Yes → Proceed to OR
      - No → Evaluate projectile trajectoy in relation to bronchus or esophagus
        - No → Observe
        - Yes → Esophogram vs. EGD and bronchoscopy to bronchus or esopagus

On "No" branch from the 5-criteria box → Stable?
- Yes → Fast Exam - Pericardial View (joins right branch)
- No → Fast Exam - Pericardial View
  - Negative → Massive hemothorax? → Consider other injury - abdomen, spinal chord. Consider formal ECHO.
  - Positive → Proceed to OR Consider intraoperative EGD and Bronchoscopy

Proceed to OR Consider intraoperative EGD and Bronchoscopy → Proceed to OR → Select incision ☆

"Patient undergoing CPR / No signs of life" branch:
- CPR < 15 minutes?
  - Yes → ED Thoracotomy
    - Tamponade → Repair Heart
    - Thoracic Hemorrhage → Control
    - Extrathoracic Hemorrhage → Aortic Cross Clamp
    - → SBP > 70 mmHg?
      - Yes → OR for Definitve Repair
      - No → Death
  - No → Death

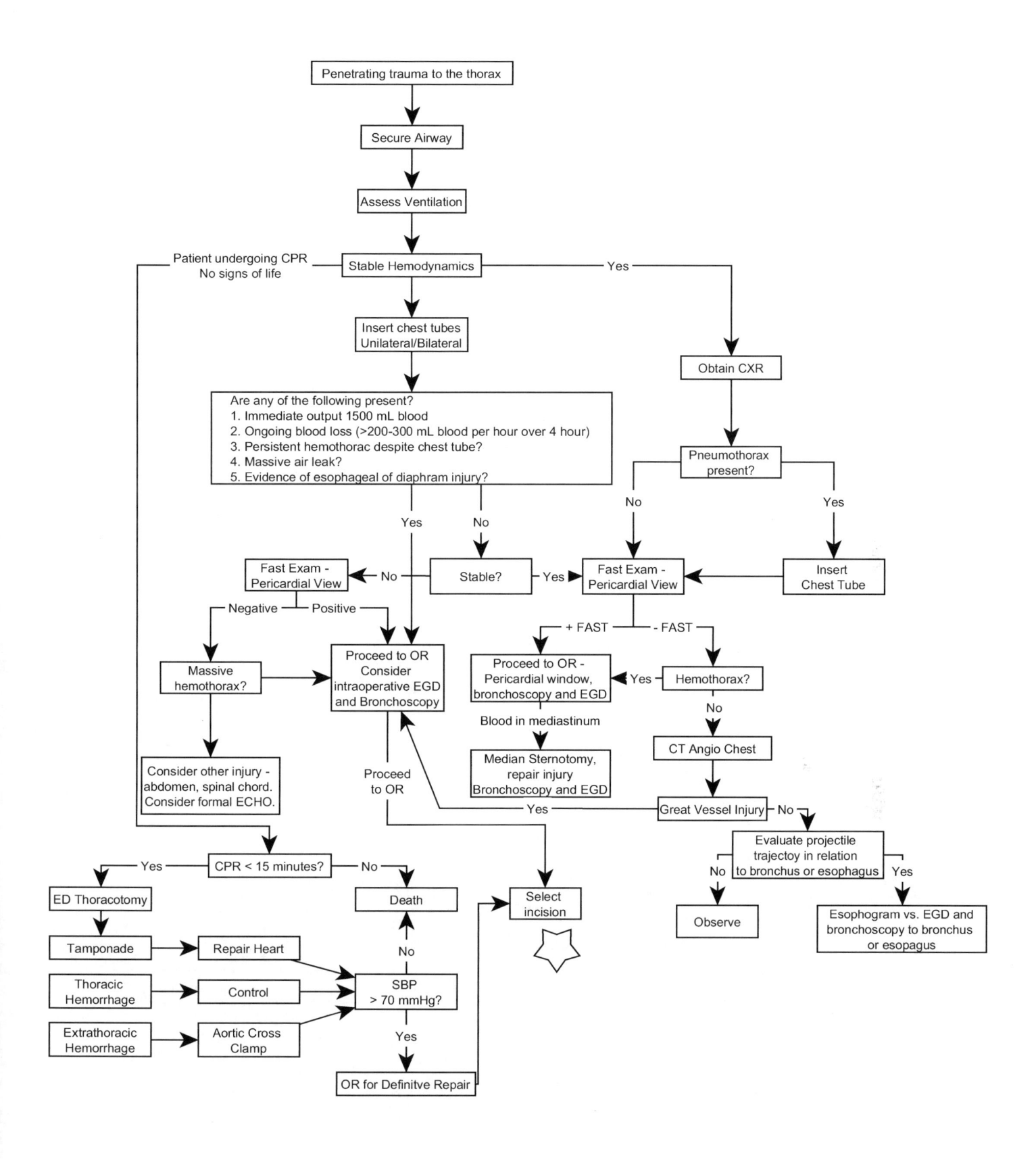

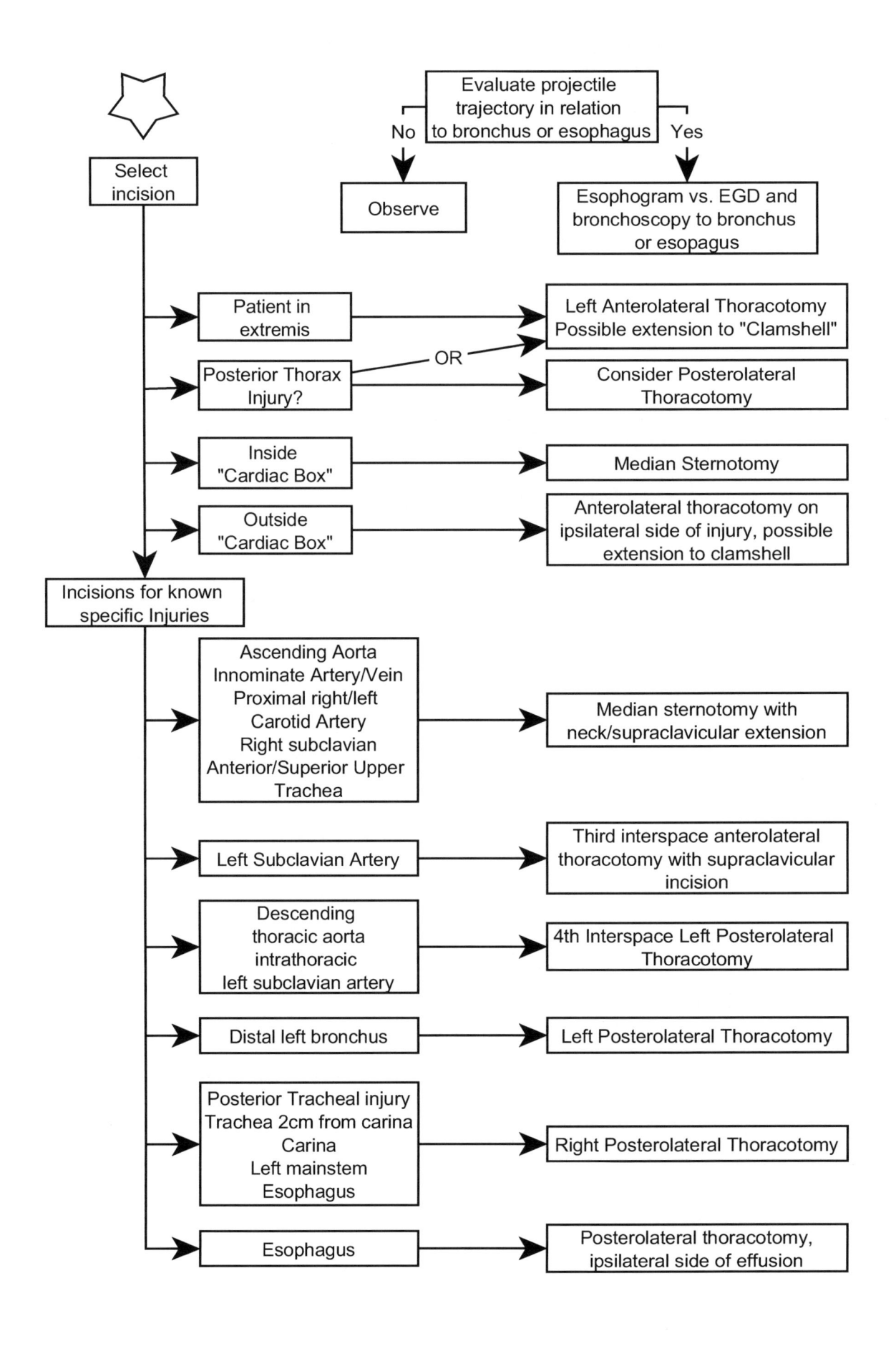

```
                                    ┌─────────────────────────┐
                                    │ Evaluate projectile     │
                                    │ trajectory in relation  │
                               No   │ to bronchus or esophagus│  Yes
                          ┌─────────┴─────────────────────────┴─────────┐
                          ▼                                             ▼
                      ┌────────┐                      ┌──────────────────────────┐
                      │Observe │                      │ Esophogram vs. EGD and   │
                      └────────┘                      │ bronchoscopy to bronchus │
    ☆                                                 │      or esopagus         │
                                                      └──────────────────────────┘
```

Select incision

- **Patient in extremis** → Left Anterolateral Thoracotomy Possible extension to "Clamshell"
- **Posterior Thorax Injury?** —OR→ (Left Anterolateral Thoracotomy...) / Consider Posterolateral Thoracotomy
- **Inside "Cardiac Box"** → Median Sternotomy
- **Outside "Cardiac Box"** → Anterolateral thoracotomy on ipsilateral side of injury, possible extension to clamshell

Incisions for known specific Injuries

- **Ascending Aorta, Innominate Artery/Vein, Proximal right/left Carotid Artery, Right subclavian, Anterior/Superior Upper Trachea** → Median sternotomy with neck/supraclavicular extension
- **Left Subclavian Artery** → Third interspace anterolateral thoracotomy with supraclavicular incision
- **Descending thoracic aorta, intrathoracic left subclavian artery** → 4th Interspace Left Posterolateral Thoracotomy
- **Distal left bronchus** → Left Posterolateral Thoracotomy
- **Posterior Tracheal injury, Trachea 2cm from carina, Carina, Left mainstem, Esophagus** → Right Posterolateral Thoracotomy
- **Esophagus** → Posterolateral thoracotomy, ipsilateral side of effusion

EGD, Esophagogastroduodenoscopy; OR, Operating Room; FAST, Focused assessment with Sonography for trauma; SBP, Systolic Blood pressure

Blunt Thoracic Trauma
Reilly D. Hobbs, Kiran H. Lagisetty

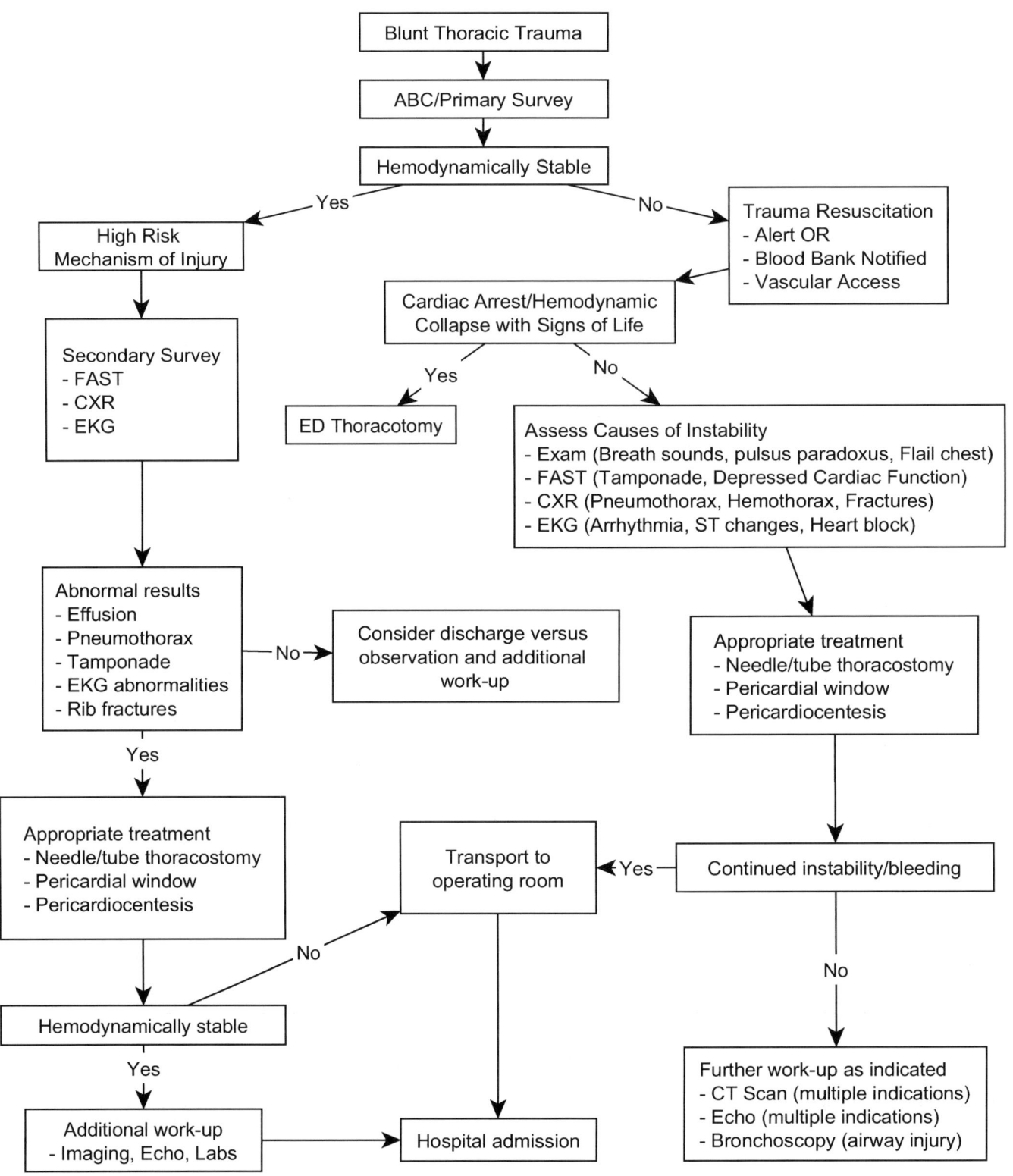

```
                    ┌─────────────────────────┐
                    │  Blunt Thoracic Trauma  │
                    └───────────┬─────────────┘
                                ▼
                    ┌─────────────────────────┐
                    │   ABC/Primary Survey    │
                    └───────────┬─────────────┘
                                ▼
                    ┌─────────────────────────┐
                    │ Hemodynamically Stable  │
                    └───┬─────────────────┬───┘
                   Yes  │                 │  No
         ┌──────────────┘                 └──────────────┐
         ▼                                               ▼
┌──────────────────┐                      ┌─────────────────────────┐
│   High Risk      │                      │  Trauma Resuscitation   │
│ Mechanism of     │                      │  - Alert OR             │
│    Injury        │                      │  - Blood Bank Notified  │
└────────┬─────────┘                      │  - Vascular Access      │
         ▼                                └───────────┬─────────────┘
┌──────────────────┐        ┌─────────────────────────┐
│ Secondary Survey │        │ Cardiac Arrest/Hemodynamic │
│  - FAST          │        │ Collapse with Signs of Life│
│  - CXR           │        └───┬─────────────────┬───────┘
│  - EKG           │        Yes │                 │ No
└────────┬─────────┘            ▼                 ▼
         │             ┌────────────────┐  ┌─────────────────────────────┐
         │             │ ED Thoracotomy │  │ Assess Causes of Instability│
         │             └────────────────┘  │ - Exam (Breath sounds,      │
         │                                 │   pulsus paradoxus, Flail)  │
         ▼                                 │ - FAST (Tamponade, Depressed│
┌──────────────────┐                       │   Cardiac Function)         │
│ Abnormal results │                       │ - CXR (Pneumothorax,        │
│  - Effusion      │                       │   Hemothorax, Fractures)    │
│  - Pneumothorax  │                       │ - EKG (Arrhythmia, ST       │
│  - Tamponade     │─No─► Consider         │   changes, Heart block)     │
│  - EKG abnorm.   │      discharge vs     └──────────────┬──────────────┘
│  - Rib fractures │      observation                     ▼
└────────┬─────────┘      and additional   ┌─────────────────────────┐
       Yes│              work-up           │  Appropriate treatment  │
         ▼                                 │  - Needle/tube thoracos.│
┌──────────────────┐                       │  - Pericardial window   │
│Appropriate treat.│                       │  - Pericardiocentesis   │
│- Needle/tube     │                       └───────────┬─────────────┘
│  thoracostomy    │                                   ▼
│- Pericardial     │   ┌──────────────┐   ┌─────────────────────────┐
│  window          │   │ Transport to │◄Yes│ Continued instability/ │
│- Pericardiocent. │   │ operating rm │    │       bleeding          │
└────────┬─────────┘   └──────┬───────┘    └───────────┬─────────────┘
         ▼                    │                      No│
┌──────────────────┐  No      │                        ▼
│ Hemodynamically  │──────────┘            ┌─────────────────────────┐
│     stable       │                       │ Further work-up as      │
└────────┬─────────┘                       │  indicated              │
       Yes│                                │ - CT Scan (multiple ind.)│
         ▼                                 │ - Echo (multiple ind.)  │
┌──────────────────┐                       │ - Bronchoscopy (airway) │
│ Additional work- │    ┌──────────────┐   └─────────────────────────┘
│     up           │───►│   Hospital   │
│- Imaging, Echo,  │    │  admission   │
│  Labs            │    └──────────────┘
└──────────────────┘
```

ABC, Airway, Breathing, Circulation; CXR, Chest X-Ray; ECHO, Echocardiogram; EKG, Electrocardiogram; FAST, Focused Assessment with Sonography in Trauma;

Endocarditis
Daniel J Weber, Tobias Deuse

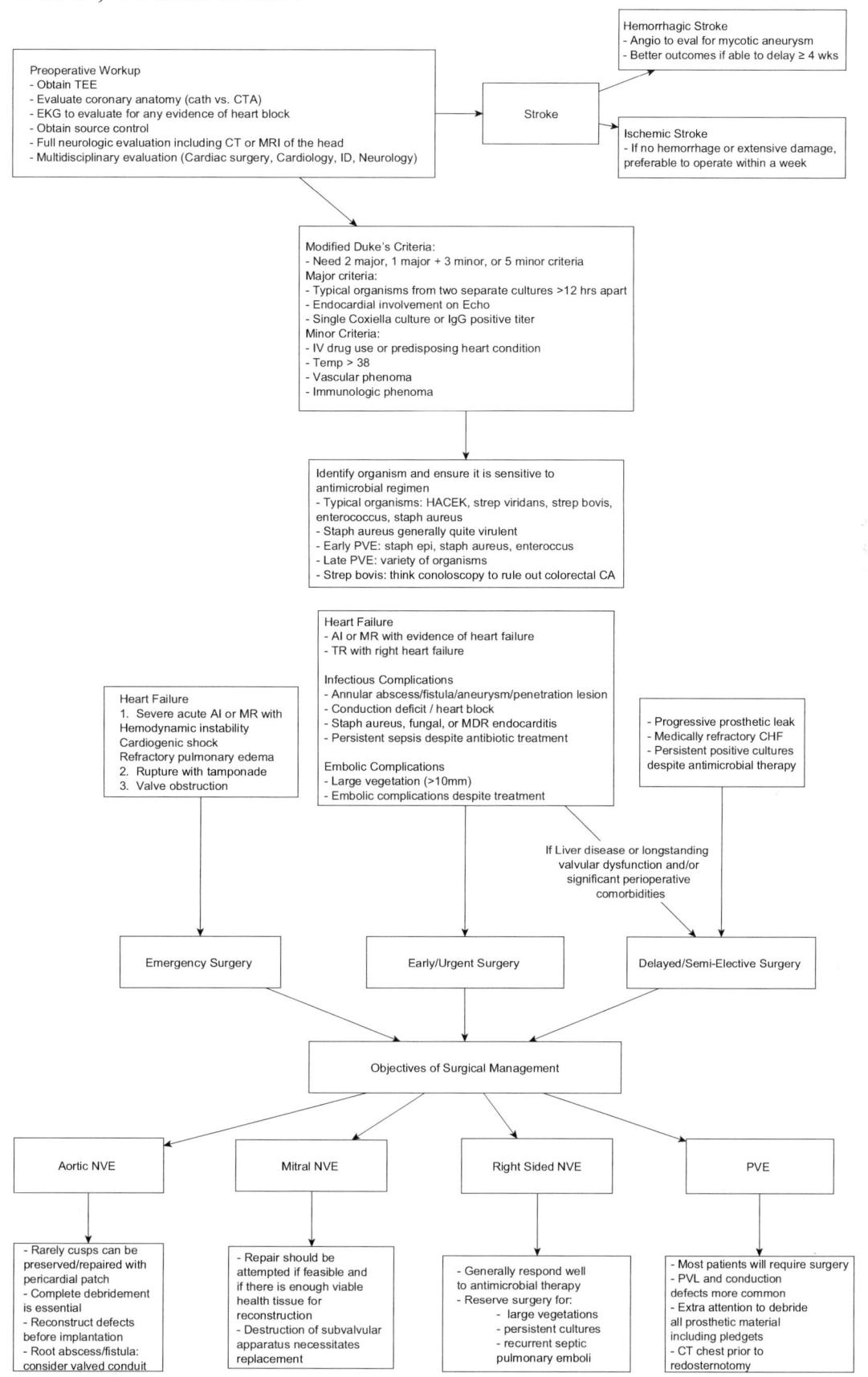

Preoperative Workup
- Obtain TEE
- Evaluate coronary anatomy (cath vs. CTA)
- EKG to evaluate for any evidence of heart block
- Obtain source control
- Full neurologic evaluation including CT or MRI of the head
- Multidisciplinary evaluation (Cardiac surgery, Cardiology, ID, Neurology)

Stroke

Hemorrhagic Stroke
- Angio to eval for mycotic aneurysm
- Better outcomes if able to delay ≥ 4 wks

Ischemic Stroke
- If no hemorrhage or extensive damage, preferable to operate within a week

Modified Duke's Criteria:
- Need 2 major, 1 major + 3 minor, or 5 minor criteria

Major criteria:
- Typical organisms from two separate cultures >12 hrs apart
- Endocardial involvement on Echo
- Single Coxiella culture or IgG positive titer

Minor Criteria:
- IV drug use or predisposing heart condition
- Temp > 38
- Vascular phenoma
- Immunologic phenoma

Identify organism and ensure it is sensitive to antimicrobial regimen
- Typical organisms: HACEK, strep viridans, strep bovis, enterococcus, staph aureus
- Staph aureus generally quite virulent
- Early PVE: staph epi, staph aureus, enterocuss
- Late PVE: variety of organisms
- Strep bovis: think conoloscopy to rule out colorectal CA

Heart Failure
1. Severe acute AI or MR with Hemodynamic instability
   Cardiogenic shock
   Refractory pulmonary edema
2. Rupture with tamponade
3. Valve obstruction

Heart Failure
- AI or MR with evidence of heart failure
- TR with right heart failure

Infectious Complications
- Annular abscess/fistula/aneurysm/penetration lesion
- Conduction deficit / heart block
- Staph aureus, fungal, or MDR endocarditis
- Persistent sepsis despite antibiotic treatment

Embolic Complications
- Large vegetation (>10mm)
- Embolic complications despite treatment

- Progressive prosthetic leak
- Medically refractory CHF
- Persistent positive cultures despite antimicrobial therapy

If Liver disease or longstanding valvular dysfunction and/or significant perioperative comorbidities

Emergency Surgery → **Early/Urgent Surgery** → **Delayed/Semi-Elective Surgery**

Objectives of Surgical Management

Aortic NVE
- Rarely cusps can be preserved/repaired with pericardial patch
- Complete debridement is essential
- Reconstruct defects before implantation
- Root abscess/fistula: consider valved conduit

Mitral NVE
- Repair should be attempted if feasible and if there is enough viable health tissue for reconstruction
- Destruction of subvalvular apparatus necessitates replacement

Right Sided NVE
- Generally respond well to antimicrobial therapy
- Reserve surgery for:
  - large vegetations
  - persistent cultures
  - recurrent septic pulmonary emboli

PVE
- Most patients will require surgery
- PVL and conduction defects more common
- Extra attention to debride all prosthetic material including pledgets
- CT chest prior to redosternotomy

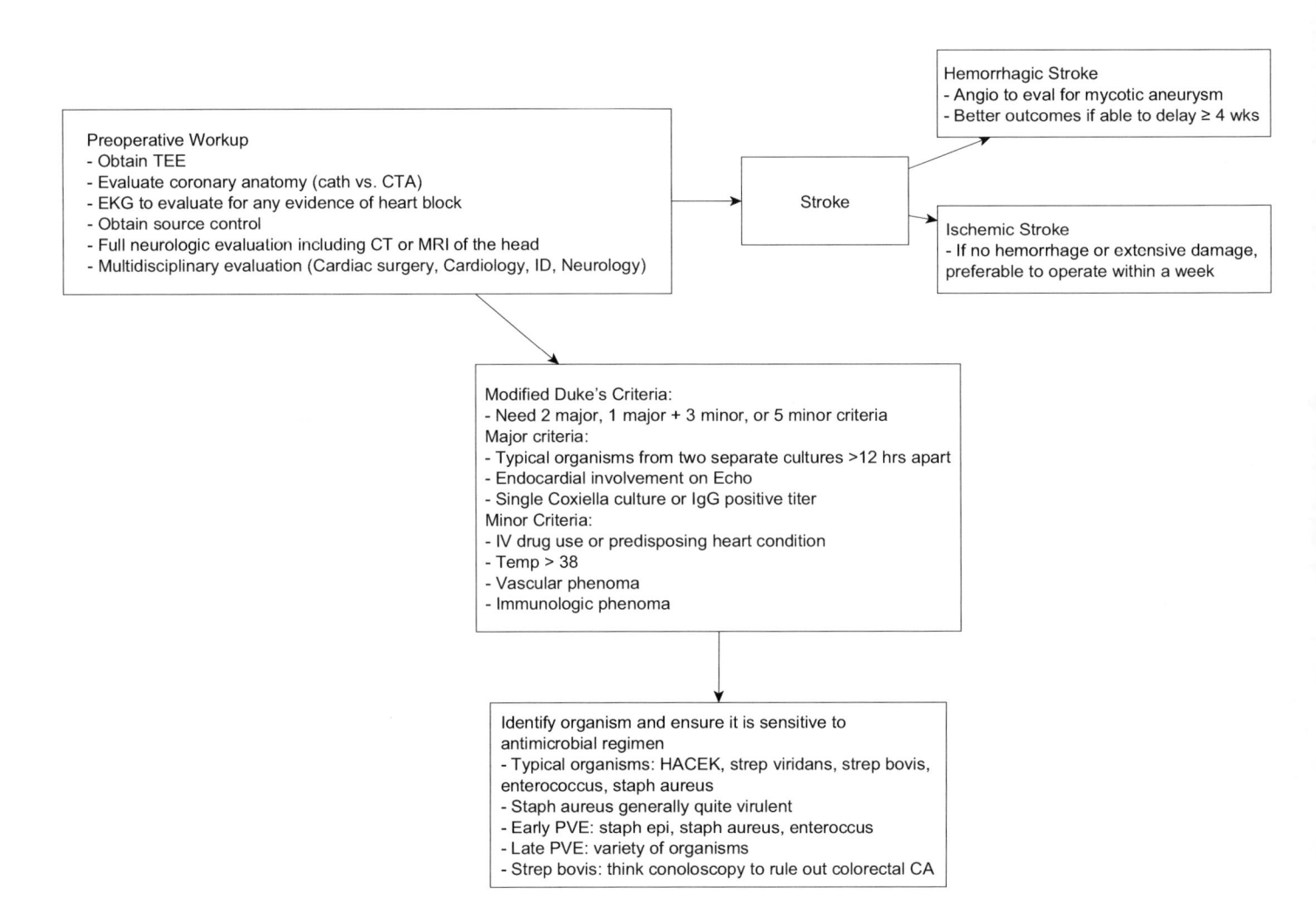

```
┌─────────────────────────────────────────────────────────────┐                    ┌──────────────────────────────────────────┐
│ Preoperative Workup                                         │                    │ Hemorrhagic Stroke                       │
│ - Obtain TEE                                                │                    │ - Angio to eval for mycotic aneurysm     │
│ - Evaluate coronary anatomy (cath vs. CTA)                  │                    │ - Better outcomes if able to delay ≥ 4 wks│
│ - EKG to evaluate for any evidence of heart block           │      ┌────────┐   └──────────────────────────────────────────┘
│ - Obtain source control                                     │─────▶│ Stroke │
│ - Full neurologic evaluation including CT or MRI of the head│      └────────┘   ┌──────────────────────────────────────────┐
│ - Multidisciplinary evaluation (Cardiac surgery, Cardiology,│                    │ Ischemic Stroke                          │
│   ID, Neurology)                                            │                    │ - If no hemorrhage or extensive damage,  │
└─────────────────────────────────────────────────────────────┘                    │   preferable to operate within a week    │
                         │                                                         └──────────────────────────────────────────┘
                         ▼
┌─────────────────────────────────────────────────────────────┐
│ Modified Duke's Criteria:                                   │
│ - Need 2 major, 1 major + 3 minor, or 5 minor criteria      │
│ Major criteria:                                             │
│ - Typical organisms from two separate cultures >12 hrs apart│
│ - Endocardial involvement on Echo                           │
│ - Single Coxiella culture or IgG positive titer             │
│ Minor Criteria:                                             │
│ - IV drug use or predisposing heart condition               │
│ - Temp > 38                                                 │
│ - Vascular phenoma                                          │
│ - Immunologic phenoma                                       │
└─────────────────────────────────────────────────────────────┘
                         │
                         ▼
┌─────────────────────────────────────────────────────────────┐
│ Identify organism and ensure it is sensitive to             │
│ antimicrobial regimen                                       │
│ - Typical organisms: HACEK, strep viridans, strep bovis,    │
│   enterococcus, staph aureus                                │
│ - Staph aureus generally quite virulent                     │
│ - Early PVE: staph epi, staph aureus, enteroccus            │
│ - Late PVE: variety of organisms                            │
│ - Strep bovis: think conoloscopy to rule out colorectal CA  │
└─────────────────────────────────────────────────────────────┘
```

Heart Failure
1. Severe acute AI or MR with Hemodynamic instability Cardiogenic shock Refractory pulmonary edema
2. Rupture with tamponade
3. Valve obstruction

Heart Failure
- AI or MR with evidence of heart failure
- TR with right heart failure

Infectious Complications
- Annular abscess/fistula/aneurysm/penetration lesion
- Conduction deficit / heart block
- Staph aureus, fungal, or MDR endocarditis
- Persistent sepsis despite antibiotic treatment

Embolic Complications
- Large vegetation (>10mm)
- Embolic complications despite treatment

- Progressive prosthetic leak
- Medically refractory CHF
- Persistent positive cultures despite antimicrobial therapy

If Liver disease or longstanding valvular dysfunction and/or significant perioperative comorbidities

↓ ↓ ↓

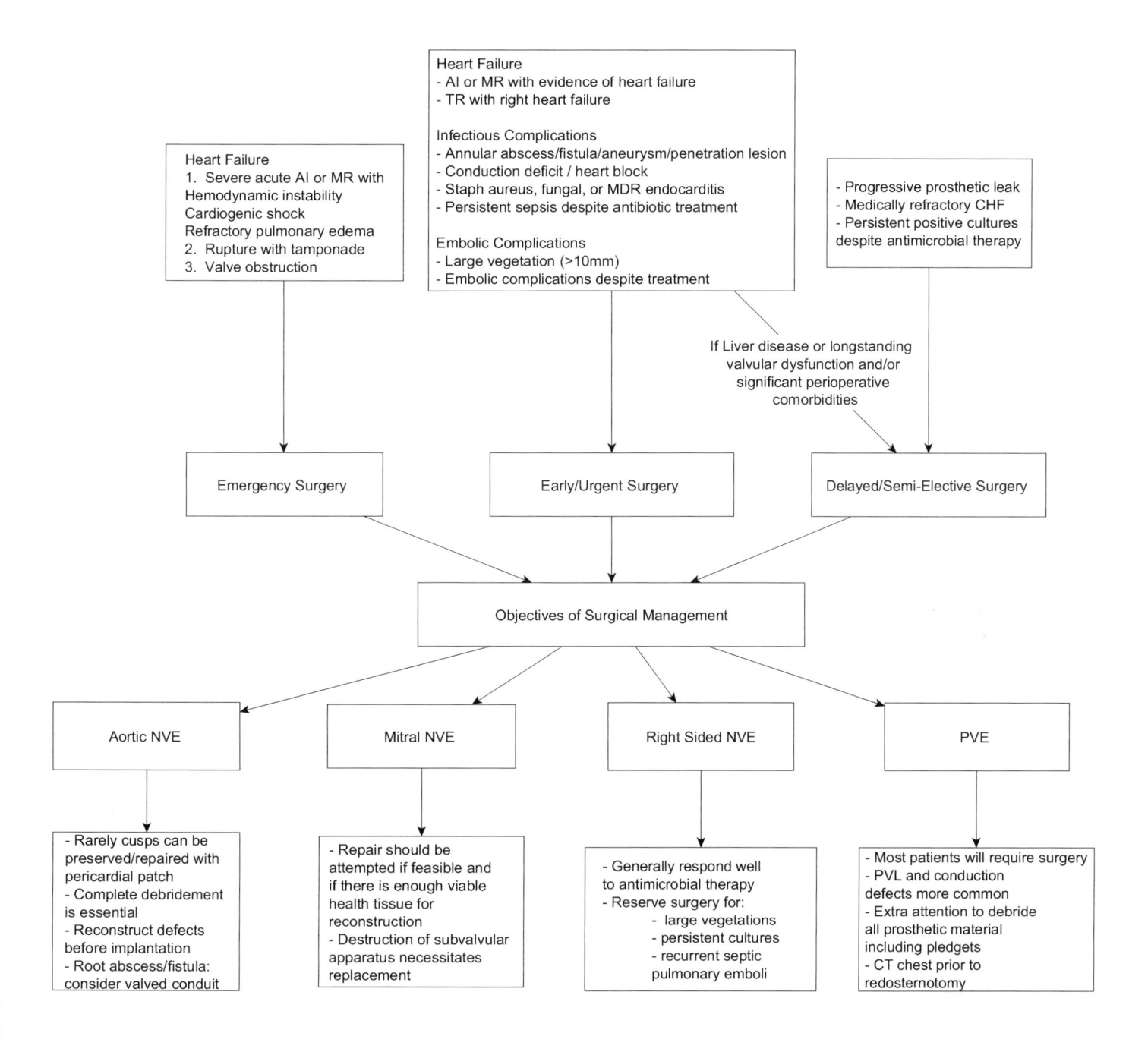

Emergency Surgery | **Early/Urgent Surgery** | **Delayed/Semi-Elective Surgery**

↓

Objectives of Surgical Management

↓ ↓ ↓ ↓

Aortic NVE | **Mitral NVE** | **Right Sided NVE** | **PVE**

Aortic NVE
- Rarely cusps can be preserved/repaired with pericardial patch
- Complete debridement is essential
- Reconstruct defects before implantation
- Root abscess/fistula: consider valved conduit

Mitral NVE
- Repair should be attempted if feasible and if there is enough viable health tissue for reconstruction
- Destruction of subvalvular apparatus necessitates replacement

Right Sided NVE
- Generally respond well to antimicrobial therapy
- Reserve surgery for:
    - large vegetations
    - persistent cultures
    - recurrent septic pulmonary emboli

PVE
- Most patients will require surgery
- PVL and conduction defects more common
- Extra attention to debride all prosthetic material including pledgets
- CT chest prior to redosternotomy

Modified Duke's Criteria:

- Need 2 major, 1 major + 3 minor, or 5 minor criteria

Major criteria:
- Typical organisms from two separate cultures >12 hrs apart
- Endocardial involvement on Echo
- Single Coxiella culture or IgG positive titer

Minor Criteria:
- IV drug use or predisposing heart condition
- Temp > 38
- Vascular phenomenon
- Immunologic phenomenon

Objectives of Surgical Management:

- Remove infected tissues
- Restore hemodynamics and valvular architecture
- Prevent embolic events
- Open/explore right atrium for those with conduction deficits
- NVE requires at least 6 weeks of post-op antimicrobial therapy
- PVE generally requires at least 8 weeks of antimicrobial therapy
- Complete removal of Pacemaker/Defibrillator system for documented infection of device or leads
- Complete removal of Pacemaker/Defibrillator system reasonable with endocarditis caused by staph aureus or fungi

AI, aortic insufficiency; HACEK, haemophilus, actinobacillus, cardiobacterium, eikenella, kingella; MDR, multi-drug resistant; MR, mitral regurgitation; NVE, native valve endocarditis; PVE, prosthetic valve endocarditis; PVL, paravalvular leak; TEE, transesophageal echocardiography

Pericardial Disease
Makato Mori, Arnar Geirsson

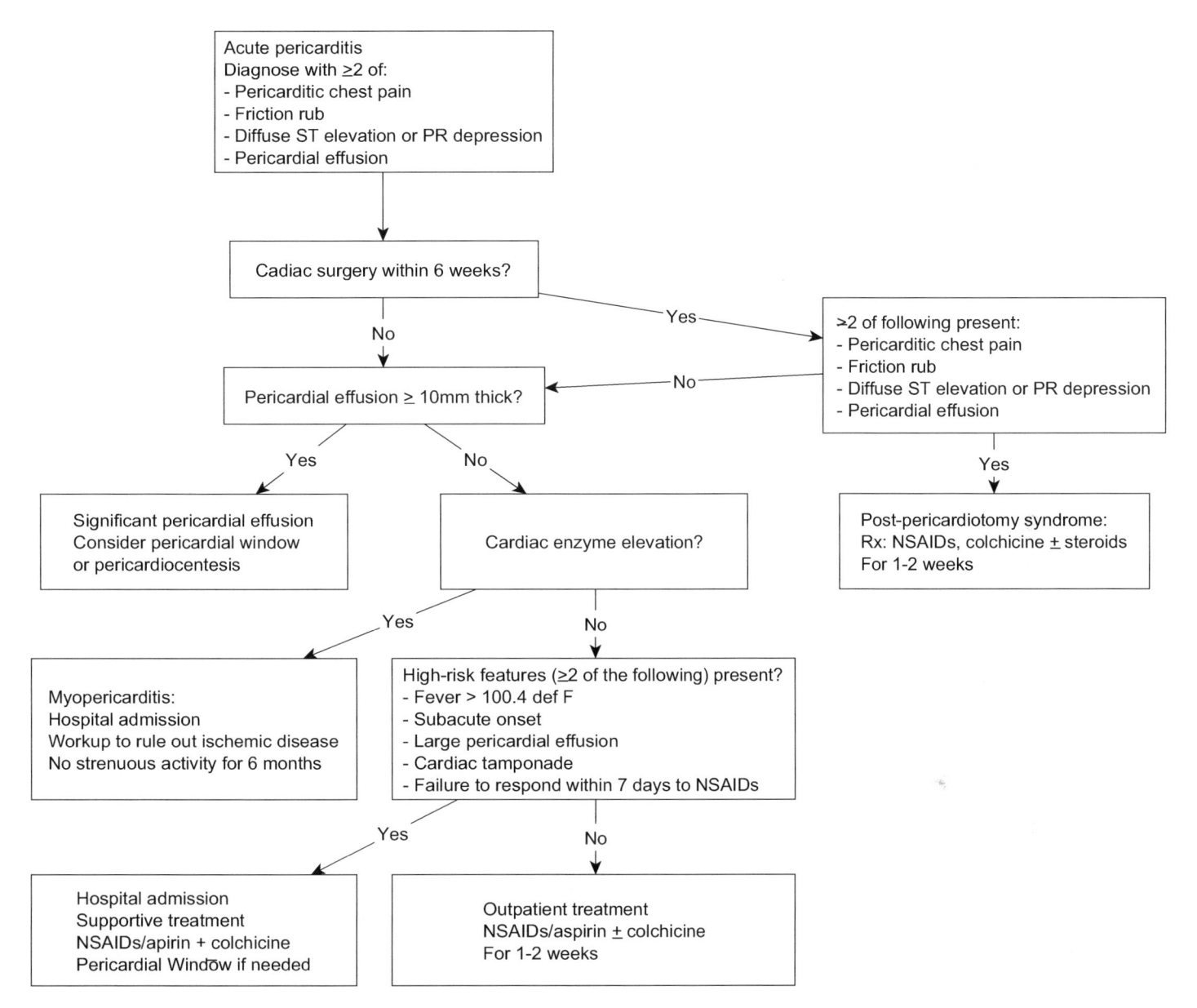

```
┌─────────────────────────────────────┐
│ Acute pericarditis                  │
│ Diagnose with ≥2 of:                │
│ - Pericarditic chest pain           │
│ - Friction rub                      │
│ - Diffuse ST elevation or PR depression │
│ - Pericardial effusion              │
└─────────────────────────────────────┘
                 │
                 ▼
     ┌───────────────────────────────┐         ┌─────────────────────────────────┐
     │ Cadiac surgery within 6 weeks?├──Yes───▶│ ≥2 of following present:         │
     └───────────────────────────────┘         │ - Pericarditic chest pain        │
                 │ No                          │ - Friction rub                   │
                 ▼                    ◀──No────│ - Diffuse ST elevation or PR depression │
     ┌───────────────────────────────┐         │ - Pericardial effusion           │
     │ Pericardial effusion ≥ 10mm thick?│     └─────────────────────────────────┘
     └───────────────────────────────┘                       │ Yes
          │ Yes         │ No                                 ▼
          ▼             ▼                          ┌─────────────────────────────┐
  ┌──────────────┐  ┌──────────────────┐           │ Post-pericardiotomy syndrome:│
  │ Significant  │  │ Cardiac enzyme   │           │ Rx: NSAIDs, colchicine ± steroids│
  │ pericardial  │  │ elevation?       │           │ For 1-2 weeks               │
  │ effusion     │  └──────────────────┘           └─────────────────────────────┘
  │ Consider     │     │ Yes    │ No
  │ pericardial  │     ▼        ▼
  │ window or    │  ┌─────────┐  ┌──────────────────────────────────┐
  │ pericardio-  │  │Myoperi- │  │ High-risk features (≥2 of the    │
  │ centesis     │  │carditis:│  │ following) present?              │
  └──────────────┘  │Hospital │  │ - Fever > 100.4 def F            │
                    │admission│  │ - Subacute onset                 │
                    │Workup to│  │ - Large pericardial effusion     │
                    │rule out │  │ - Cardiac tamponade              │
                    │ischemic │  │ - Failure to respond within 7    │
                    │disease  │  │   days to NSAIDs                 │
                    │No       │  └──────────────────────────────────┘
                    │strenuous│         │ Yes         │ No
                    │activity │         ▼             ▼
                    │for 6    │  ┌────────────┐  ┌──────────────────┐
                    │months   │  │Hospital    │  │Outpatient treatment│
                    └─────────┘  │admission   │  │NSAIDs/aspirin ±  │
                                 │Supportive  │  │colchicine         │
                                 │treatment   │  │For 1-2 weeks      │
                                 │NSAIDs/apirin│ └──────────────────┘
                                 │+ colchicine│
                                 │Pericardial │
                                 │Window if   │
                                 │needed      │
                                 └────────────┘
```

NSAIDs, Nonsteroidal Anti-inflammatory drugs

Trachea Trauma
Fatima Wilder, Sarah Minasyan

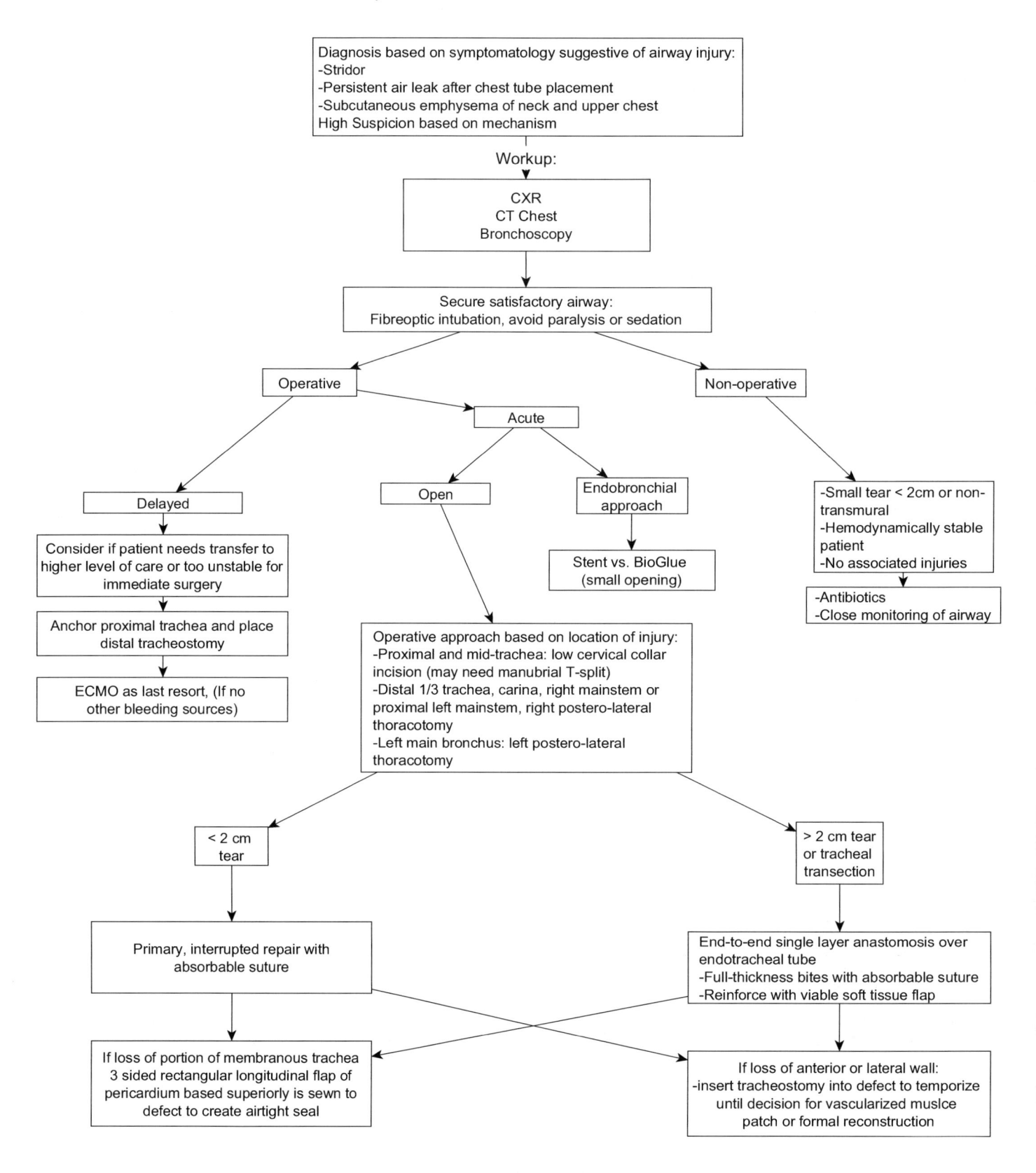

```
Diagnosis based on symptomatology suggestive of airway injury:
-Stridor
-Persistent air leak after chest tube placement
-Subcutaneous emphysema of neck and upper chest
High Suspicion based on mechanism
```

Workup:

```
CXR
CT Chest
Bronchoscopy
```

```
Secure satisfactory airway:
Fibreoptic intubation, avoid paralysis or sedation
```

Operative → **Non-operative**

Operative branches:
- **Delayed**
  - Consider if patient needs transfer to higher level of care or too unstable for immediate surgery
  - Anchor proximal trachea and place distal tracheostomy
  - ECMO as last resort, (If no other bleeding sources)
- **Acute**
  - **Open**
  - **Endobronchial approach**: Stent vs. BioGlue (small opening)

Non-operative:
- Small tear < 2cm or non-transmural
- Hemodynamically stable patient
- No associated injuries
  - Antibiotics
  - Close monitoring of airway

```
Operative approach based on location of injury:
-Proximal and mid-trachea: low cervical collar incision (may need manubrial T-split)
-Distal 1/3 trachea, carina, right mainstem or proximal left mainstem, right postero-lateral thoracotomy
-Left main bronchus: left postero-lateral thoracotomy
```

< 2 cm tear → Primary, interrupted repair with absorbable suture

> 2 cm tear or tracheal transection → End-to-end single layer anastomosis over endotracheal tube
- Full-thickness bites with absorbable suture
- Reinforce with viable soft tissue flap

If loss of portion of membranous trachea 3 sided rectangular longitudinal flap of pericardium based superiorly is sewn to defect to create airtight seal

If loss of anterior or lateral wall:
- insert tracheostomy into defect to temporize until decision for vascularized muslce patch or formal reconstruction

Trachea Tumors
Fatima Wilder, Sarah Minasyan

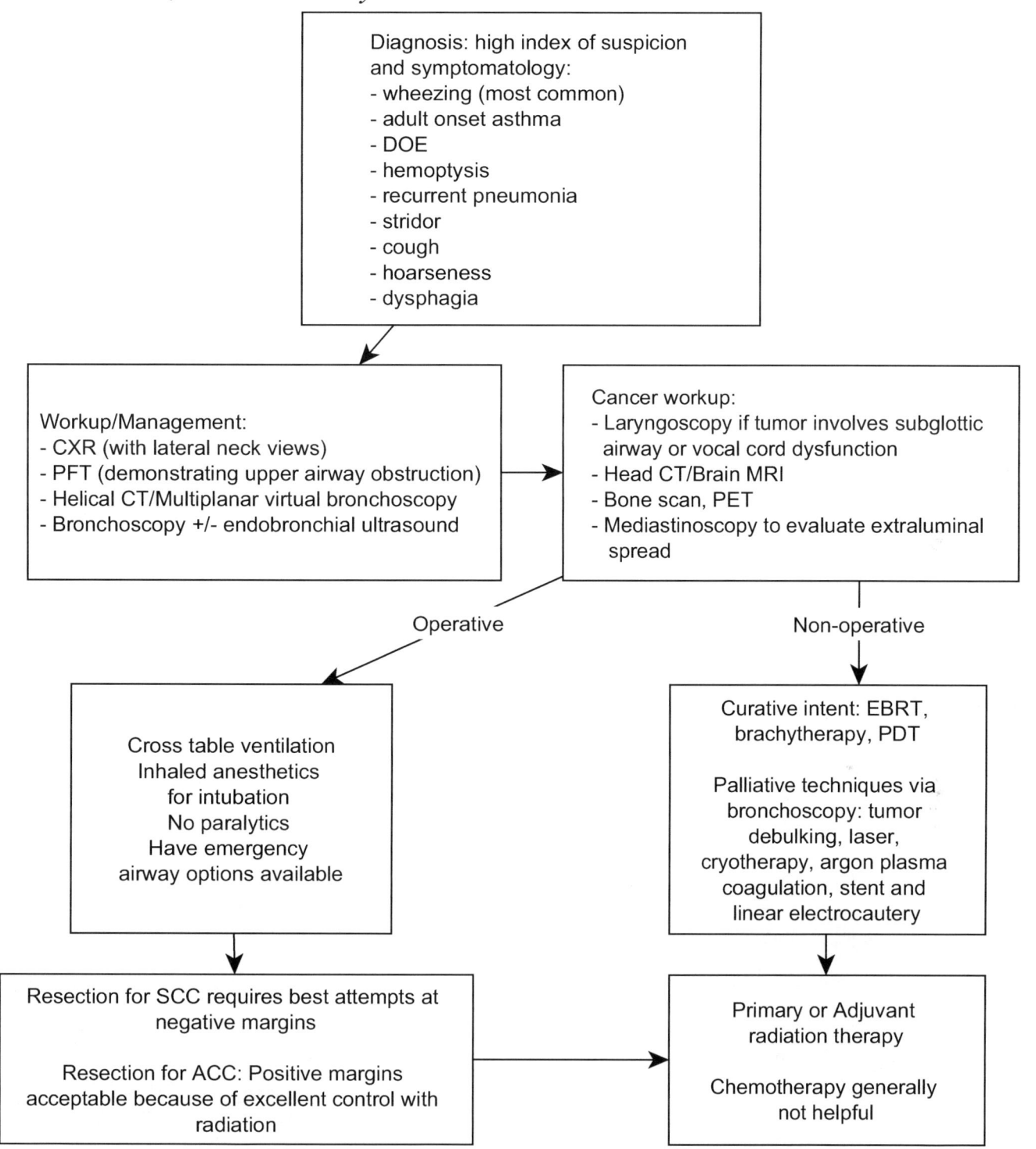

```
┌─────────────────────────────────────────┐
│ Diagnosis: high index of suspicion      │
│ and symptomatology:                     │
│ - wheezing (most common)                │
│ - adult onset asthma                    │
│ - DOE                                   │
│ - hemoptysis                            │
│ - recurrent pneumonia                   │
│ - stridor                               │
│ - cough                                 │
│ - hoarseness                            │
│ - dysphagia                             │
└─────────────────────────────────────────┘
                    │
                    ▼
┌──────────────────────────────────────────┐     ┌──────────────────────────────────────┐
│ Workup/Management:                       │     │ Cancer workup:                       │
│ - CXR (with lateral neck views)          │     │ - Laryngoscopy if tumor involves     │
│ - PFT (demonstrating upper airway        │ ──▶ │   subglottic airway or vocal cord    │
│   obstruction)                           │     │   dysfunction                        │
│ - Helical CT/Multiplanar virtual         │     │ - Head CT/Brain MRI                  │
│   bronchoscopy                           │     │ - Bone scan, PET                     │
│ - Bronchoscopy +/- endobronchial         │     │ - Mediastinoscopy to evaluate        │
│   ultrasound                             │     │   extraluminal spread                │
└──────────────────────────────────────────┘     └──────────────────────────────────────┘
                        Operative  ◀──────────┘         │ Non-operative
                            │                           │
                            ▼                           ▼
┌──────────────────────────────┐        ┌──────────────────────────────────┐
│ Cross table ventilation      │        │ Curative intent: EBRT,           │
│ Inhaled anesthetics          │        │ brachytherapy, PDT               │
│ for intubation               │        │                                  │
│ No paralytics                │        │ Palliative techniques via        │
│ Have emergency               │        │ bronchoscopy: tumor              │
│ airway options available     │        │ debulking, laser,                │
└──────────────────────────────┘        │ cryotherapy, argon plasma        │
                │                       │ coagulation, stent and           │
                ▼                       │ linear electrocautery            │
┌─────────────────────────────────────┐ └──────────────────────────────────┘
│ Resection for SCC requires best     │                 │
│ attempts at negative margins        │                 ▼
│                                     │   ┌──────────────────────────────┐
│ Resection for ACC: Positive margins │──▶│ Primary or Adjuvant          │
│ acceptable because of excellent     │   │ radiation therapy            │
│ control with radiation              │   │                              │
└─────────────────────────────────────┘   │ Chemotherapy generally       │
                                          │ not helpful                  │
                                          └──────────────────────────────┘
```

Differential (Most common tracheal tumors):
Benign: Squamous papilloma, Pleomorphic Adenoma, or Benign cartilaginous tumors
Malignant: Squamous Cell carcinoma (SCC) or Adenoid cystic carcinoma (ACC)
*Refer to Algorithm 1B for details on surgical resection
EBRT = External Beam Radiation Therapy, PDT = Photodynamic Therapy, DOE = Dyspnea on exertion

Tracheal Stenosis
Fatima Wilder, Sarah Minasyan

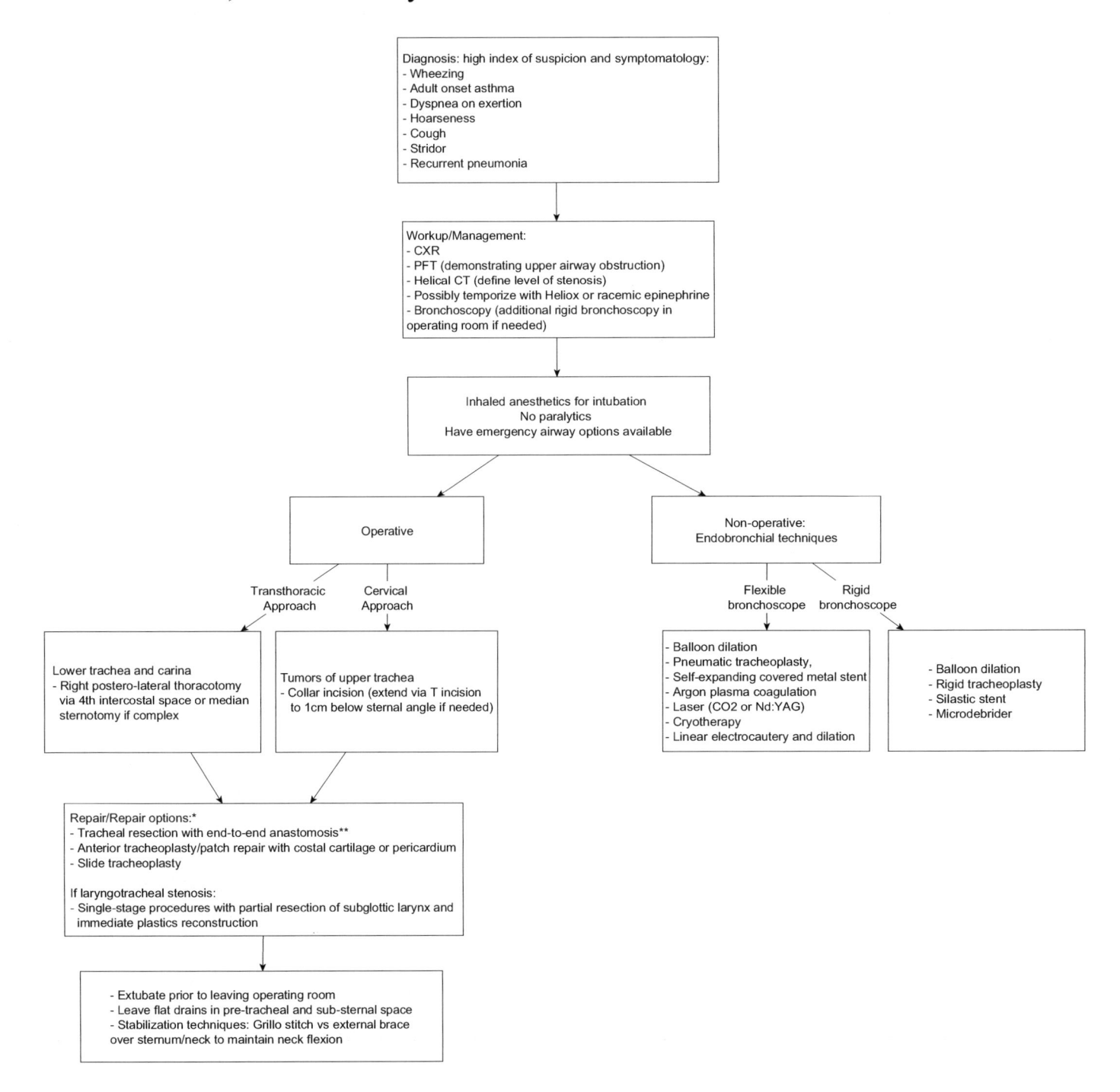

```
┌─────────────────────────────────────────────┐
│ Diagnosis: high index of suspicion and      │
│ symptomatology:                             │
│  - Wheezing                                 │
│  - Adult onset asthma                       │
│  - Dyspnea on exertion                      │
│  - Hoarseness                               │
│  - Cough                                    │
│  - Stridor                                  │
│  - Recurrent pneumonia                      │
└─────────────────────────────────────────────┘
                      │
                      ▼
┌─────────────────────────────────────────────┐
│ Workup/Management:                          │
│  - CXR                                      │
│  - PFT (demonstrating upper airway          │
│    obstruction)                             │
│  - Helical CT (define level of stenosis)    │
│  - Possibly temporize with Heliox or        │
│    racemic epinephrine                      │
│  - Bronchoscopy (additional rigid           │
│    bronchoscopy in operating room if needed)│
└─────────────────────────────────────────────┘
                      │
                      ▼
┌─────────────────────────────────────────────┐
│   Inhaled anesthetics for intubation        │
│   No paralytics                             │
│   Have emergency airway options available   │
└─────────────────────────────────────────────┘
              │                    │
              ▼                    ▼
      ┌─────────────┐      ┌──────────────────┐
      │  Operative  │      │  Non-operative:  │
      │             │      │  Endobronchial   │
      │             │      │  techniques      │
      └─────────────┘      └──────────────────┘
```

Operative branch:
- Transthoracic Approach: Lower trachea and carina
  - Right postero-lateral thoracotomy via 4th intercostal space or median sternotomy if complex
- Cervical Approach: Tumors of upper trachea
  - Collar incision (extend via T incision to 1cm below sternal angle if needed)

Repair/Repair options:*
- Tracheal resection with end-to-end anastomosis**
- Anterior tracheoplasty/patch repair with costal cartilage or pericardium
- Slide tracheoplasty

If laryngotracheal stenosis:
- Single-stage procedures with partial resection of subglottic larynx and immediate plastics reconstruction

Post-op:
- Extubate prior to leaving operating room
- Leave flat drains in pre-tracheal and sub-sternal space
- Stabilization techniques: Grillo stitch vs external brace over sternum/neck to maintain neck flexion

Non-operative branch:

Flexible bronchoscope:
- Balloon dilation
- Pneumatic tracheoplasty,
- Self-expanding covered metal stent
- Argon plasma coagulation
- Laser (CO2 or Nd:YAG)
- Cryotherapy
- Linear electrocautery and dilation

Rigid bronchoscope:
- Balloon dilation
- Rigid tracheoplasty
- Silastic stent
- Microdebrider

*Aim for dissection close to the tracheal wall or the scar to avoid injury to RLN which lies in TE groove; no need to expose the nerves

**Maneuvers to minimize tension: flexion of neck and mobilization of pre-tracheal plane – avoiding lateral blood supply to trachea; Montgomery suprahyoid laryngeal release; Right hilar and inferior pulmonary ligament release

⌘Airway control options:
- Suspended laryngoscope (Primarily for subglottic and proximal tracheal stenosis), rigid bronchoscope, endotracheal tube or LMA (laryngeal mask airway);
- Ventilate w/ intermittent apnea or jet techniques during procedure

Common Causes of Tracheal Stenosis
- Focal Inflammation
- Systemic Inflammation
- Infection
- Dynamic collapse (e.g. malacia)
- Malignancy

Pulmonary Nodules
Stephanie G. Worrell, Andrew C. Chang

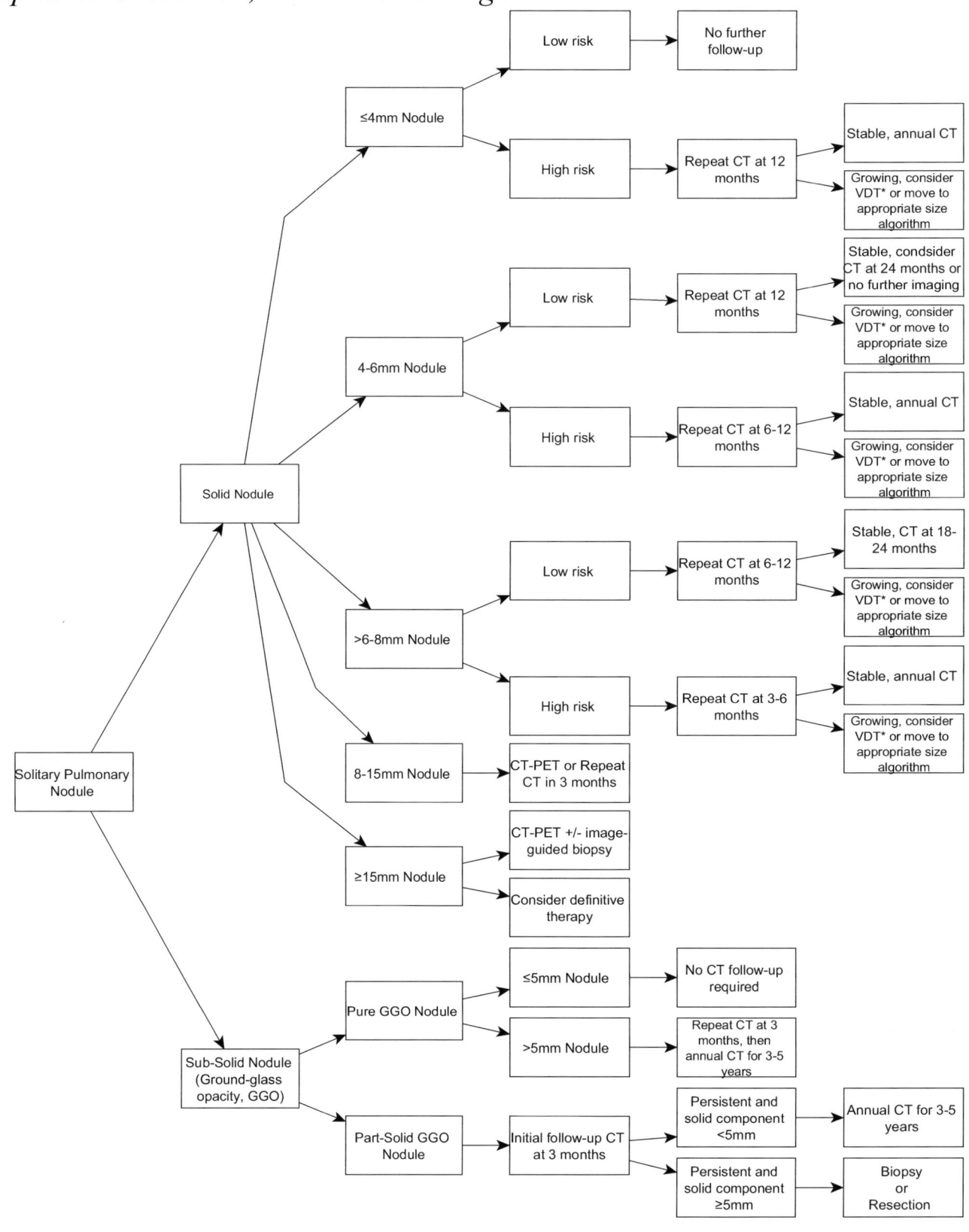

```
Solitary Pulmonary Nodule
├── Solid Nodule
│   ├── ≤4mm Nodule
│   │   ├── Low risk → No further follow-up
│   │   └── High risk → Repeat CT at 12 months
│   │       ├── Stable, annual CT
│   │       └── Growing, consider VDT* or move to appropriate size algorithm
│   ├── 4-6mm Nodule
│   │   ├── Low risk → Repeat CT at 12 months
│   │   │   ├── Stable, condsider CT at 24 months or no further imaging
│   │   │   └── Growing, consider VDT* or move to appropriate size algorithm
│   │   └── High risk → Repeat CT at 6-12 months
│   │       ├── Stable, annual CT
│   │       └── Growing, consider VDT* or move to appropriate size algorithm
│   ├── >6-8mm Nodule
│   │   ├── Low risk → Repeat CT at 6-12 months
│   │   │   ├── Stable, CT at 18-24 months
│   │   │   └── Growing, consider VDT* or move to appropriate size algorithm
│   │   └── High risk → Repeat CT at 3-6 months
│   │       ├── Stable, annual CT
│   │       └── Growing, consider VDT* or move to appropriate size algorithm
│   ├── 8-15mm Nodule → CT-PET or Repeat CT in 3 months
│   └── ≥15mm Nodule
│       ├── CT-PET +/- image-guided biopsy
│       └── Consider definitive therapy
└── Sub-Solid Nodule (Ground-glass opacity, GGO)
    ├── Pure GGO Nodule
    │   ├── ≤5mm Nodule → No CT follow-up required
    │   └── >5mm Nodule → Repeat CT at 3 months, then annual CT for 3-5 years
    └── Part-Solid GGO Nodule → Initial follow-up CT at 3 months
        ├── Persistent and solid component <5mm → Annual CT for 3-5 years
        └── Persistent and solid component ≥5mm → Biopsy or Resection
```

118

A solitary pulmonary nodule is defined as a discrete, rounded opacity less than or equal to 3 cm in diameter that is surrounded by lung parenchyma.

A low risk patient has no or minimal (<20 pack-year) smoking history or other known risk factors. A high-risk patient has a history of smoking or of other known risk factors. Known risk factors include advanced age, first degree relative with lung cancer, personal history of malignancy greater than 5 years prior to nodule detection, or exposure to asbestos, radon, or uranium (2,3)

All follow-up CT scans should be performed at low dose, unless evaluating the mediastinum or lymph nodes. All annual low dose CTs should be continued until the patient is no longer a candidate for definitive therapy (4).

Volume-Doubling time (VDT) is the number of days in which a nodule doubles in volume. Using the British Thoracic Society guidelines, a solid nodule with a VDT ≤ 400 days increases the risk of malignancy and requires further work-up and consideration of definitive management. A nodule with a VDT of 400-600 days should be considered for further surveillance versus biopsy based on patient preference (5).

Pleural Effusion
Catherine Bixby, Kirk McMurtry

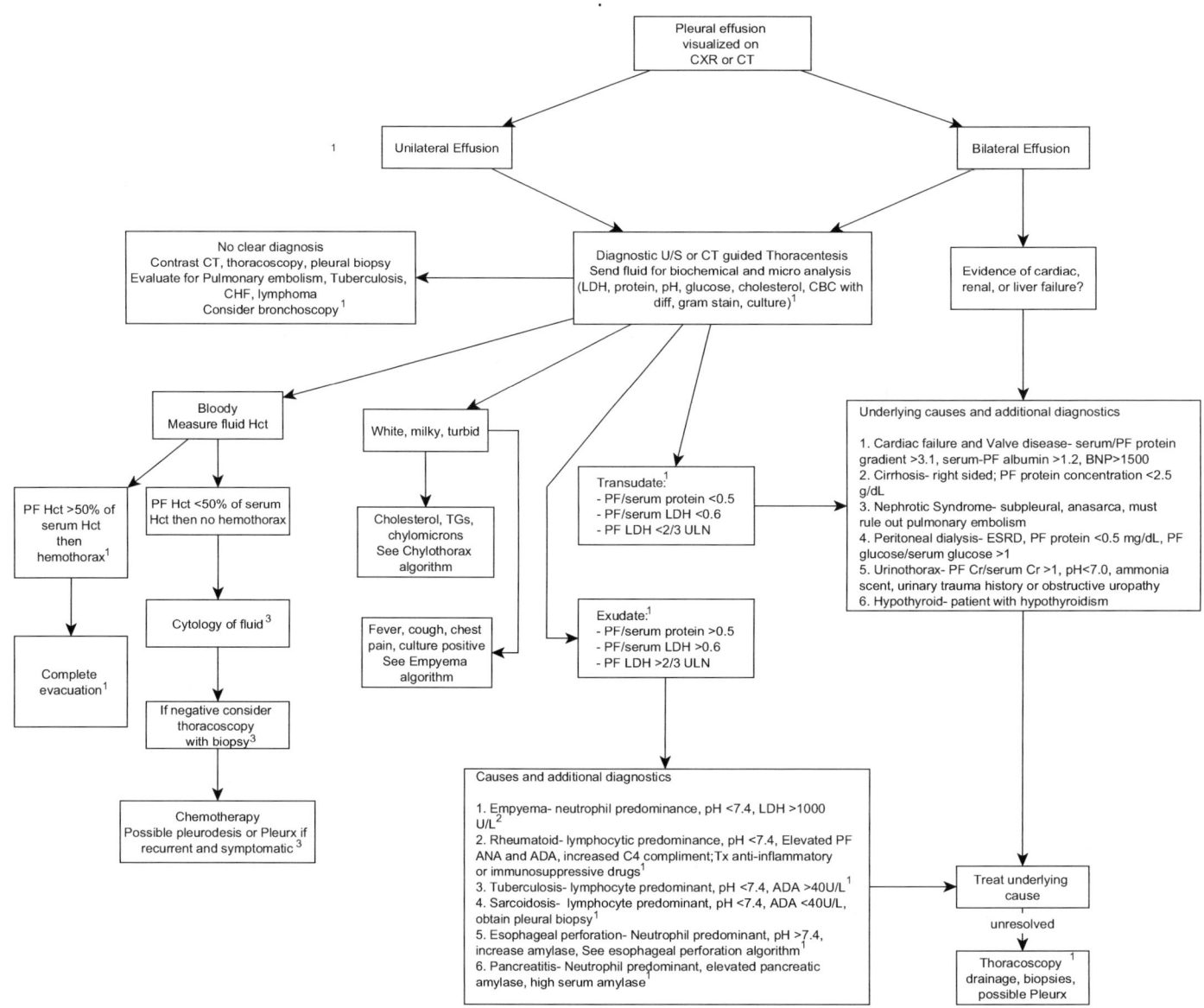

```
                    Pleural effusion
                    visualized on
                     CXR or CT
                    /            \
           Unilateral Effusion   Bilateral Effusion
```

Unilateral Effusion → Diagnostic U/S or CT guided Thoracentesis. Send fluid for biochemical and micro analysis (LDH, protein, pH, glucose, cholesterol, CBC with diff, gram stain, culture)[1]

No clear diagnosis
Contrast CT, thoracoscopy, pleural biopsy
Evaluate for Pulmonary embolism, Tuberculosis, CHF, lymphoma
Consider bronchoscopy[1]

Bloody — Measure fluid Hct
- PF Hct >50% of serum Hct then hemothorax[1] → Complete evacuation[1]
- PF Hct <50% of serum Hct then no hemothorax → Cytology of fluid[3] → If negative consider thoracoscopy with biopsy[3] → Chemotherapy, Possible pleurodesis or Pleurx if recurrent and symptomatic[3]

White, milky, turbid
- Cholesterol, TGs, chylomicrons — See Chylothorax algorithm
- Fever, cough, chest pain, culture positive — See Empyema algorithm

Transudate:[1]
- PF/serum protein <0.5
- PF/serum LDH <0.6
- PF LDH <2/3 ULN

Exudate:[1]
- PF/serum protein >0.5
- PF/serum LDH >0.6
- PF LDH >2/3 ULN

Causes and additional diagnostics
1. Empyema- neutrophil predominance, pH <7.4, LDH >1000 U/L[2]
2. Rheumatoid- lymphocytic predominance, pH <7.4, Elevated PF ANA and ADA, increased C4 compliment; Tx anti-inflammatory or immunosuppressive drugs[1]
3. Tuberculosis- lymphocyte predominant, pH <7.4, ADA >40U/L[1]
4. Sarcoidosis- lymphocyte predominant, pH <7.4, ADA <40U/L, obtain pleural biopsy[1]
5. Esophageal perforation- Neutrophil predominant, pH >7.4, increase amylase, See esophageal perforation algorithm[1]
6. Pancreatitis- Neutrophil predominant, elevated pancreatic amylase, high serum amylase[1]

Bilateral Effusion → Evidence of cardiac, renal, or liver failure?

Underlying causes and additional diagnostics
1. Cardiac failure and Valve disease- serum/PF protein gradient >3.1, serum-PF albumin >1.2, BNP>1500
2. Cirrhosis- right sided; PF protein concentration <2.5 g/dL
3. Nephrotic Syndrome- subpleural, anasarca, must rule out pulmonary embolism
4. Peritoneal dialysis- ESRD, PF protein <0.5 mg/dL, PF glucose/serum glucose >1
5. Urinothorax- PF Cr/serum Cr >1, pH<7.0, ammonia scent, urinary trauma history or obstructive uropathy
6. Hypothyroid- patient with hypothyroidism

Treat underlying cause → unresolved → Thoracoscopy drainage, biopsies, possible Pleurx[1]

CHF- Congestive heart failure, U/S- ultrasound, LDH- lactate dehydrogenase, Hct- Hematocrit, TGs- triglycerides, PF- pleural fluid, ESRD- end stage renal disease, ADA- Adenosine deaminase, ANA- Anti-nucleic acid

Bronchopulmonary Carcinoid
Caitlin Harrington, Brandon Tieu

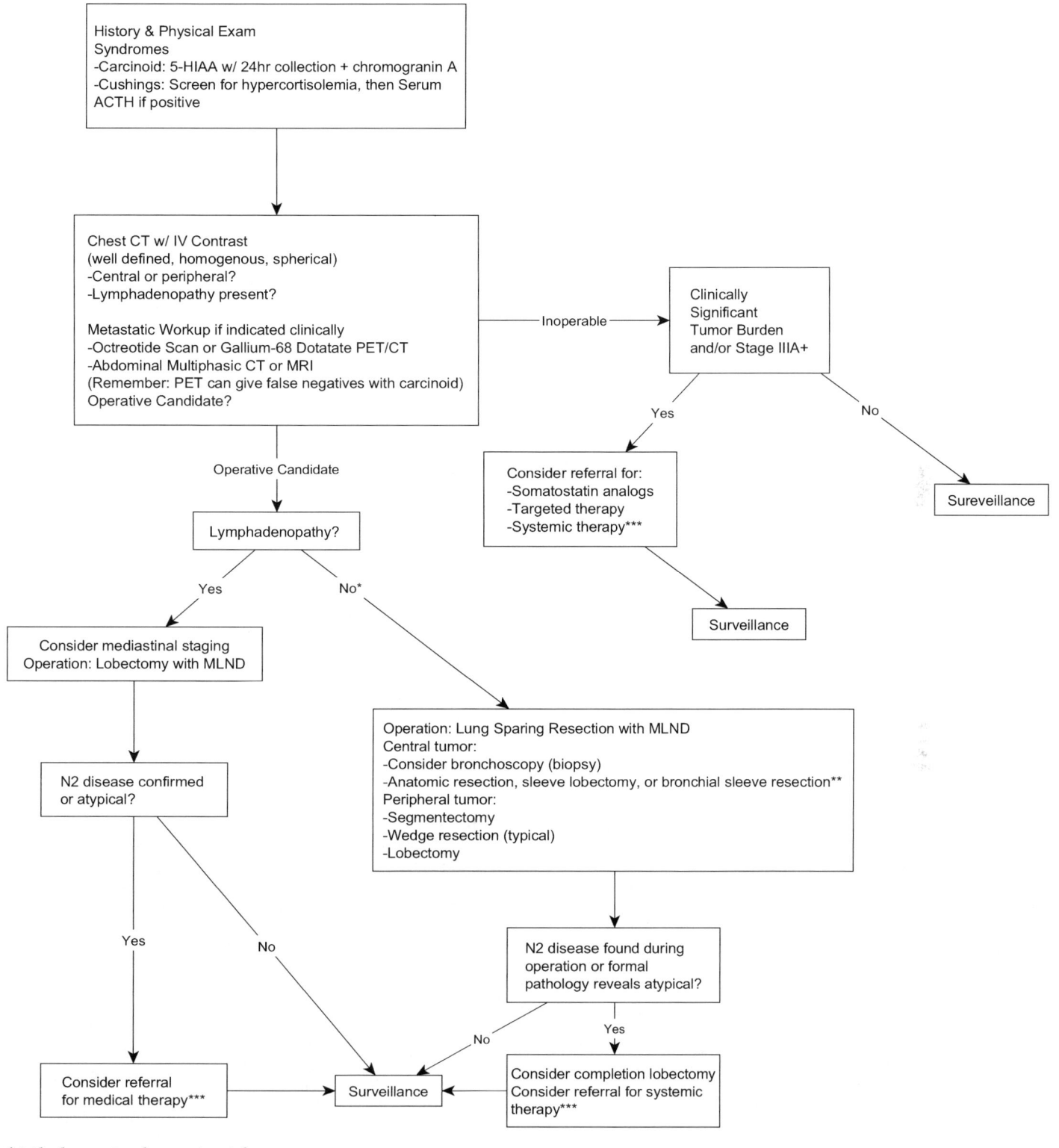

```
┌─────────────────────────────────────┐
│ History & Physical Exam             │
│ Syndromes                           │
│ -Carcinoid: 5-HIAA w/ 24hr          │
│  collection + chromogranin A        │
│ -Cushings: Screen for               │
│  hypercortisolemia, then Serum      │
│  ACTH if positive                   │
└─────────────────┬───────────────────┘
                  ↓
┌─────────────────────────────────────┐                    ┌──────────────┐
│ Chest CT w/ IV Contrast             │                    │ Clinically   │
│ (well defined, homogenous,          │                    │ Significant  │
│ spherical)                          │                    │ Tumor Burden │
│ -Central or peripheral?             │──Inoperable───────→│ and/or Stage │
│ -Lymphadenopathy present?           │                    │ IIIA+        │
│                                     │                    └──┬────────┬──┘
│ Metastatic Workup if indicated      │                    Yes│        │No
│ clinically                          │                       ↓        ↓
│ -Octreotide Scan or Gallium-68      │              ┌──────────────┐  ┌──────────────┐
│  Dotatate PET/CT                    │              │Consider      │  │ Sureveillance│
│ -Abdominal Multiphasic CT or MRI    │              │referral for: │  └──────────────┘
│ (Remember: PET can give false       │              │-Somatostatin │
│  negatives with carcinoid)          │              │ analogs      │
│ Operative Candidate?                │              │-Targeted     │
└─────────────────┬───────────────────┘              │ therapy      │
                  │Operative Candidate               │-Systemic     │
                  ↓                                  │ therapy***   │
┌─────────────────────┐                              └──────┬───────┘
│ Lymphadenopathy?    │                                     ↓
└──┬──────────────┬───┘                             ┌──────────────┐
Yes│              │No*                              │ Surveillance │
   ↓              ↓                                 └──────────────┘
┌──────────────┐  ┌──────────────────────────────────────────────────────┐
│Consider      │  │ Operation: Lung Sparing Resection with MLND          │
│mediastinal   │  │ Central tumor:                                       │
│staging       │  │ -Consider bronchoscopy (biopsy)                      │
│Operation:    │  │ -Anatomic resection, sleeve lobectomy, or bronchial  │
│Lobectomy     │  │  sleeve resection**                                  │
│with MLND     │  │ Peripheral tumor:                                    │
└──────┬───────┘  │ -Segmentectomy                                       │
       ↓          │ -Wedge resection (typical)                           │
┌──────────────┐  │ -Lobectomy                                           │
│ N2 disease   │  └──────────────────────┬───────────────────────────────┘
│ confirmed    │                         ↓
│ or atypical? │              ┌──────────────────────┐
└──┬────────┬──┘              │ N2 disease found     │
Yes│        │No               │ during operation or  │
   │        │                 │ formal pathology     │
   │        │                 │ reveals atypical?    │
   │        │                 └──┬────────────────┬──┘
   ↓        ↓                  No│              Yes│
┌──────────┐                     ↓                 ↓
│Consider  │  ┌──────────────┐  ┌──────────────────────────┐
│referral  │  │ Surveillance │←─│Consider completion       │
│for       │  └──────────────┘  │lobectomy                 │
│medical   │                    │Consider referral for     │
│therapy***│                    │systemic therapy***       │
└──────────┘                    └──────────────────────────┘
```

*Likely typical carcinoid
**Lung sparing resection preferred over pneumonectomy
***Limited data for efficacy
MLND = Mediastinal lymph node dissection

Small Cell Carcinoma
Julie Stortz, Vincent Daniel

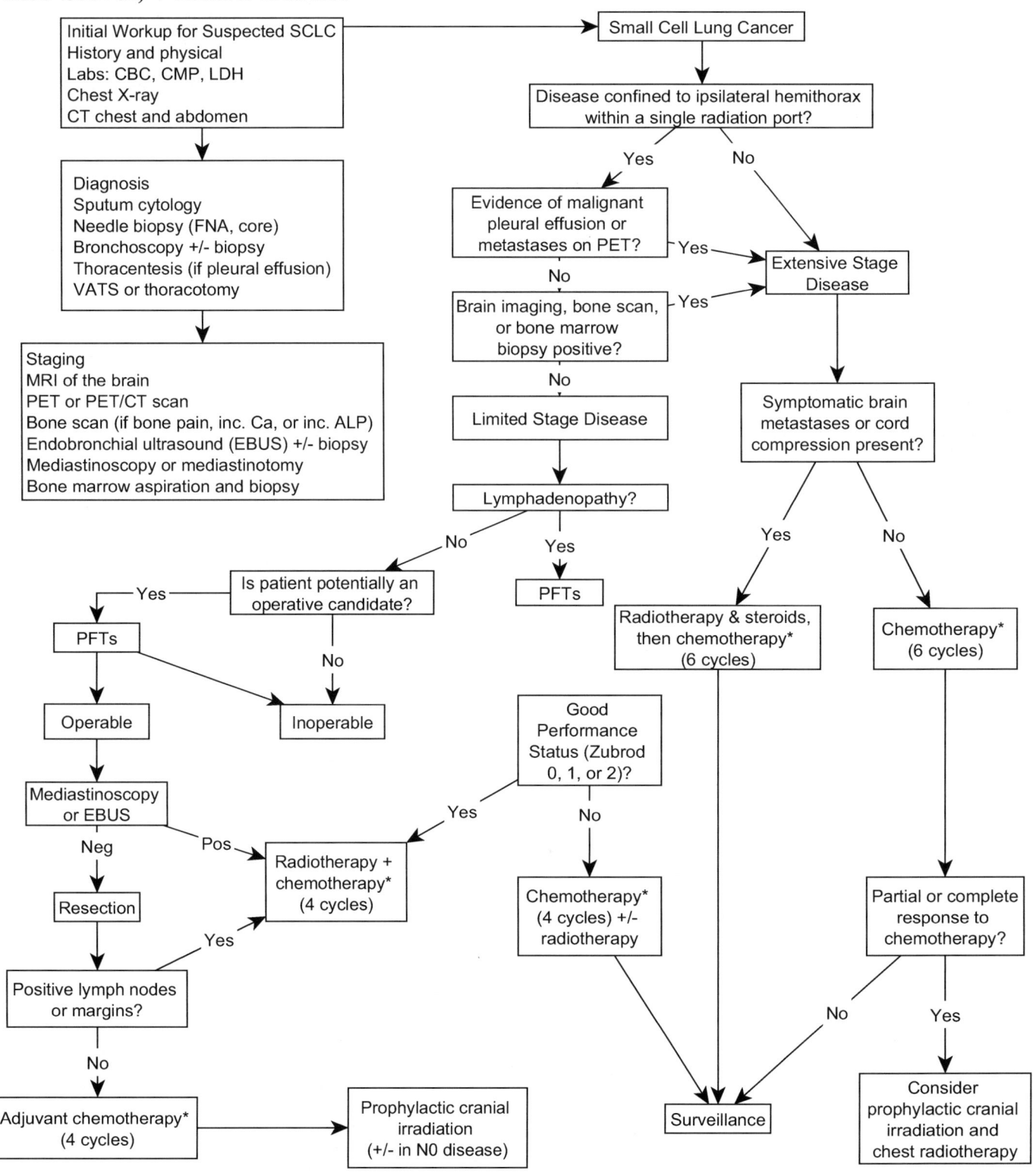

```
┌─────────────────────────────────┐                              ┌─────────────────────────┐
│ Initial Workup for Suspected SCLC│─────────────────────────────→│ Small Cell Lung Cancer  │
│ History and physical             │                              └─────────────────────────┘
│ Labs: CBC, CMP, LDH              │                                        │
│ Chest X-ray                      │                                        ▼
│ CT chest and abdomen             │                    ┌──────────────────────────────────────┐
└─────────────────────────────────┘                    │ Disease confined to ipsilateral       │
                │                                       │ hemithorax within a single radiation  │
                ▼                                       │ port?                                 │
┌─────────────────────────────────┐                    └──────────────────────────────────────┘
│ Diagnosis                        │                              Yes ↙        ↘ No
│ Sputum cytology                  │                  ┌─────────────────────┐
│ Needle biopsy (FNA, core)        │                  │ Evidence of         │
│ Bronchoscopy +/- biopsy          │                  │ malignant pleural   │──Yes──┐
│ Thoracentesis (if pleural effus.)│                  │ effusion or         │       │
│ VATS or thoracotomy              │                  │ metastases on PET?  │       ▼
└─────────────────────────────────┘                  └─────────────────────┘   ┌──────────────┐
                │                                              │ No             │ Extensive    │
                ▼                                              ▼          Yes──→│ Stage        │
┌─────────────────────────────────┐                  ┌─────────────────────┐   │ Disease      │
│ Staging                          │                  │ Brain imaging, bone │   └──────────────┘
│ MRI of the brain                 │                  │ scan, or bone marrow│           │
│ PET or PET/CT scan               │                  │ biopsy positive?    │           ▼
│ Bone scan (if bone pain, inc. Ca,│                  └─────────────────────┘   ┌──────────────┐
│  or inc. ALP)                    │                              │ No          │ Symptomatic  │
│ Endobronchial ultrasound (EBUS)  │                              ▼             │ brain        │
│  +/- biopsy                      │                  ┌─────────────────────┐   │ metastases   │
│ Mediastinoscopy or mediastinotomy│                  │ Limited Stage       │   │ or cord      │
│ Bone marrow aspiration and biopsy│                  │ Disease             │   │ compression  │
└─────────────────────────────────┘                  └─────────────────────┘   │ present?     │
                                                                 │              └──────────────┘
                                                                 ▼                Yes ↙    ↘ No
                                                      ┌─────────────────────┐
                                                      │ Lymphadenopathy?    │
                                                      └─────────────────────┘
                                         No ↙                   ↘ Yes
                          ┌─────────────────────┐                  ▼
                          │ Is patient          │             ┌────────┐
              ←──Yes──────│ potentially an      │             │ PFTs   │
              │           │ operative candidate?│             └────────┘
              ▼           └─────────────────────┘                  │
         ┌────────┐              │ No                              ▼
         │ PFTs   │              ▼                        ┌─────────────────────┐   ┌─────────────────┐
         └────────┘         ┌────────────┐                │ Radiotherapy &      │   │ Chemotherapy*   │
              │             │ Inoperable │                │ steroids, then      │   │ (6 cycles)      │
              ▼             └────────────┘                │ chemotherapy*       │   └─────────────────┘
         ┌──────────┐                                     │ (6 cycles)          │           │
         │ Operable │                                     └─────────────────────┘           ▼
         └──────────┘                 ┌─────────────────────┐                      ┌─────────────────┐
              │                       │ Good Performance    │                      │ Partial or      │
              ▼                       │ Status (Zubrod      │                      │ complete        │
       ┌────────────────┐             │ 0, 1, or 2)?        │                      │ response to     │
       │ Mediastinoscopy│             └─────────────────────┘                      │ chemotherapy?   │
       │ or EBUS        │            Yes ↙            ↘ No                         └─────────────────┘
       └────────────────┘     ┌───────────────┐   ┌─────────────────┐                No ↙      ↘ Yes
         Neg ↙    ↘ Pos       │ Radiotherapy +│   │ Chemotherapy*   │
    ┌──────────┐              │ chemotherapy* │   │ (4 cycles) +/-  │
    │Resection │              │ (4 cycles)    │   │ radiotherapy    │
    └──────────┘              └───────────────┘   └─────────────────┘
         │  ──Yes──→                                                                         ┌─────────────────┐
         ▼                                                                                   │ Consider        │
   ┌──────────────────┐                                                                      │ prophylactic    │
   │ Positive lymph   │                                                                      │ cranial         │
   │ nodes or margins?│                                                                      │ irradiation and │
   └──────────────────┘                                                                      │ chest           │
         │ No                                                                                │ radiotherapy    │
         ▼                                                                                   └─────────────────┘
   ┌──────────────────┐    ┌──────────────────┐                     ┌──────────────┐
   │ Adjuvant         │───→│ Prophylactic     │                     │ Surveillance │
   │ chemotherapy*    │    │ cranial          │                     └──────────────┘
   │ (4 cycles)       │    │ irradiation      │
   └──────────────────┘    │ (+/- in N0 dis.) │
                           └──────────────────┘
```

*Chemotherapy consists of platinum & etoposide

Surgical Management of Early Stage Non-Small Cell Lung Cancer
Michael A. Archer, Eric S. Lambright

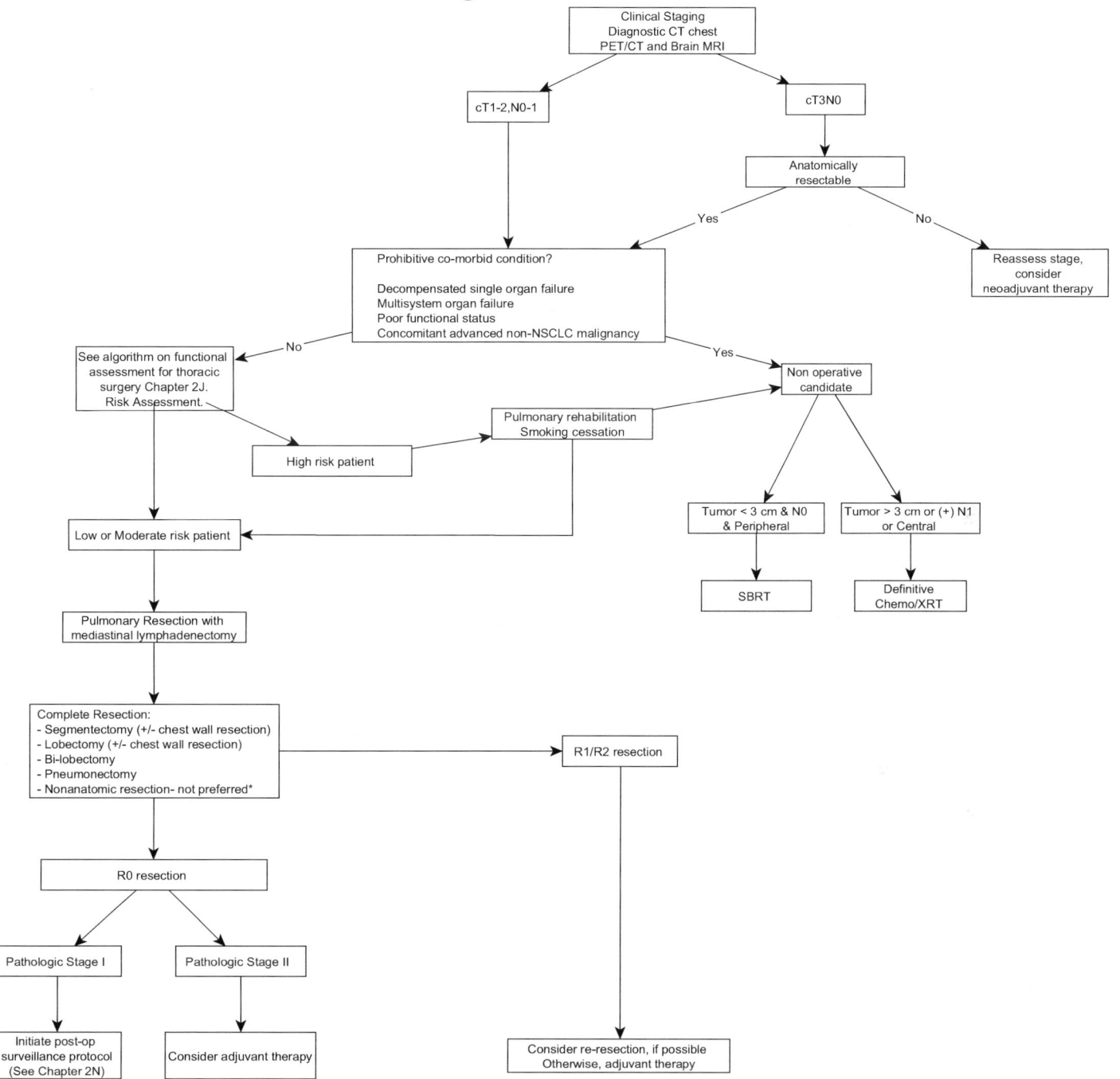

```
                    Clinical Staging
                    Diagnostic CT chest
                    PET/CT and Brain MRI
                    /              \
              cT1-2,N0-1          cT3N0
                                    |
                              Anatomically
                               resectable
                              /         \
                           Yes           No
                                          \
                                       Reassess stage,
                                         consider
                                      neoadjuvant therapy

        Prohibitive co-morbid condition?
          Decompensated single organ failure
          Multisystem organ failure
          Poor functional status
          Concomitant advanced non-NSCLC malignancy
        /                                    \
      No                                     Yes
      |                                       |
  See algorithm on functional          Non operative
  assessment for thoracic              candidate
  surgery Chapter 2J.                  /          \
  Risk Assessment.          Tumor < 3 cm & N0   Tumor > 3 cm or (+) N1
      |                      & Peripheral        or Central
      |                           |                   |
  High risk patient ─ Pulmonary rehabilitation    Definitive
                      Smoking cessation           Chemo/XRT
                           |
                         SBRT

  Low or Moderate risk patient
      |
  Pulmonary Resection with
  mediastinal lymphadenectomy
      |
  Complete Resection:
   - Segmentectomy (+/- chest wall resection)
   - Lobectomy (+/- chest wall resection)
   - Bi-lobectomy
   - Pneumonectomy
   - Nonanatomic resection- not preferred*
      |                                  \
  R0 resection                         R1/R2 resection
   /         \                              |
  Pathologic   Pathologic            Consider re-resection, if possible
  Stage I      Stage II              Otherwise, adjuvant therapy
    |             |
  Initiate     Consider
  post-op      adjuvant
  surveillance therapy
  protocol
  (See Chapter 2N)
```

Nonanatomic resection with mediastinal lymphadenectomy may be considered for patients with small tumors and marginal physiologic reserve in whom the operative risk of anatomic resection outweighs the potential survival benefit. The decision should be made as part of a multidisciplinary approach that considers surgical and radiation modalities.

ppoFEV1 – predicted post-operative forced expiratory volume, ppoDLCO – predicted post-operative diffusion limiting capacity of carbon monoxide; CPET – cardiopulmonary exercise testing; R0 – negative microscopic margins / R1 – positive microscopic margins, / R2 – positive macroscopic margins

Locally Advanced Lung Cancer
Barry Gibney, Michael Jaklitsch

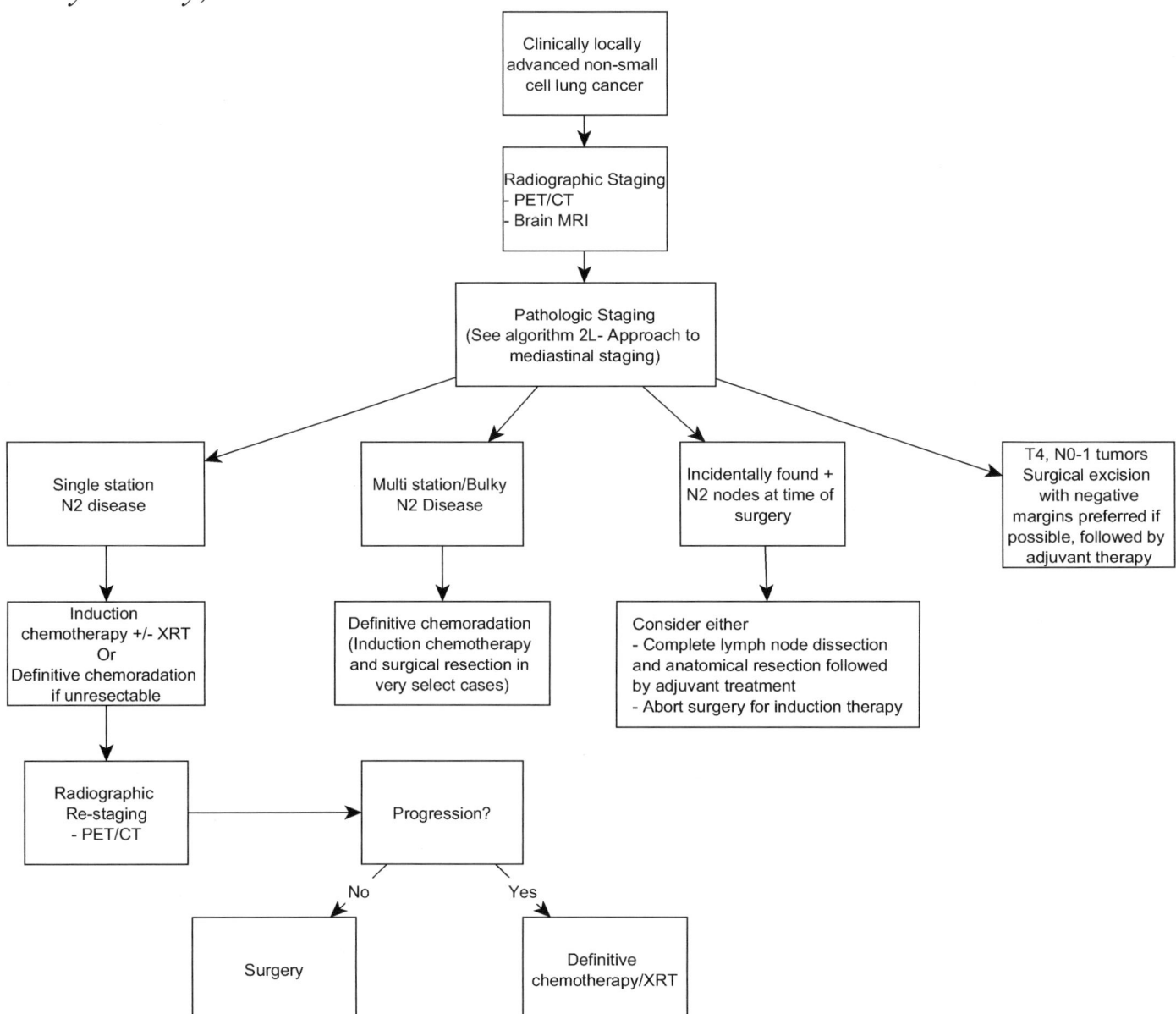

```
                    ┌─────────────────────┐
                    │ Clinically locally  │
                    │ advanced non-small  │
                    │ cell lung cancer    │
                    └──────────┬──────────┘
                               ▼
                    ┌─────────────────────┐
                    │ Radiographic Staging│
                    │ - PET/CT            │
                    │ - Brain MRI         │
                    └──────────┬──────────┘
                               ▼
                    ┌─────────────────────────┐
                    │ Pathologic Staging      │
                    │ (See algorithm 2L-      │
                    │ Approach to mediastinal │
                    │ staging)                │
                    └─────────────────────────┘
```

Branches from Pathologic Staging:

- **Single station N2 disease** → Induction chemotherapy +/- XRT Or Definitive chemoradation if unresectable → Radiographic Re-staging - PET/CT → Progression?
  - No → Surgery
  - Yes → Definitive chemotherapy/XRT
- **Multi station/Bulky N2 Disease** → Definitive chemoradation (Induction chemotherapy and surgical resection in very select cases)
- **Incidentally found + N2 nodes at time of surgery** → Consider either
  - Complete lymph node dissection and anatomical resection followed by adjuvant treatment
  - Abort surgery for induction therapy
- **T4, N0-1 tumors** Surgical excision with negative margins preferred if possible, followed by adjuvant therapy

Stage IIIA: T1-2, N2; T3, N1-2; T4, N0-1
T4 tumors- Size >7 cm, invasion of diaphragm, mediastinum, heart, great vessels, trachea, recurrent laryngeal nerve, esophagus, vertebral body, carina or tumor in ipsilateral lobe from primary

Stage IV Lung Cancer
Daniel E. Mansour, Robert E. Merritt

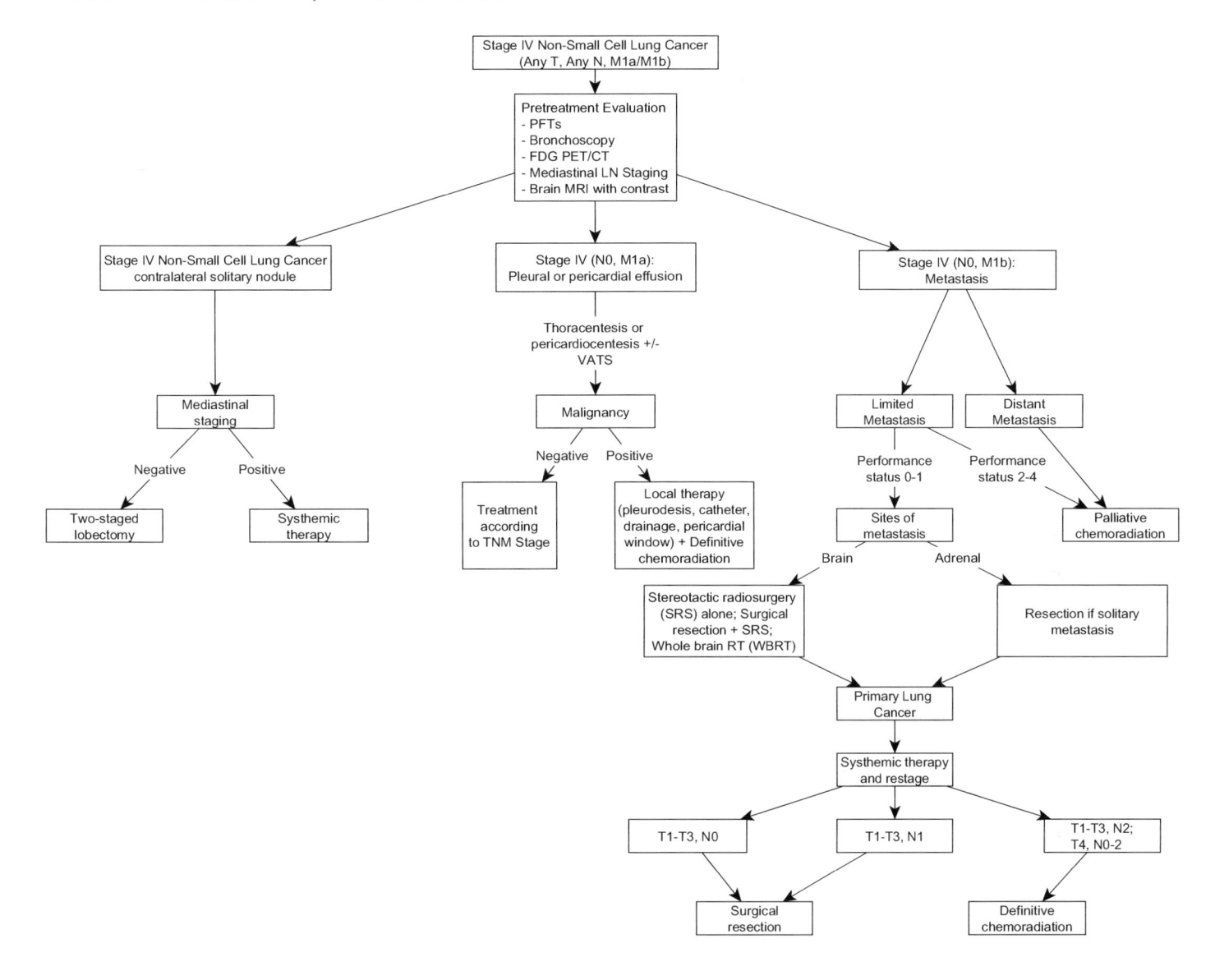

```
┌─────────────────────────────────────┐
│ Stage IV Non-Small Cell Lung Cancer │
│      (Any T, Any N, M1a/M1b)        │
└─────────────────────────────────────┘
                  │
                  ▼
┌─────────────────────────────────────┐
│       Pretreatment Evaluation       │
│  - PFTs                             │
│  - Bronchoscopy                     │
│  - FDG PET/CT                       │
│  - Mediastinal LN Staging           │
│  - Brain MRI with contrast          │
└─────────────────────────────────────┘
```

Branch 1: Stage IV Non-Small Cell Lung Cancer contralateral solitary nodule → Mediastinal staging
- Negative → Two-staged lobectomy
- Positive → Systhemic therapy

Branch 2: Stage IV (N0, M1a): Pleural or pericardial effusion → Thoracentesis or pericardiocentesis +/- VATS → Malignancy
- Negative → Treatment according to TNM Stage
- Positive → Local therapy (pleurodesis, catheter, drainage, pericardial window) + Definitive chemoradiation

Branch 3: Stage IV (N0, M1b): Metastasis
- Limited Metastasis → Performance status 0-1 → Sites of metastasis
  - Brain → Stereotactic radiosurgery (SRS) alone; Surgical resection + SRS; Whole brain RT (WBRT)
  - Adrenal → Resection if solitary metastasis
  → Primary Lung Cancer → Systhemic therapy and restage
    - T1-T3, N0 → Surgical resection
    - T1-T3, N1 → Surgical resection
    - T1-T3, N2; T4, N0-2 → Definitive chemoradiation
- Distant Metastasis → Performance status 2-4 → Palliative chemoradiation

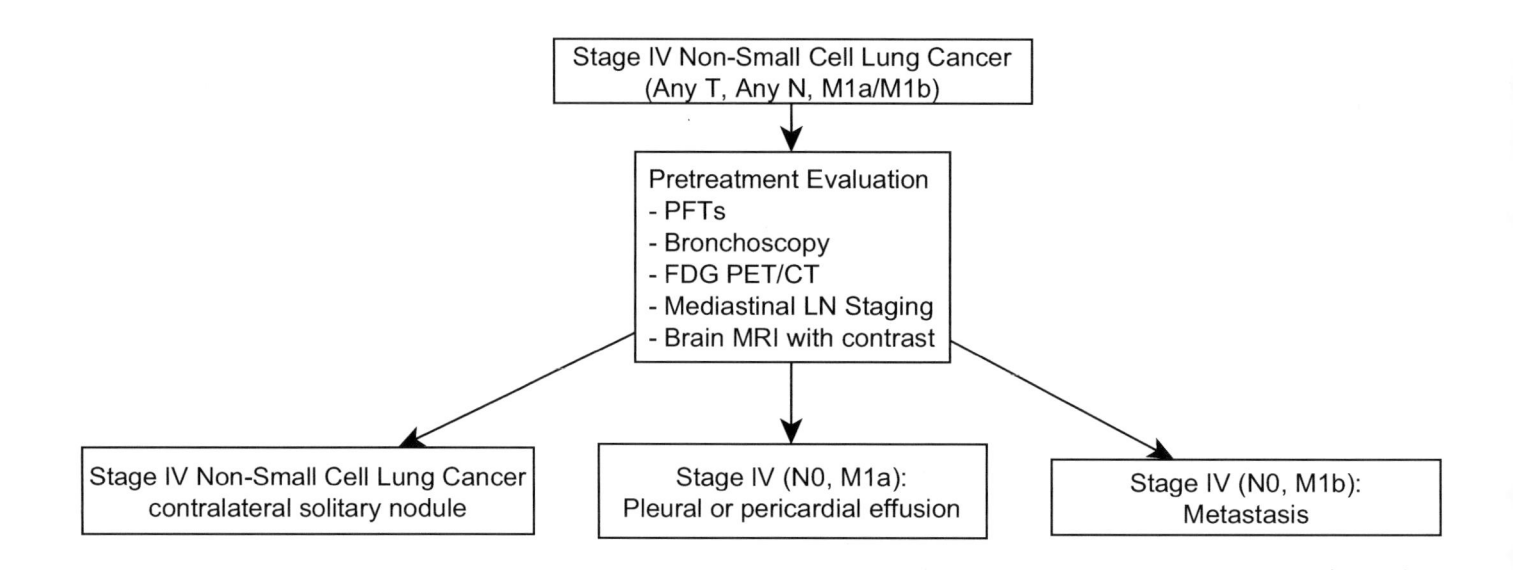

```
┌─────────────────────────────────────┐
│ Stage IV Non-Small Cell Lung Cancer │
│      (Any T, Any N, M1a/M1b)        │
└─────────────────────────────────────┘
                  │
                  ▼
┌─────────────────────────────────────┐
│      Pretreatment Evaluation        │
│      - PFTs                         │
│      - Bronchoscopy                 │
│      - FDG PET/CT                   │
│      - Mediastinal LN Staging       │
│      - Brain MRI with contrast      │
└─────────────────────────────────────┘
        │             │              │
        ▼             ▼              ▼
┌──────────────────┐ ┌──────────────────┐ ┌──────────────────┐
│ Stage IV Non-    │ │ Stage IV (N0,    │ │ Stage IV (N0,    │
│ Small Cell Lung  │ │ M1a): Pleural or │ │ M1b):            │
│ Cancer           │ │ pericardial      │ │ Metastasis       │
│ contralateral    │ │ effusion         │ │                  │
│ solitary nodule  │ │                  │ │                  │
└──────────────────┘ └──────────────────┘ └──────────────────┘
```

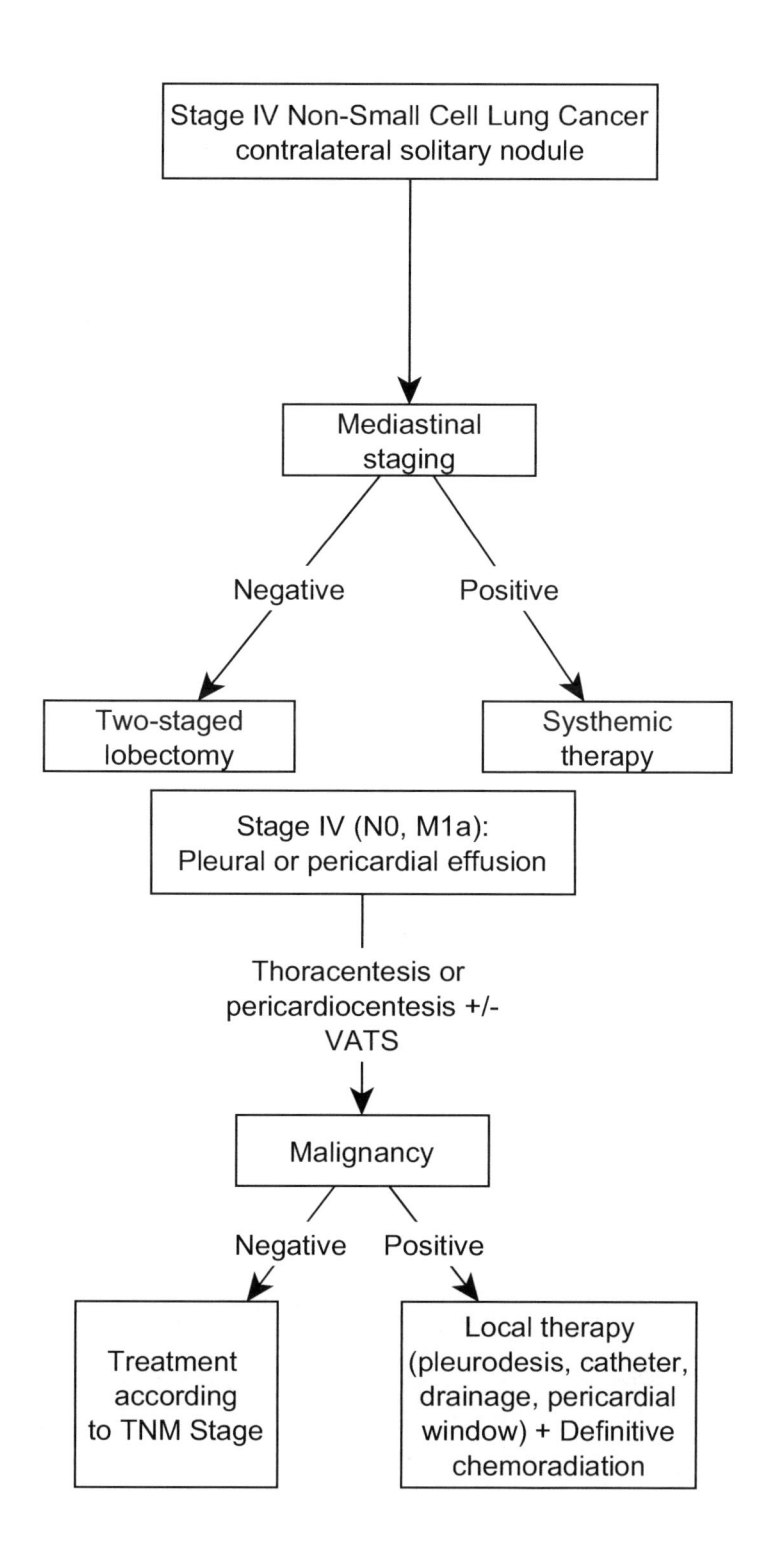

```
┌─────────────────────────────┐
│ Stage IV Non-Small Cell Lung Cancer │
│   contralateral solitary nodule      │
└─────────────────────────────┘
                │
                ▼
        ┌───────────────┐
        │  Mediastinal  │
        │    staging    │
        └───────────────┘
           ╱         ╲
      Negative      Positive
         ╱             ╲
┌───────────────┐   ┌───────────────┐
│  Two-staged   │   │   Systhemic   │
│   lobectomy   │   │    therapy    │
└───────────────┘   └───────────────┘
```

┌─────────────────────────────┐
│   Stage IV (N0, M1a):   │
│ Pleural or pericardial effusion │
└─────────────────────────────┘
                │
        Thoracentesis or
        pericardiocentesis +/-
              VATS
                ▼
        ┌───────────────┐
        │   Malignancy │
        └───────────────┘
           ╱   ╲
      Negative   Positive
         ╱   ╲
┌───────────────┐   ┌─────────────────────────┐
│ Treatment   │   │ Local therapy   │
│ according   │   │ (pleurodesis, catheter, │
│ to TNM Stage │   │ drainage, pericardial   │
│   │   │ window) + Definitive   │
│   │   │ chemoradiation   │
└───────────────┘   └─────────────────────────┘

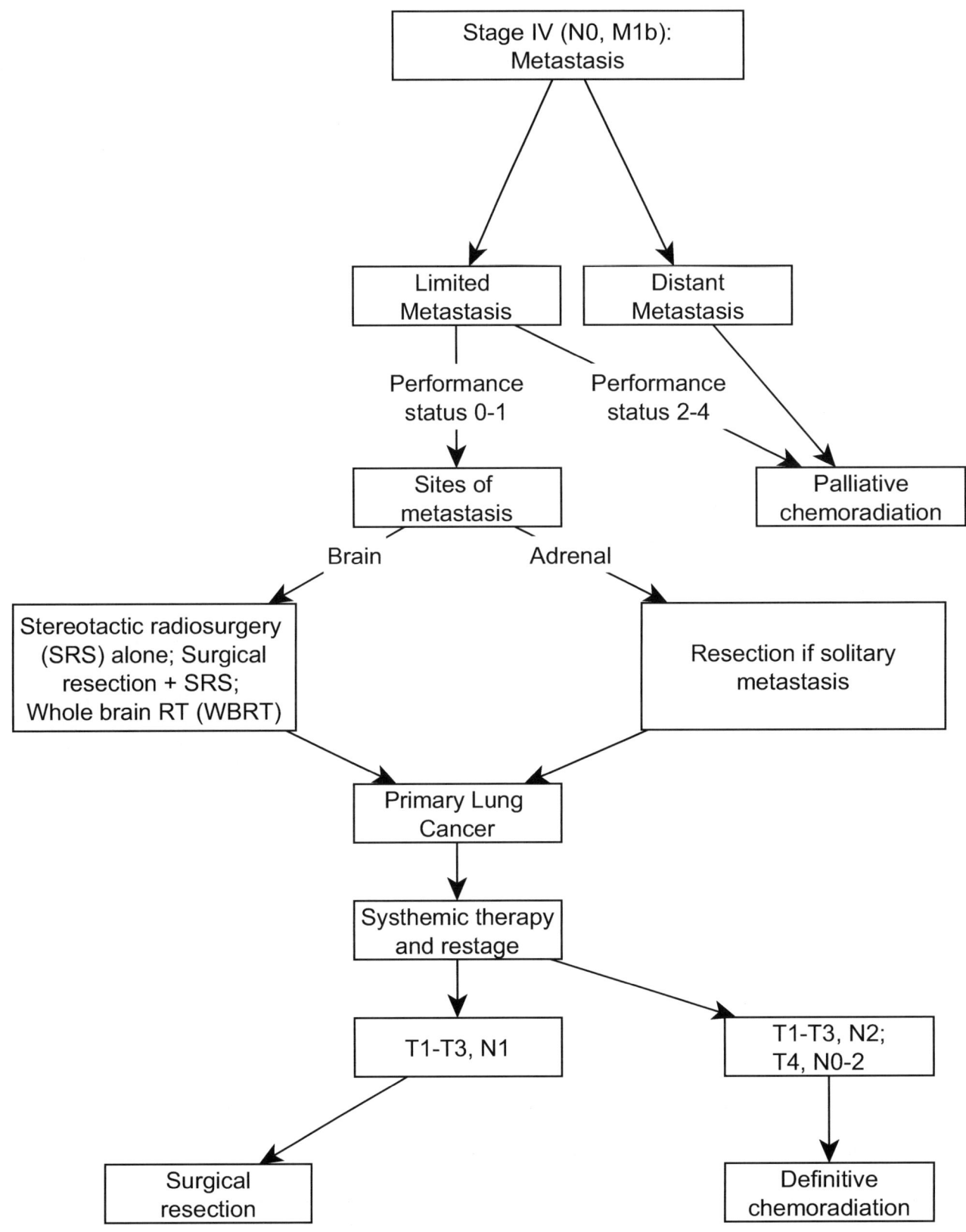

```
                    ┌─────────────────────┐
                    │  Stage IV (N0, M1b):│
                    │     Metastasis      │
                    └─────────────────────┘
                         ↙            ↘
              ┌──────────┐           ┌──────────┐
              │ Limited  │           │ Distant  │
              │Metastasis│           │Metastasis│
              └──────────┘           └──────────┘
```

- Limited Metastasis → Performance status 0-1 → Sites of metastasis
- Limited Metastasis / Distant Metastasis → Performance status 2-4 → Palliative chemoradiation

Sites of metastasis:
- Brain → Stereotactic radiosurgery (SRS) alone; Surgical resection + SRS; Whole brain RT (WBRT)
- Adrenal → Resection if solitary metastasis

→ Primary Lung Cancer → Systhemic therapy and restage

- T1-T3, N1 → Surgical resection
- T1-T3, N2; T4, N0-2 → Definitive chemoradiation

Refer to AJCC 8th Edition of the TNM Classification for Lung Cancer; T, Tumor Size; N, Lymph Nodes involved; M, describes metastasis; PFTs, pulmonary function tests; VATS; video assisted thoracoscopic surgery

Physiologic Assessment for Thoracic Surgery
Meghan Halub, Christopher Komanapalli

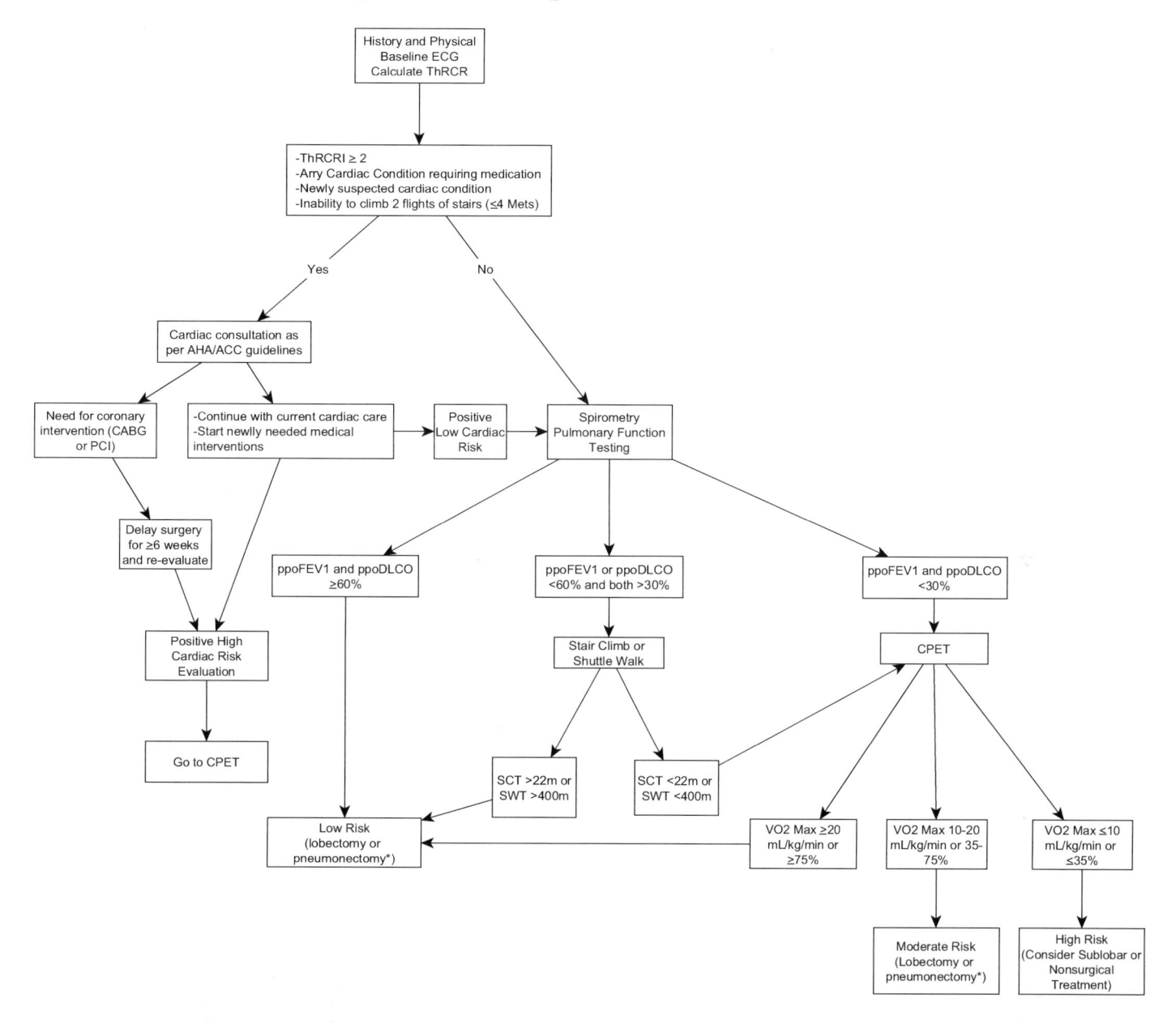

```
┌─────────────────────────┐
│ History and Physical    │
│ Baseline ECG            │
│ Calculate ThRCR         │
└───────────┬─────────────┘
            ▼
┌─────────────────────────────────────────────┐
│ -ThRCRI ≥ 2                                 │
│ -Any Cardiac Condition requiring medication │
│ -Newly suspected cardiac condition          │
│ -Inability to climb 2 flights of stairs     │
│  (≤4 Mets)                                  │
└──────┬───────────────────────────┬──────────┘
       │ Yes                    No │
       ▼                           │
┌──────────────────────┐           │
│ Cardiac consultation │           │
│ as per AHA/ACC       │           │
│ guidelines           │           │
└──┬────────────────┬──┘           │
   ▼                ▼              │
┌──────────┐  ┌──────────────┐  ┌──────────┐   ┌──────────────┐
│ Need for │  │-Continue with│  │ Positive │──▶│ Spirometry   │
│ coronary │  │ current      │──▶│ Low      │   │ Pulmonary    │
│ interv.  │  │ cardiac care │  │ Cardiac  │   │ Function     │
│ (CABG    │  │-Start newly  │  │ Risk     │   │ Testing      │
│ or PCI)  │  │ needed med.  │  └──────────┘   └──────────────┘
└────┬─────┘  │ interventions│
     │        └──────┬───────┘
     ▼               │
┌──────────────┐     │
│ Delay surgery│     │
│ for ≥6 weeks │     │
│ and re-eval. │     │
└──────┬───────┘     │
       ▼             ▼
┌──────────────────────┐
│ Positive High        │
│ Cardiac Risk         │
│ Evaluation           │
└──────────┬───────────┘
           ▼
    ┌─────────────┐
    │ Go to CPET  │
    └─────────────┘
```

Spirometry PFT branches:
- ppoFEV1 and ppoDLCO ≥60% → Low Risk (lobectomy or pneumonectomy*)
- ppoFEV1 or ppoDLCO <60% and both >30% → Stair Climb or Shuttle Walk
  - SCT >22m or SWT >400m → Low Risk (lobectomy or pneumonectomy*)
  - SCT <22m or SWT <400m → CPET
- ppoFEV1 and ppoDLCO <30% → CPET

CPET:
- VO2 Max ≥20 mL/kg/min or ≥75% → Low Risk (lobectomy or pneumonectomy*)
- VO2 Max 10-20 mL/kg/min or 35-75% → Moderate Risk (Lobectomy or pneumonectomy*)
- VO2 Max ≤10 mL/kg/min or ≤35% → High Risk (Consider Sublobar or Nonsurgical Treatment)

AHA/ACC, American Heart Association/American College of Cardiology; CABG, Coronary Artery Bypass Graft; CPET, Cardiopulmonary Exercise Testing; DLCO, Carbon Monoxide Diffusion Capacity; FEV1, Forced Expiratory Volume in 1 Second; PCI, Percutaneous Intervention; PPO, Percent Predicted Postoperative Lung Function; ThRCRI, Thoracic Revised Cardiac Risk Index; TTE, Transthoracic Echocardiogram; SCT, Stair Climbing Test; SWT, Shuttle Walk Test; VO2, Maximum Oxygen Consumption;

"Superior Sulcus Tumors
Sudhan Nagarajan, Andrew Kaufman

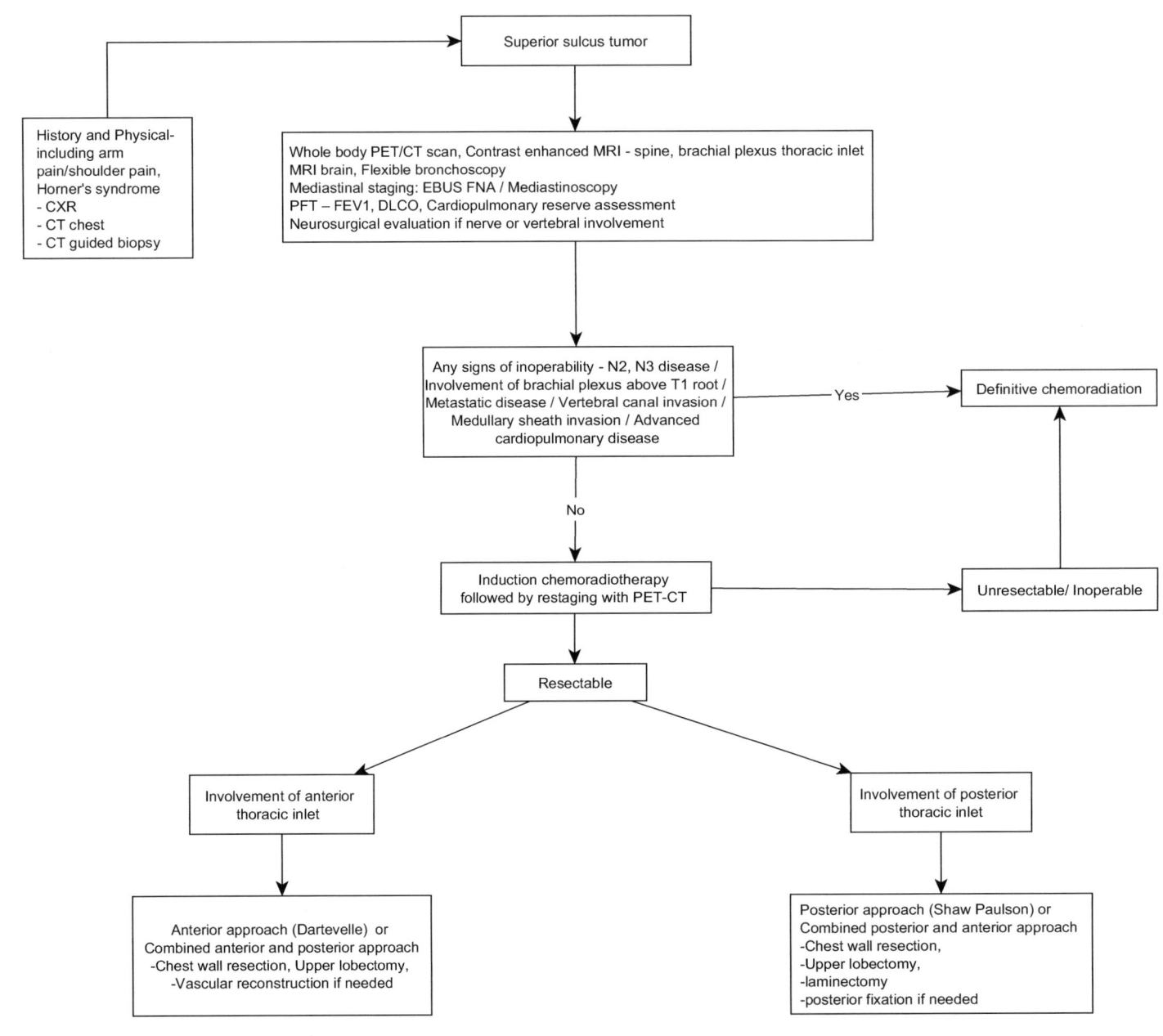

```
                                    ┌──────────────────────┐
                                    │ Superior sulcus tumor│
                                    └──────────┬───────────┘
                                               │
┌──────────────────────┐                       ▼
│ History and Physical-│   ┌─────────────────────────────────────────────────────────────┐
│ including arm        │   │ Whole body PET/CT scan, Contrast enhanced MRI - spine,      │
│ pain/shoulder pain,  │   │ brachial plexus thoracic inlet                              │
│ Horner's syndrome    │   │ MRI brain, Flexible bronchoscopy                            │
│ - CXR                │   │ Mediastinal staging: EBUS FNA / Mediastinoscopy             │
│ - CT chest           │   │ PFT – FEV1, DLCO, Cardiopulmonary reserve assessment        │
│ - CT guided biopsy   │   │ Neurosurgical evaluation if nerve or vertebral involvement  │
└──────────────────────┘   └─────────────────────────────────────────────────────────────┘
                                               │
                                               ▼
                        ┌──────────────────────────────────────────┐
                        │ Any signs of inoperability - N2, N3      │         ┌─────────────────────────┐
                        │ disease / Involvement of brachial plexus │──Yes──▶│ Definitive chemoradiation│
                        │ above T1 root / Metastatic disease /     │         └─────────────────────────┘
                        │ Vertebral canal invasion / Medullary     │                    ▲
                        │ sheath invasion / Advanced               │                    │
                        │ cardiopulmonary disease                  │                    │
                        └──────────────────┬───────────────────────┘                    │
                                          No                                            │
                                           ▼                                            │
                        ┌──────────────────────────────────────────┐        ┌──────────────────────┐
                        │ Induction chemoradiotherapy              │───────▶│ Unresectable/        │
                        │ followed by restaging with PET-CT        │        │ Inoperable           │
                        └──────────────────┬───────────────────────┘        └──────────────────────┘
                                           ▼
                                  ┌────────────────┐
                                  │   Resectable   │
                                  └───┬────────┬───┘
                        ┌─────────────┘        └─────────────┐
                        ▼                                    ▼
            ┌─────────────────────┐              ┌─────────────────────┐
            │ Involvement of      │              │ Involvement of      │
            │ anterior thoracic   │              │ posterior thoracic  │
            │ inlet               │              │ inlet               │
            └──────────┬──────────┘              └──────────┬──────────┘
                       ▼                                    ▼
         ┌────────────────────────────┐        ┌─────────────────────────────┐
         │ Anterior approach          │        │ Posterior approach (Shaw    │
         │ (Dartevelle) or            │        │ Paulson) or Combined        │
         │ Combined anterior and      │        │ posterior and anterior      │
         │ posterior approach         │        │ approach                    │
         │ -Chest wall resection,     │        │ -Chest wall resection,      │
         │ Upper lobectomy,           │        │ -Upper lobectomy,           │
         │ -Vascular reconstruction   │        │ -laminectomy                │
         │  if needed                 │        │ -posterior fixation if      │
         │                            │        │  needed                     │
         └────────────────────────────┘        └─────────────────────────────┘
```

Non-small cell cancer of the apex of the lung located in the costovertebral gutter and can involve structures within or near the thoracic inlet.

CXR, Chest X ray; CT, Computed tomography; PET, Positron emission tomography; MRI, Magnetic resonance imaging; EBUS, Endobronchial ultrasound; FNA, Fine needle aspiration; PFT, Pulmonary function test; FEV1, Forced expiratory volume in one second; DLCO, Diffusion capacity of lung for carbon monoxide; N2,N3 – mediastinal nodal disease; T1, first thoracic;

Mediastinal Staging for Non-Small Cell Lung Cancer
Smarika Shrestha, Michael Flored Reed

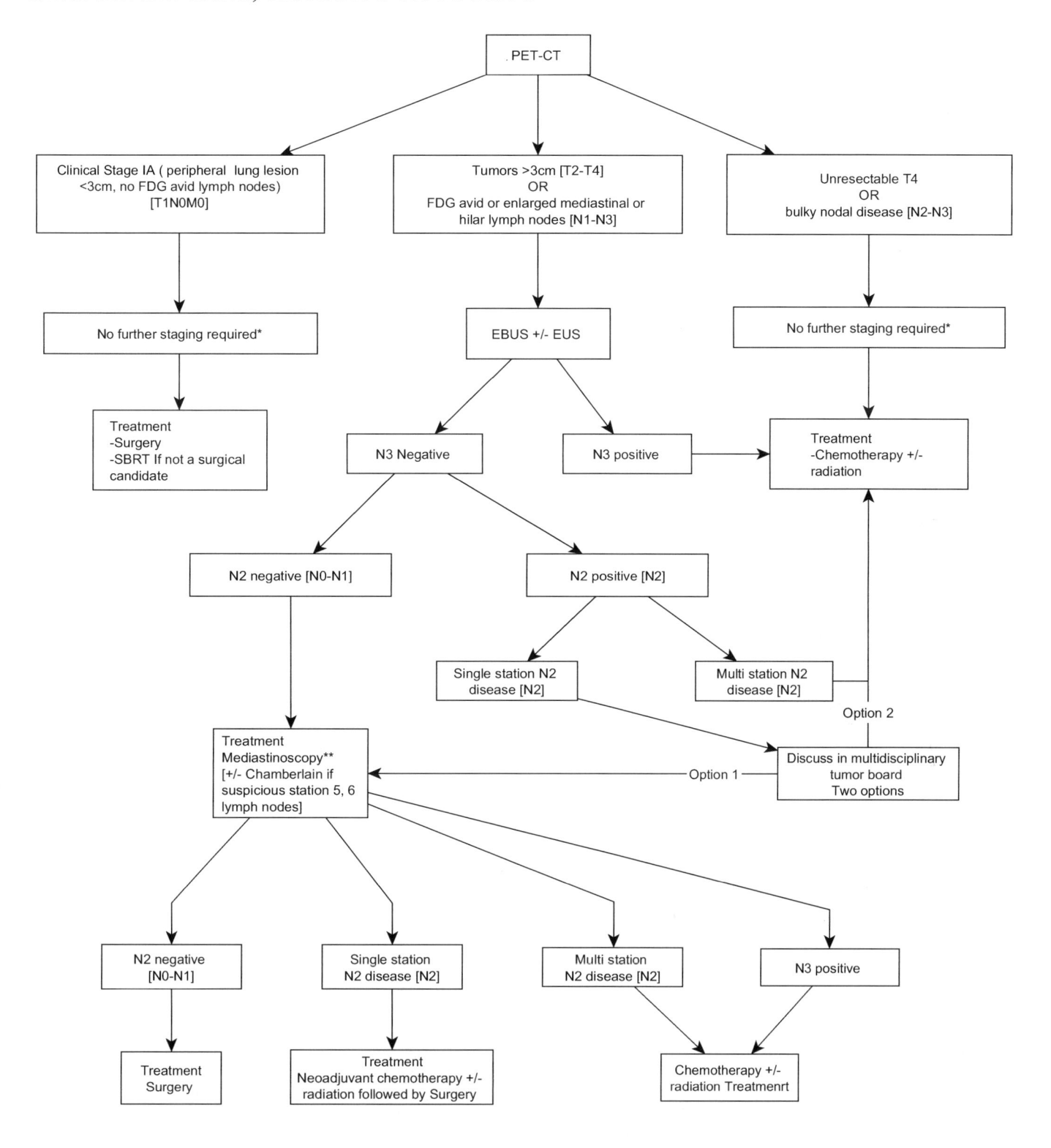

```
                                    PET-CT
            ┌───────────────────────┼───────────────────────┐
            ▼                       ▼                       ▼
  Clinical Stage IA        Tumors >3cm [T2-T4]        Unresectable T4
  (peripheral lung lesion           OR                      OR
  <3cm, no FDG avid        FDG avid or enlarged     bulky nodal disease
  lymph nodes)             mediastinal or hilar          [N2-N3]
  [T1N0M0]                 lymph nodes [N1-N3]
            │                       │                       │
            ▼                       ▼                       ▼
  No further staging         EBUS +/- EUS           No further staging
  required*                                         required*
            │                  ┌────┴────┐                  │
            ▼                  ▼         ▼                  ▼
  Treatment              N3 Negative  N3 positive   Treatment
  -Surgery                    │           │         -Chemotherapy +/-
  -SBRT If not a              │           └────────► radiation
  surgical candidate          │
                       ┌──────┴──────┐
                       ▼             ▼
               N2 negative      N2 positive [N2]
               [N0-N1]               │
                       │         ┌───┴───┐
                       │         ▼       ▼
                       │    Single      Multi station
                       │    station N2  N2 disease [N2]
                       │    disease [N2]
                       ▼
  Treatment Mediastinoscopy**     ◄── Option 1 ── Discuss in
  [+/- Chamberlain if suspicious                  multidisciplinary
  station 5, 6 lymph nodes]                       tumor board
                                                  Two options
       ┌──────┬───────┴────┬──────────┐                Option 2
       ▼      ▼            ▼          ▼
  N2 neg  Single      Multi station   N3 positive
  [N0-N1] station N2  N2 disease [N2]
          disease [N2]
       │      │            │          │
       ▼      ▼            ▼          ▼
  Treatment  Treatment        Chemotherapy +/-
  Surgery    Neoadjuvant      radiation Treatmenrt
             chemotherapy +/-
             radiation followed
             by Surgery
```

131

* There is a low likelihood of involvement with tumors <1 cm or purely non-solid tumors <3 cm
**Mediastinoscopy is not required but up to the discretion of a thoracic surgeon if there is a negative EBUS, but strongly recommend if discordant information (positive imaging but negative EBUS)

Pulmonary Metastatectomy
Sudhan Nagarajan, Andrew Kaufman

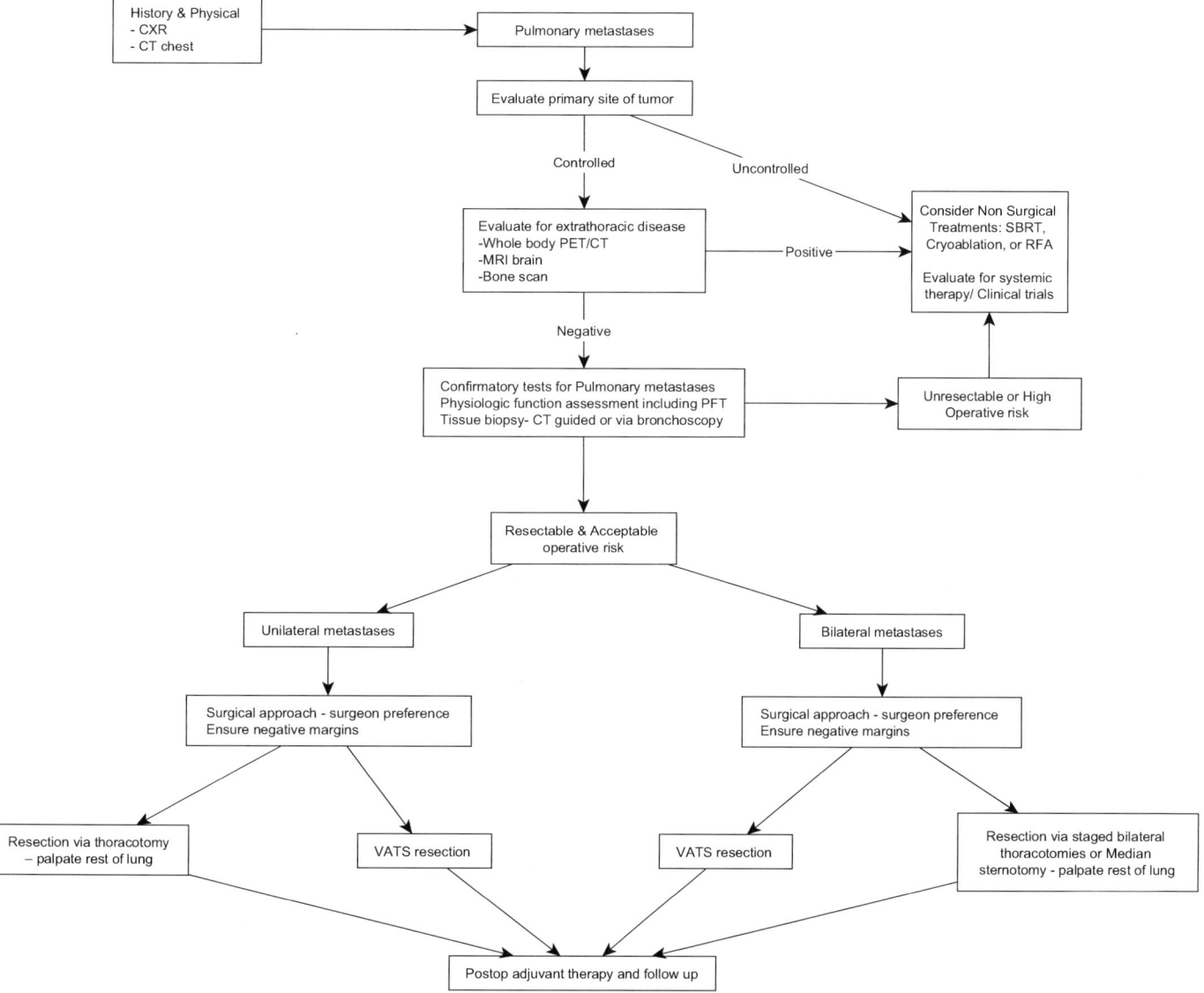

```
History & Physical
- CXR                    →    Pulmonary metastases
- CT chest                            ↓
                         Evaluate primary site of tumor
                          ↓ Controlled     ↘ Uncontrolled
         Evaluate for extrathoracic disease              Consider Non Surgical
         -Whole body PET/CT              ─Positive→      Treatments: SBRT,
         -MRI brain                                      Cryoablation, or RFA
         -Bone scan
                          ↓ Negative                     Evaluate for systemic
         Confirmatory tests for Pulmonary metastases     therapy/ Clinical trials
         Physiologic function assessment including PFT
         Tissue biopsy- CT guided or via bronchoscopy → Unresectable or High
                          ↓                              Operative risk
              Resectable & Acceptable
                 operative risk
              ↙                    ↘
      Unilateral metastases      Bilateral metastases
              ↓                        ↓
      Surgical approach - surgeon preference
      Ensure negative margins
```

Resection via thoracotomy – palpate rest of lung | VATS resection | VATS resection | Resection via staged bilateral thoracotomies or Median sternotomy - palpate rest of lung

Postop adjuvant therapy and follow up

Lung metastases from Soft tissue sarcomas and colorectal cancer compared to melanomas have better survival after Metastatectomy

CXR, Chest X ray; CT, Computed tomography; PET, Positron emission tomography; MRI, Magnetic resonance imaging; RFA, Radiofrequency ablation; SBRT, Stereotactic body radiation therapy; PFT, Pulmonary function test; VATS, Video assisted thoracoscopic surgery

Postoperative Surveillance for Lung Cancer
Syed Razi, Nestor Villamizar

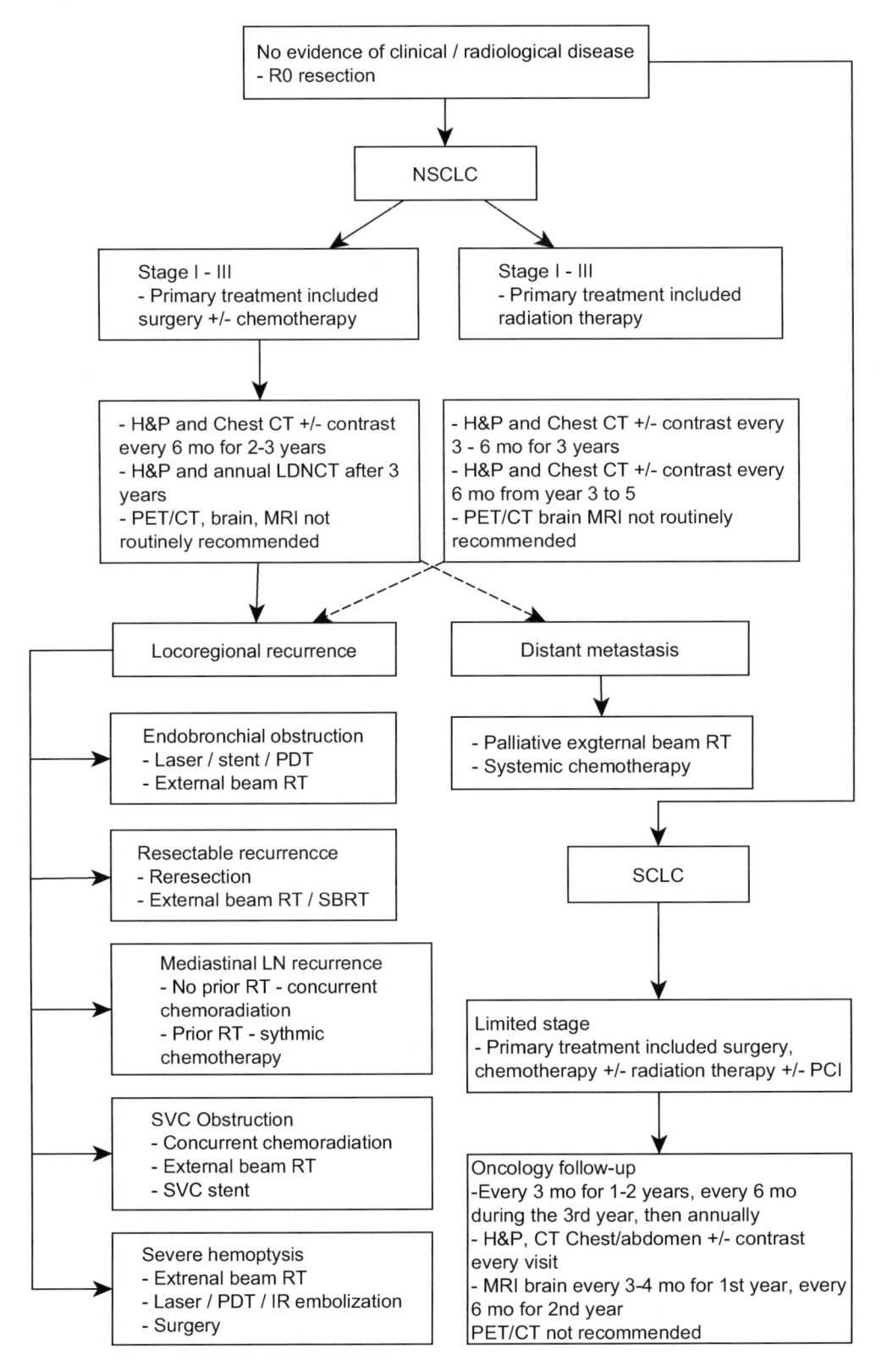

```
┌─────────────────────────────────────┐
│ No evidence of clinical / radiological disease │
│ - R0 resection                      │
└─────────────────┬───────────────────┘
                  ▼
            ┌──────────┐
            │  NSCLC   │
            └─────┬────┘
          ┌───────┴────────┐
          ▼                ▼
┌──────────────────┐  ┌──────────────────┐
│ Stage I - III    │  │ Stage I - III    │
│ - Primary treatment │ - Primary treatment │
│ included surgery  │  │ included         │
│ +/- chemotherapy │  │ radiation therapy│
└────────┬─────────┘  └────────┬─────────┘
         ▼                     ▼
┌──────────────────────┐  ┌──────────────────────┐
│ - H&P and Chest CT   │  │ - H&P and Chest CT   │
│   +/- contrast every │  │   +/- contrast every │
│   6 mo for 2-3 years │  │   3 - 6 mo for 3 yrs │
│ - H&P and annual     │  │ - H&P and Chest CT   │
│   LDNCT after 3 yrs  │  │   +/- contrast every │
│ - PET/CT, brain, MRI │  │   6 mo from yr 3 to 5│
│   not routinely rec. │  │ - PET/CT brain MRI   │
│                      │  │   not routinely rec. │
└──────────────────────┘  └──────────────────────┘
```

- Locoregional recurrence
  - Endobronchial obstruction
    - Laser / stent / PDT
    - External beam RT
  - Resectable recurrencce
    - Reresection
    - External beam RT / SBRT
  - Mediastinal LN recurrence
    - No prior RT - concurrent chemoradiation
    - Prior RT - sythmic chemotherapy
  - SVC Obstruction
    - Concurrent chemoradiation
    - External beam RT
    - SVC stent
  - Severe hemoptysis
    - Extrenal beam RT
    - Laser / PDT / IR embolization
    - Surgery

- Distant metastasis
  - Palliative exgternal beam RT
  - Systemic chemotherapy

SCLC

Limited stage
- Primary treatment included surgery, chemotherapy +/- radiation therapy +/- PCI

Oncology follow-up
- Every 3 mo for 1-2 years, every 6 mo during the 3rd year, then annually
- H&P, CT Chest/abdomen +/- contrast every visit
- MRI brain every 3-4 mo for 1st year, every 6 mo for 2nd year
PET/CT not recommended

NSCLC, non-small cell lung cancer; SCLC, small cell lung cancer; PDT, photodynamic therapy; RT, radiation therapy; LN, lymph node; SVC, superior vena cava; SBRT, stereotactic body radiation therapy

Pulmonary Tuberculosis
Parth Amin

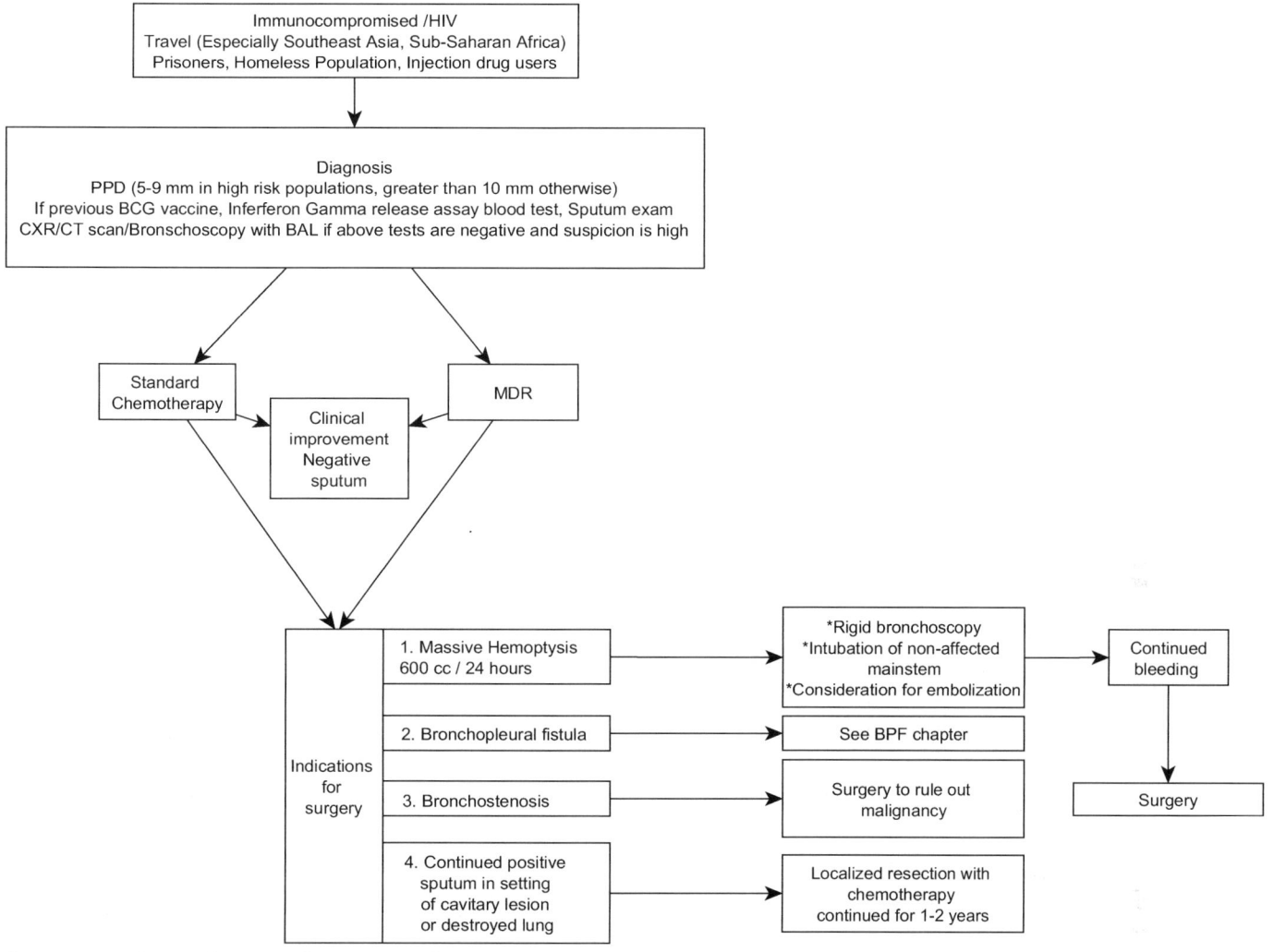

```
┌─────────────────────────────────────────────────┐
│ Immunocompromised /HIV                          │
│ Travel (Especially Southeast Asia, Sub-Saharan  │
│ Africa)                                         │
│ Prisoners, Homeless Population, Injection drug  │
│ users                                           │
└─────────────────────────────────────────────────┘
                        │
                        ▼
┌─────────────────────────────────────────────────────────────┐
│ Diagnosis                                                   │
│ PPD (5-9 mm in high risk populations, greater than 10 mm    │
│ otherwise)                                                  │
│ If previous BCG vaccine, Inferferon Gamma release assay     │
│ blood test, Sputum exam                                     │
│ CXR/CT scan/Bronschoscopy with BAL if above tests are       │
│ negative and suspicion is high                              │
└─────────────────────────────────────────────────────────────┘
```

- Standard Chemotherapy → Clinical improvement Negative sputum ← MDR

Indications for surgery:
1. Massive Hemoptysis 600 cc / 24 hours → *Rigid bronchoscopy, *Intubation of non-affected mainstem, *Consideration for embolization → Continued bleeding → Surgery
2. Bronchopleural fistula → See BPF chapter
3. Bronchostenosis → Surgery to rule out malignancy
4. Continued positive sputum in setting of cavitary lesion or destroyed lung → Localized resection with chemotherapy continued for 1-2 years

Overview chemotherapy for active disease
1st line drugs: Isoniazid, Rifampin, Ethambutol, Pyrazinamide
2nd line drugs: Cycloserine, Amikacin, Streptomycin, Capreomycin

MDR – multidrug resistant
PPD – purified protein derivative

Interstitial Lung Disease
Clauden Louis, Christian Peyre

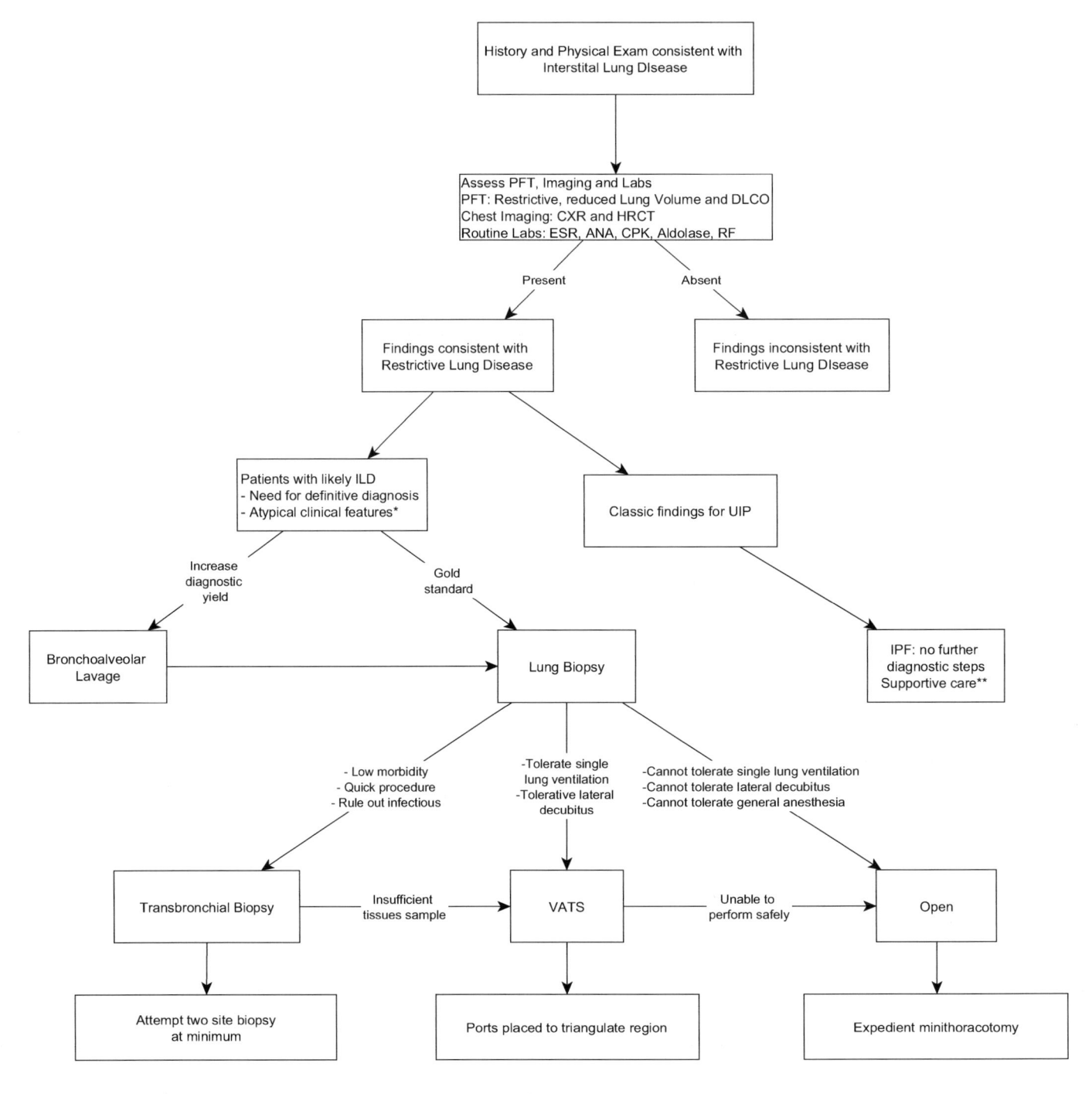

```
History and Physical Exam consistent with
          Interstitial Lung Disease
                    │
                    ▼
Assess PFT, Imaging and Labs
PFT: Restrictive, reduced Lung Volume and DLCO
Chest Imaging: CXR and HRCT
Routine Labs: ESR, ANA, CPK, Aldolase, RF
            │                    │
         Present               Absent
            ▼                    ▼
   Findings consistent with   Findings inconsistent with
   Restrictive Lung Disease   Restrictive Lung Disease
        │           │
        ▼           ▼
Patients with likely ILD      Classic findings for UIP
- Need for definitive                │
  diagnosis                          ▼
- Atypical clinical features*   IPF: no further
                                diagnostic steps
                                Supportive care**
   Increase        Gold
   diagnostic     standard
   yield
     ▼              ▼
Bronchoalveolar → Lung Biopsy
   Lavage
            │
   ┌────────┼────────────────┐
Low morbidity  Tolerate single   Cannot tolerate single lung ventilation
Quick procedure lung ventilation Cannot tolerate lateral decubitus
Rule out       Tolerative lateral Cannot tolerate general anesthesia
infectious     decubitus
     ▼              ▼                    ▼
Transbronchial → VATS →              Open
  Biopsy     Insufficient  Unable to
             tissues sample perform safely
     ▼              ▼                    ▼
Attempt two site   Ports placed to    Expedient
biopsy at minimum  triangulate region minithoracotomy
```

* = <50 age, fever, wt. loss, extrapulmonary manifestations
** = O2, pulmonary rehabilitation, vaccines
PFT: pulmonary function test; BAL bronchoalveolar lavage; IPF: Idiopathic Pulmonary Fibrosis; UIP: Usual Interstitial Pneumonia, DLCO: Diffusing Lung Capacity for Carbon Monoxide, ILD: Interstitial Lung Disease

Lung Volume Reduction Surgery
Clauden Louis, Christian Peyre

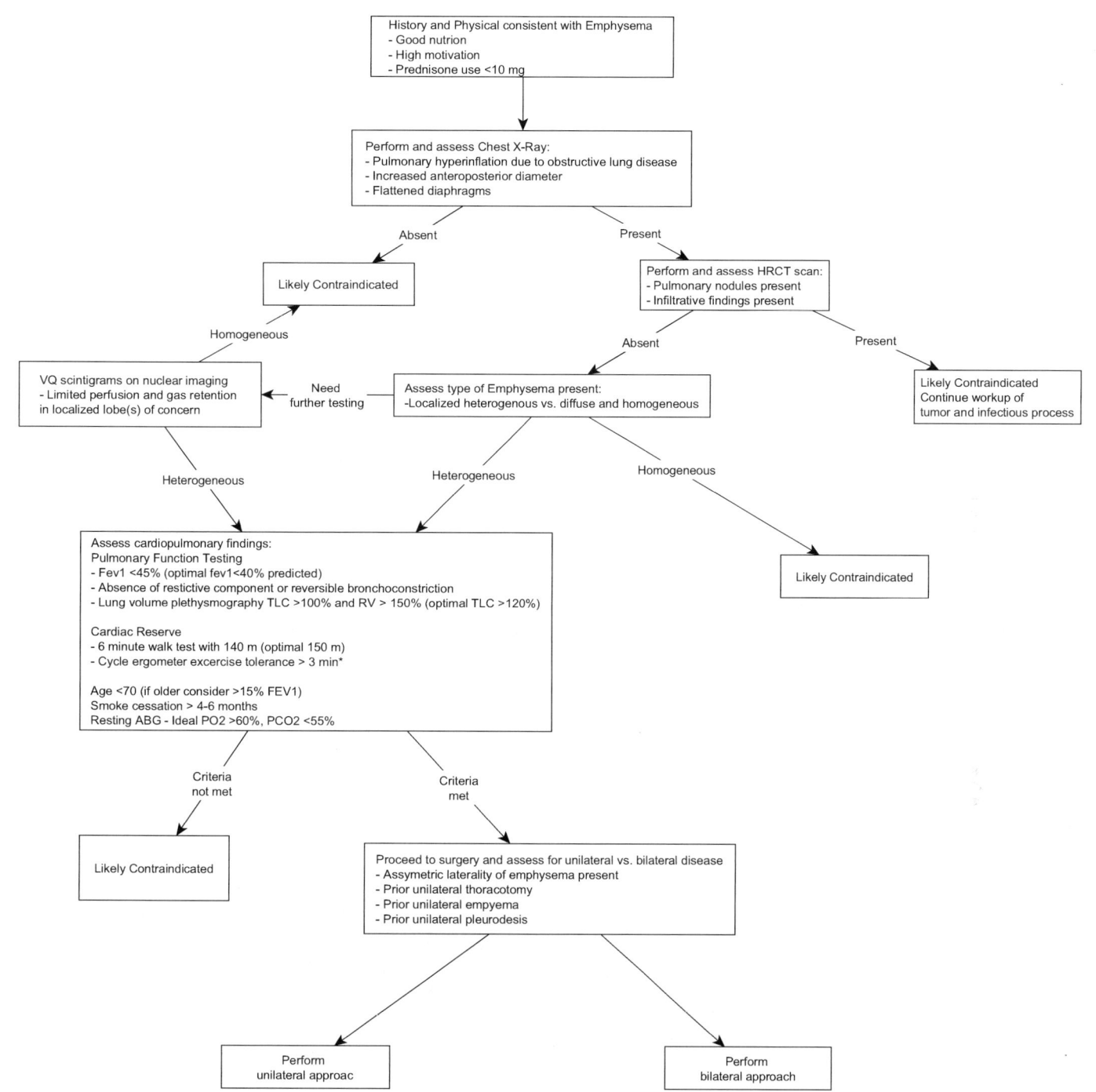

```
                    ┌─────────────────────────────────────┐
                    │ History and Physical consistent with │
                    │          Emphysema                   │
                    │  - Good nutrion                      │
                    │  - High motivation                   │
                    │  - Prednisone use <10 mg             │
                    └─────────────────┬───────────────────┘
                                      ▼
                    ┌─────────────────────────────────────┐
                    │ Perform and assess Chest X-Ray:     │
                    │  - Pulmonary hyperinflation due to  │
                    │    obstructive lung disease         │
                    │  - Increased anteroposterior diameter│
                    │  - Flattened diaphragms             │
                    └──────┬──────────────────────┬───────┘
                   Absent  │                      │ Present
                           ▼                      ▼
              ┌────────────────────┐   ┌──────────────────────────┐
              │ Likely             │   │ Perform and assess HRCT  │
              │ Contraindicated    │   │ scan:                    │
              └────────▲───────────┘   │ - Pulmonary nodules      │
                       │               │   present                │
           Homogeneous │               │ - Infiltrative findings  │
                       │               │   present                │
                       │               └──────┬──────────────┬────┘
                       │                Absent│              │Present
                       │                      ▼              ▼
    ┌──────────────────┴──┐  Need   ┌────────────────────┐  ┌──────────────────┐
    │ VQ scintigrams on   │◄─further│ Assess type of     │  │ Likely           │
    │ nuclear imaging     │ testing │ Emphysema present: │  │ Contraindicated  │
    │ - Limited perfusion │         │ -Localized         │  │ Continue workup  │
    │   and gas retention │         │  heterogenous vs.  │  │ of tumor and     │
    │   in localized      │         │  diffuse and       │  │ infectious       │
    │   lobe(s) of concern│         │  homogeneous       │  │ process          │
    └──────────┬──────────┘         └──────┬────────┬────┘  └──────────────────┘
   Heterogeneous│              Heterogeneous│        │Homogeneous
               │                           │        ▼
               │                           │   ┌──────────────────┐
               │                           │   │ Likely           │
               │                           │   │ Contraindicated  │
               │                           │   └──────────────────┘
               ▼                           ▼
    ┌─────────────────────────────────────────────┐
    │ Assess cardiopulmonary findings:            │
    │ Pulmonary Function Testing                  │
    │ - Fev1 <45% (optimal fev1<40% predicted)    │
    │ - Absence of restictive component or        │
    │   reversible bronchoconstriction            │
    │ - Lung volume plethysmography TLC >100%     │
    │   and RV > 150% (optimal TLC >120%)         │
    │                                             │
    │ Cardiac Reserve                             │
    │ - 6 minute walk test with 140 m             │
    │   (optimal 150 m)                           │
    │ - Cycle ergometer excercise tolerance > 3 min*│
    │                                             │
    │ Age <70 (if older consider >15% FEV1)       │
    │ Smoke cessation > 4-6 months                │
    │ Resting ABG - Ideal PO2 >60%, PCO2 <55%     │
    └──────┬───────────────────────────┬──────────┘
    Criteria│                   Criteria│
    not met │                       met │
            ▼                           ▼
    ┌──────────────────┐   ┌──────────────────────────────────┐
    │ Likely           │   │ Proceed to surgery and assess    │
    │ Contraindicated  │   │ for unilateral vs. bilateral     │
    └──────────────────┘   │ disease                          │
                           │ - Assymetric laterality of       │
                           │   emphysema present              │
                           │ - Prior unilateral thoracotomy   │
                           │ - Prior unilateral empyema       │
                           │ - Prior unilateral pleurodesis   │
                           └──────┬──────────────────┬────────┘
                                  ▼                  ▼
                        ┌──────────────────┐ ┌──────────────────┐
                        │ Perform          │ │ Perform          │
                        │ unilateral approac│ │ bilateral approach│
                        └──────────────────┘ └──────────────────┘
```

* = *3 minutes of unloading pedaling in exercise tolerance testing*
FEV1, forced expiratory volume in 1 second; HRCT, high-resolution computed tomography; RV, residual volume; TLC, total lung capacity.

Evaluation and Approach to Lung Transplant
Pauline Go, John Keech

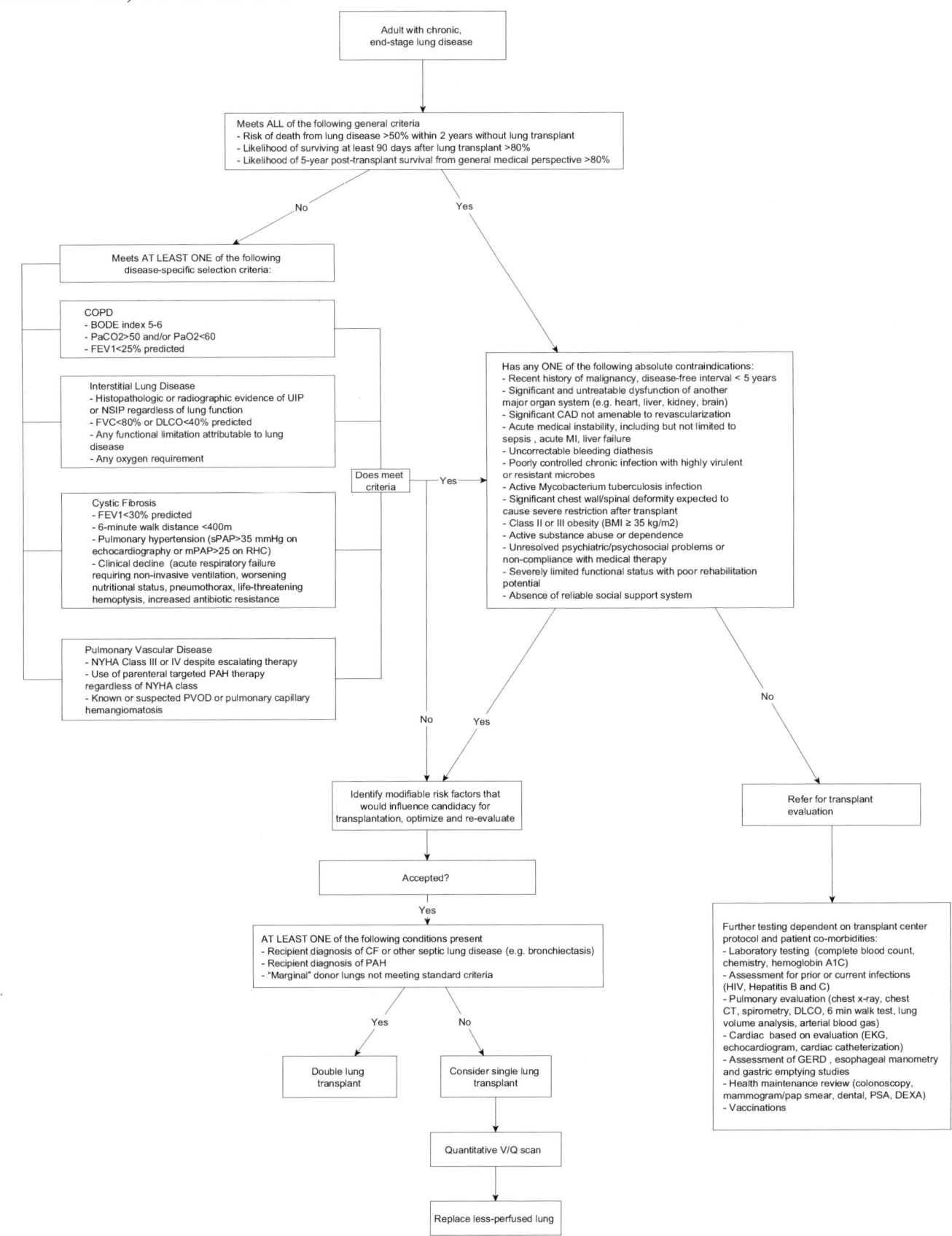

```
                    ┌─────────────────────────┐
                    │ Adult with chronic,     │
                    │ end-stage lung disease  │
                    └───────────┬─────────────┘
                                ▼
        ┌──────────────────────────────────────────────────┐
        │ Meets ALL of the following general criteria      │
        │ - Risk of death from lung disease >50% within    │
        │   2 years without lung transplant                │
        │ - Likelihood of surviving at least 90 days       │
        │   after lung transplant >80%                     │
        │ - Likelihood of 5-year post-transplant survival  │
        │   from general medical perspective >80%          │
        └──────────────────────────────────────────────────┘
                   No │           │ Yes
                      ▼           ▼
```

Meets AT LEAST ONE of the following disease-specific selection criteria:

COPD
- BODE index 5-6
- PaCO2>50 and/or PaO2<60
- FEV1<25% predicted

Interstitial Lung Disease
- Histopathologic or radiographic evidence of UIP or NSIP regardless of lung function
- FVC<80% or DLCO<40% predicted
- Any functional limitation attributable to lung disease
- Any oxygen requirement

Cystic Fibrosis
- FEV1<30% predicted
- 6-minute walk distance <400m
- Pulmonary hypertension (sPAP>35 mmHg on echocardiography or mPAP>25 on RHC)
- Clinical decline (acute respiratory failure requiring non-invasive ventilation, worsening nutritional status, pneumothorax, life-threatening hemoptysis, increased antibiotic resistance

Pulmonary Vascular Disease
- NYHA Class III or IV despite escalating therapy
- Use of parenteral targeted PAH therapy regardless of NYHA class
- Known or suspected PVOD or pulmonary capillary hemangiomatosis

Does meet criteria → Yes →

Has any ONE of the following absolute contraindications:
- Recent history of malignancy, disease-free interval < 5 years
- Significant and untreatable dysfunction of another major organ system (e.g. heart, liver, kidney, brain)
- Significant CAD not amenable to revascularization
- Acute medical instability, including but not limited to sepsis, acute MI, liver failure
- Uncorrectable bleeding diathesis
- Poorly controlled chronic infection with highly virulent or resistant microbes
- Active Mycobacterium tuberculosis infection
- Significant chest wall/spinal deformity expected to cause severe restriction after transplant
- Class II or III obesity (BMI ≥ 35 kg/m2)
- Active substance abuse or dependence
- Unresolved psychiatric/psychosocial problems or non-compliance with medical therapy
- Severely limited functional status with poor rehabilitation potential
- Absence of reliable social support system

No → **Identify modifiable risk factors that would influence candidacy for transplantation, optimize and re-evaluate**

Yes (from contraindications) → same box above

Accepted? → Yes →

AT LEAST ONE of the following conditions present
- Recipient diagnosis of CF or other septic lung disease (e.g. bronchiectasis)
- Recipient diagnosis of PAH
- "Marginal" donor lungs not meeting standard criteria

Yes → **Double lung transplant**

No → **Consider single lung transplant** → **Quantitative V/Q scan** → **Replace less-perfused lung**

(From general criteria Yes, No contraindications) No → **Refer for transplant evaluation** →

Further testing dependent on transplant center protocol and patient co-morbidities:
- Laboratory testing (complete blood count, chemistry, hemoglobin A1C)
- Assessment for prior or current infections (HIV, Hepatitis B and C)
- Pulmonary evaluation (chest x-ray, chest CT, spirometry, DLCO, 6 min walk test, lung volume analysis, arterial blood gas)
- Cardiac based on evaluation (EKG, echocardiogram, cardiac catheterization)
- Assessment of GERD, esophageal manometry and gastric emptying studies
- Health maintenance review (colonoscopy, mammogram/pap smear, dental, PSA, DEXA)
- Vaccinations

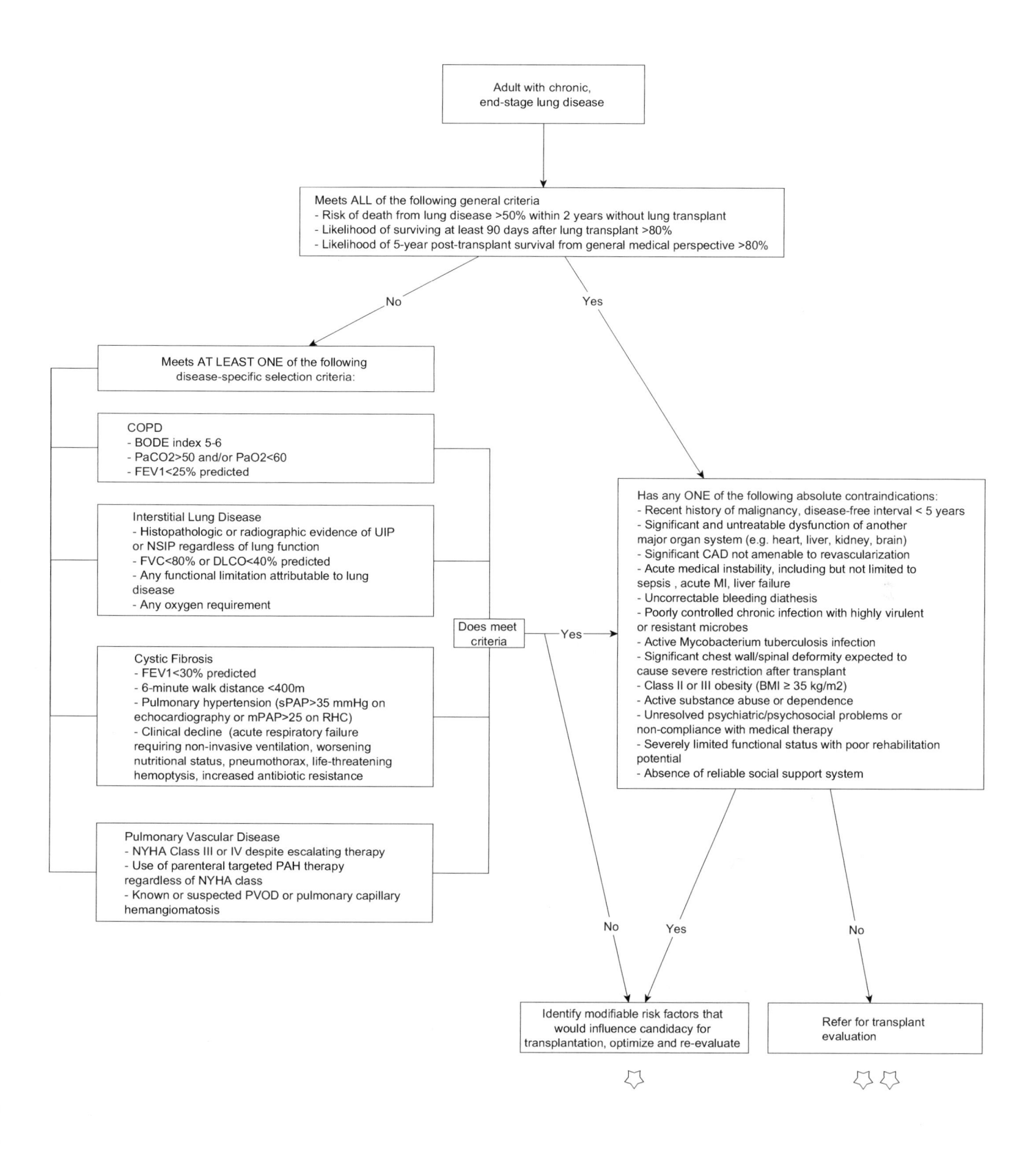

```
┌─────────────────────────────┐
│   Adult with chronic,       │
│   end-stage lung disease    │
└─────────────┬───────────────┘
              │
              ▼
┌─────────────────────────────────────────────────────────┐
│ Meets ALL of the following general criteria             │
│ - Risk of death from lung disease >50% within 2 years   │
│   without lung transplant                               │
│ - Likelihood of surviving at least 90 days after lung   │
│   transplant >80%                                       │
│ - Likelihood of 5-year post-transplant survival from    │
│   general medical perspective >80%                      │
└─────────────────────────────────────────────────────────┘
```

No → Meets AT LEAST ONE of the following disease-specific selection criteria:

COPD
- BODE index 5-6
- PaCO2>50 and/or PaO2<60
- FEV1<25% predicted

Interstitial Lung Disease
- Histopathologic or radiographic evidence of UIP or NSIP regardless of lung function
- FVC<80% or DLCO<40% predicted
- Any functional limitation attributable to lung disease
- Any oxygen requirement

Cystic Fibrosis
- FEV1<30% predicted
- 6-minute walk distance <400m
- Pulmonary hypertension (sPAP>35 mmHg on echocardiography or mPAP>25 on RHC)
- Clinical decline (acute respiratory failure requiring non-invasive ventilation, worsening nutritional status, pneumothorax, life-threatening hemoptysis, increased antibiotic resistance

Pulmonary Vascular Disease
- NYHA Class III or IV despite escalating therapy
- Use of parenteral targeted PAH therapy regardless of NYHA class
- Known or suspected PVOD or pulmonary capillary hemangiomatosis

Does meet criteria — **Yes** →

Yes (from general criteria) →

Has any ONE of the following absolute contraindications:
- Recent history of malignancy, disease-free interval < 5 years
- Significant and untreatable dysfunction of another major organ system (e.g. heart, liver, kidney, brain)
- Significant CAD not amenable to revascularization
- Acute medical instability, including but not limited to sepsis, acute MI, liver failure
- Uncorrectable bleeding diathesis
- Poorly controlled chronic infection with highly virulent or resistant microbes
- Active Mycobacterium tuberculosis infection
- Significant chest wall/spinal deformity expected to cause severe restriction after transplant
- Class II or III obesity (BMI ≥ 35 kg/m2)
- Active substance abuse or dependence
- Unresolved psychiatric/psychosocial problems or non-compliance with medical therapy
- Severely limited functional status with poor rehabilitation potential
- Absence of reliable social support system

No / **Yes** → Identify modifiable risk factors that would influence candidacy for transplantation, optimize and re-evaluate

No → Refer for transplant evaluation

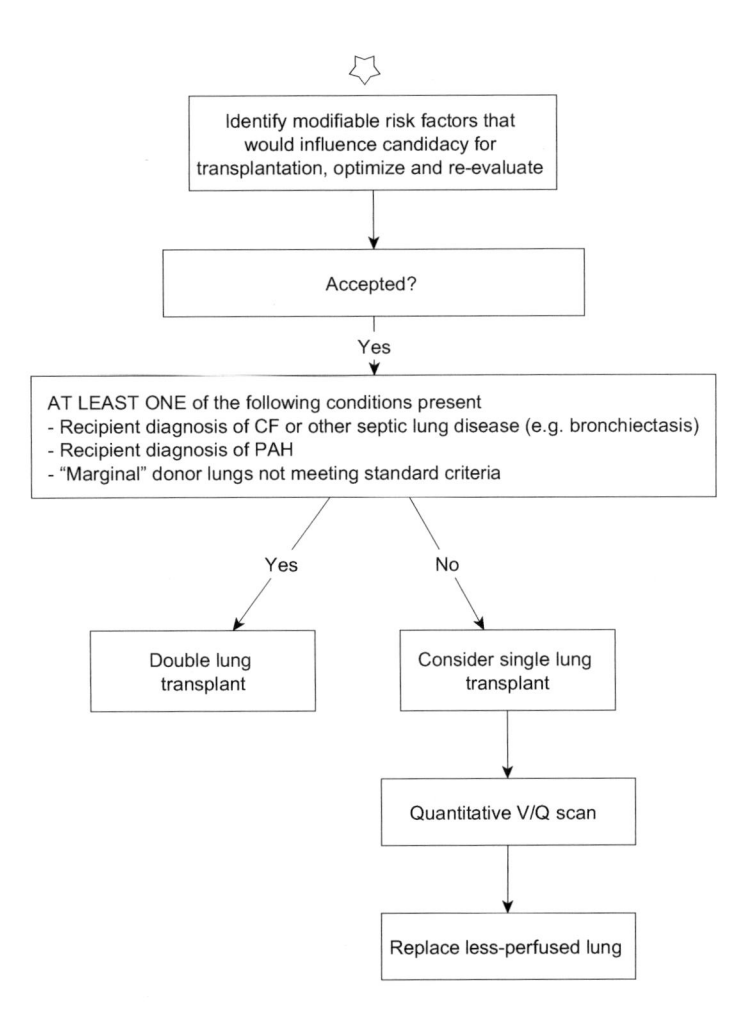

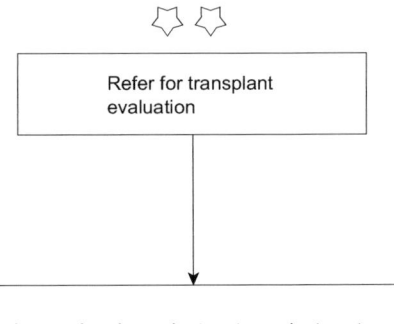

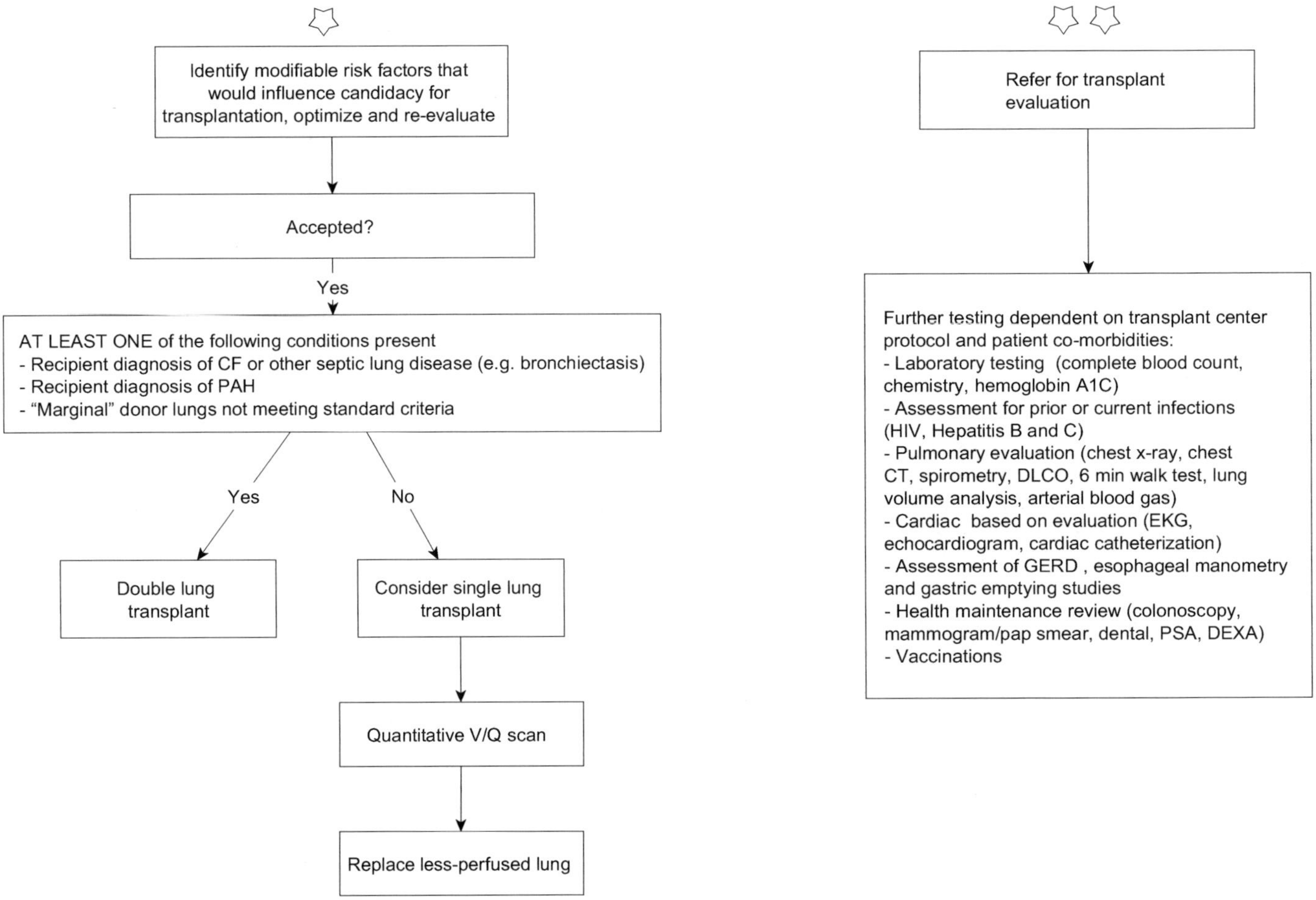

```
                    ☆                                          ☆ ☆
        ┌──────────────────────────┐                  ┌──────────────────┐
        │ Identify modifiable risk │                  │ Refer for        │
        │ factors that would       │                  │ transplant       │
        │ influence candidacy for  │                  │ evaluation       │
        │ transplantation, optimize│                  └────────┬─────────┘
        │ and re-evaluate          │                           │
        └────────────┬─────────────┘                           ▼
                     ▼                            ┌──────────────────────────────┐
        ┌──────────────────────────┐              │ Further testing dependent on │
        │       Accepted?          │              │ transplant center protocol   │
        └────────────┬─────────────┘              │ and patient co-morbidities:  │
                    Yes                           │ - Laboratory testing         │
                     ▼                            │ (complete blood count,       │
┌──────────────────────────────────────────────┐  │ chemistry, hemoglobin A1C)   │
│ AT LEAST ONE of the following conditions     │  │ - Assessment for prior or    │
│ present                                      │  │ current infections           │
│ - Recipient diagnosis of CF or other septic  │  │ (HIV, Hepatitis B and C)     │
│   lung disease (e.g. bronchiectasis)         │  │ - Pulmonary evaluation       │
│ - Recipient diagnosis of PAH                 │  │ (chest x-ray, chest CT,      │
│ - "Marginal" donor lungs not meeting         │  │ spirometry, DLCO, 6 min walk │
│   standard criteria                          │  │ test, lung volume analysis,  │
└──────────────────────────────────────────────┘  │ arterial blood gas)          │
         │Yes                    │No              │ - Cardiac based on           │
         ▼                       ▼                │ evaluation (EKG,             │
   ┌──────────────┐       ┌──────────────┐        │ echocardiogram, cardiac      │
   │ Double lung  │       │ Consider     │        │ catheterization)             │
   │ transplant   │       │ single lung  │        │ - Assessment of GERD,        │
   └──────────────┘       │ transplant   │        │ esophageal manometry and     │
                          └──────┬───────┘        │ gastric emptying studies     │
                                 ▼                │ - Health maintenance review  │
                          ┌──────────────┐        │ (colonoscopy, mammogram/pap  │
                          │ Quantitative │        │ smear, dental, PSA, DEXA)    │
                          │ V/Q scan     │        │ - Vaccinations               │
                          └──────┬───────┘        └──────────────────────────────┘
                                 ▼
                          ┌──────────────┐
                          │ Replace      │
                          │ less-perfused│
                          │ lung         │
                          └──────────────┘
```

Empyema
Catherine Bixby, Kirk McMurtry

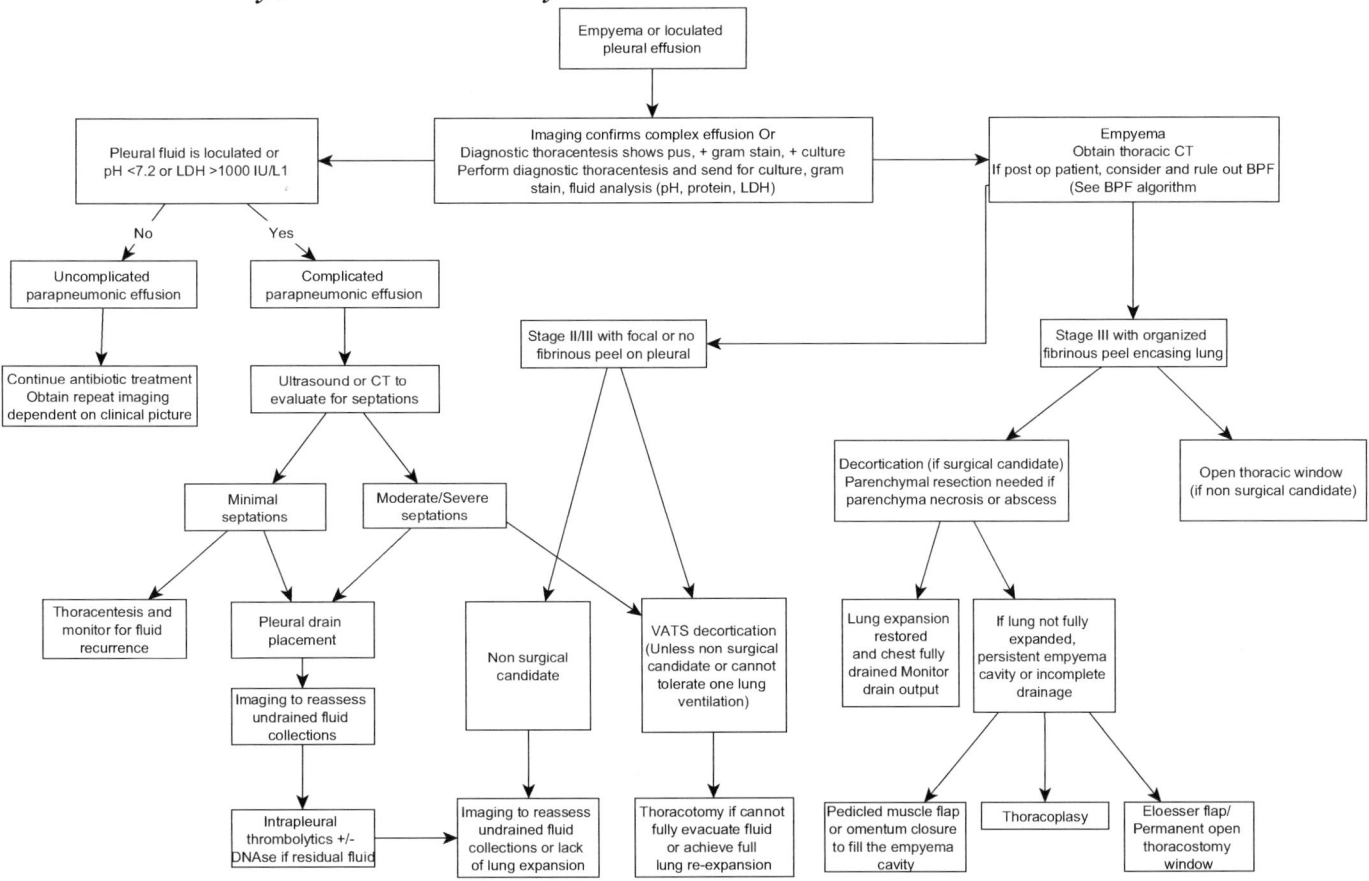

```
                          ┌─────────────────────────┐
                          │ Empyema or loculated    │
                          │ pleural effusion        │
                          └───────────┬─────────────┘
                                      ▼
┌──────────────────────┐  ┌──────────────────────────────────────────────────┐  ┌──────────────────────────────┐
│ Pleural fluid is     │◄─│ Imaging confirms complex effusion Or             │─►│ Empyema                      │
│ loculated or         │  │ Diagnostic thoracentesis shows pus, + gram       │  │ Obtain thoracic CT           │
│ pH <7.2 or LDH       │  │ stain, + culture                                 │  │ If post op patient, consider │
│ >1000 IU/L1          │  │ Perform diagnostic thoracentesis and send for    │  │ and rule out BPF             │
│                      │  │ culture, gram stain, fluid analysis (pH,         │  │ (See BPF algorithm)          │
│                      │  │ protein, LDH)                                    │  │                              │
└──┬────────────────┬──┘  └──────────────────────────────────────────────────┘  └──────────────┬───────────────┘
  No              Yes                                                                          ▼
   ▼                ▼                    ┌────────────────────────────────┐       ┌──────────────────────────────┐
┌──────────┐  ┌──────────────┐           │ Stage II/III with focal or no  │◄──────│ Stage III with organized     │
│Uncompli- │  │ Complicated  │           │ fibrinous peel on pleural      │       │ fibrinous peel encasing lung │
│cated     │  │ parapneumonic│           └──────────────┬─────────────────┘       └──────────────┬───────────────┘
│parapneu- │  │ effusion     │                          │                                        │
│monic     │  └──────┬───────┘                          │                                        │
│effusion  │         ▼                                  │                                        │
└────┬─────┘  ┌──────────────┐                          │                          ┌─────────────┴──────────────┐
     ▼        │ Ultrasound   │                          │                          ▼                            ▼
┌──────────┐  │ or CT to     │                          │            ┌──────────────────────────┐   ┌────────────────────┐
│Continue  │  │ evaluate for │                          │            │ Decortication (if        │   │ Open thoracic      │
│antibiotic│  │ septations   │                          │            │ surgical candidate)      │   │ window (if non     │
│treatment │  └──┬────────┬──┘                          │            │ Parenchymal resection    │   │ surgical candidate)│
│Obtain    │     ▼        ▼                             │            │ needed if parenchyma     │   └────────────────────┘
│repeat    │ ┌────────┐ ┌────────────┐                  │            │ necrosis or abscess      │
│imaging   │ │Minimal │ │Moderate/   │                  │            └──────────┬───────────────┘
│dependent │ │septa-  │ │Severe      │                  │                       │
│on clini- │ │tions   │ │septations  │                  │              ┌────────┴────────┐
│cal       │ └───┬────┘ └─────┬──────┘                  │              ▼                 ▼
│picture   │     ▼            ▼                         ▼      ┌───────────────┐  ┌──────────────┐
└──────────┘ ┌───────┐  ┌───────────┐          ┌──────────────┐│Lung expansion │  │If lung not   │
             │Thora- │  │Pleural    │  ┌───────│VATS          ││restored and   │  │fully expanded│
             │cente- │  │drain      │  │       │decortication ││chest fully    │  │persistent    │
             │sis and│  │placement  │  │       │(Unless non   ││drained Monitor│  │empyema cavity│
             │monitor│  └─────┬─────┘  │       │surgical      ││drain output   │  │or incomplete │
             │for    │        ▼        │       │candidate or  │└───────────────┘  │drainage      │
             │fluid  │  ┌───────────┐  │       │cannot        │                   └──────┬───────┘
             │recur- │  │Imaging to │  │       │tolerate one  │                          │
             │rence  │  │reassess   │  │       │lung          │            ┌─────────────┼─────────────┐
             └───────┘  │undrained  │  │       │ventilation)  │            ▼             ▼             ▼
                        │fluid      │  │       └──────┬───────┘     ┌─────────────┐ ┌──────────┐ ┌──────────────┐
                        │collections│  ▼              │             │Pedicled     │ │Thoraco-  │ │Eloesser flap/│
                        └─────┬─────┘┌───────────┐    │             │muscle flap  │ │plasty    │ │Permanent open│
                              ▼      │Non        │    │             │or omentum   │ │          │ │thoracostomy  │
                        ┌───────────┐│surgical   │    │             │closure to   │ │          │ │window        │
                        │Intrapleur-││candidate  │    │             │fill the     │ │          │ │              │
                        │al thrombo-│└─────┬─────┘    │             │empyema      │ │          │ │              │
                        │lytics +/- │      ▼          ▼             │cavity       │ │          │ │              │
                        │DNAse if   │┌────────────┐┌──────────────┐ └─────────────┘ └──────────┘ └──────────────┘
                        │residual   ││Imaging to  ││Thoracotomy if│
                        │fluid      ││reassess    ││cannot fully  │
                        └───────────┘│undrained   ││evacuate fluid│
                                     │fluid       ││or achieve    │
                                     │collections ││full lung     │
                                     │or lack of  ││re-expansion  │
                                     │lung        │└──────────────┘
                                     │expansion   │
                                     └────────────┘
```

141

Spontaneous Pneumothorax
Jennifer Burg, Paul Schipper

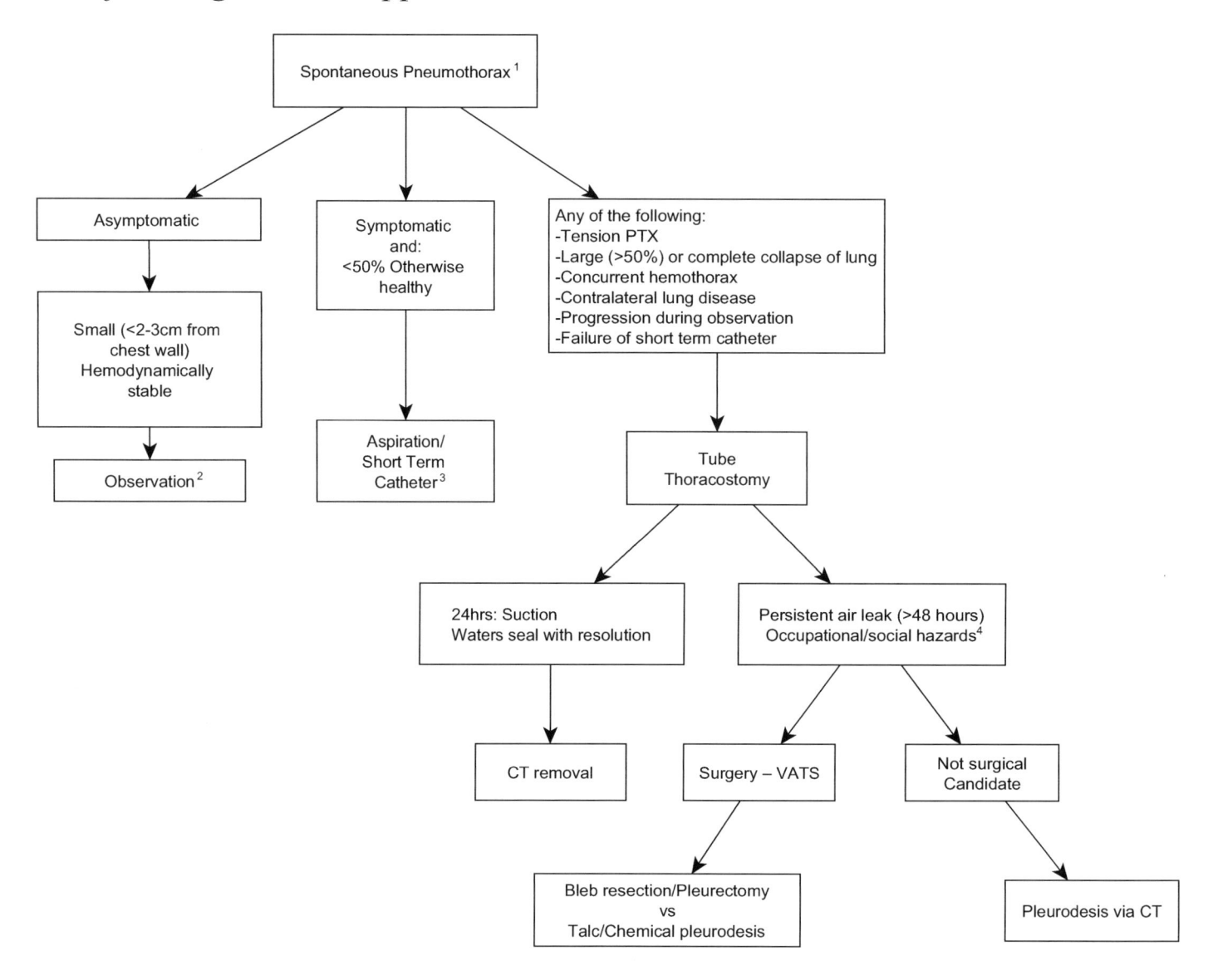

```
                          ┌─────────────────────────────┐
                          │ Spontaneous Pneumothorax [1]│
                          └─────────────────────────────┘
                 ┌────────────────┼──────────────────────────┐
                 ▼                ▼                          ▼
        ┌──────────────┐  ┌──────────────┐   ┌─────────────────────────────────┐
        │ Asymptomatic │  │ Symptomatic  │   │ Any of the following:           │
        └──────────────┘  │ and:         │   │ -Tension PTX                    │
                 │        │ <50% Otherwise│  │ -Large (>50%) or complete       │
                 ▼        │ healthy      │   │  collapse of lung               │
        ┌──────────────┐  └──────────────┘   │ -Concurrent hemothorax          │
        │ Small (<2-3cm│         │           │ -Contralateral lung disease     │
        │  from chest  │         ▼           │ -Progression during observation │
        │  wall)       │  ┌──────────────┐   │ -Failure of short term catheter │
        │ Hemodynamic- │  │ Aspiration/  │   └─────────────────────────────────┘
        │ ally stable  │  │ Short Term   │                  │
        └──────────────┘  │ Catheter [3] │                  ▼
                 │        └──────────────┘         ┌──────────────┐
                 ▼                                 │    Tube      │
        ┌──────────────┐                           │ Thoracostomy │
        │ Observation[2]│                          └──────────────┘
        └──────────────┘                     ┌────────────┴─────────────┐
                                             ▼                          ▼
                                  ┌──────────────────┐   ┌──────────────────────────┐
                                  │ 24hrs: Suction   │   │ Persistent air leak      │
                                  │ Waters seal with │   │ (>48 hours)              │
                                  │ resolution       │   │ Occupational/social      │
                                  └──────────────────┘   │ hazards [4]              │
                                           │             └──────────────────────────┘
                                           ▼                 │              │
                                  ┌──────────────┐           ▼              ▼
                                  │ CT removal   │   ┌──────────────┐  ┌──────────────┐
                                  └──────────────┘   │Surgery – VATS│  │Not surgical  │
                                                     └──────────────┘  │  Candidate   │
                                                           │           └──────────────┘
                                                           ▼                  │
                                         ┌────────────────────────────┐       ▼
                                         │ Bleb resection/Pleurectomy │ ┌──────────────┐
                                         │            vs              │ │Pleurodesis   │
                                         │ Talc/Chemical pleurodesis  │ │   via CT     │
                                         └────────────────────────────┘ └──────────────┘
```

PTX: Pneumothorax; VATS: Video-assisted thoracoscopic Surgery; CT: chest tube
1: If diagnosed via CXR, consider CT scan to evaluate for underlying disease
2: ED observation followed by CXR to evaluate for progression. Observation requires close follow up and discussion of risks/benefits.
3: Placement of catheter with aspiration of PTX. Catheter left in place attached to pleur-vac or Heimlich valve until serial CXRs show resolution without recurrence (Vallee et al)
4: Patients with occupational risk (SCUBA divers, pilots) or who live in or travel to isolated areas

Post-pneumonectomy Bronchopleural Fistula
Justin Watson, Brandon Tieu

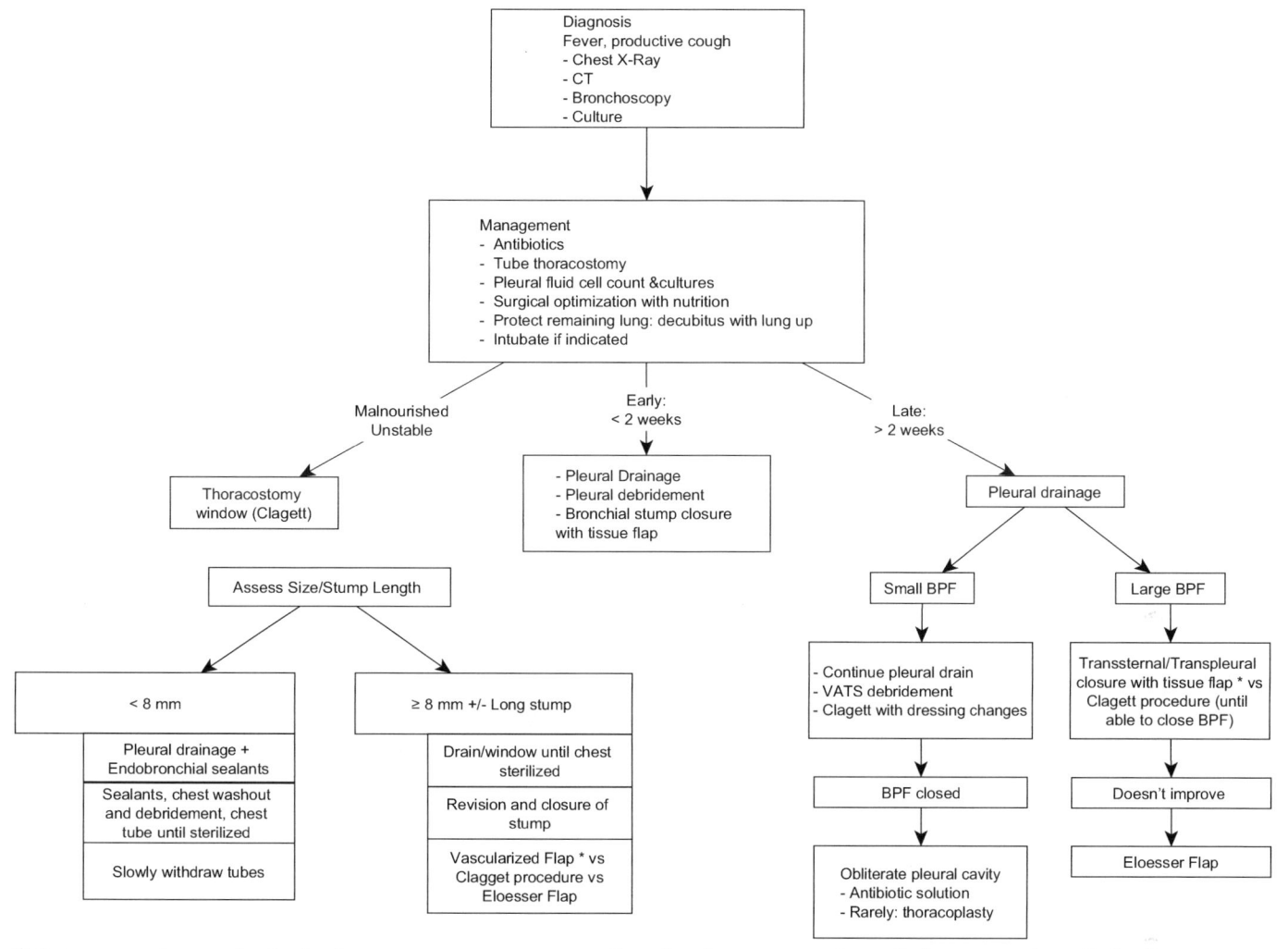

```
┌─────────────────────────────┐
│ Diagnosis                   │
│ Fever, productive cough     │
│  - Chest X-Ray              │
│  - CT                       │
│  - Bronchoscopy             │
│  - Culture                  │
└──────────────┬──────────────┘
               ▼
┌─────────────────────────────────────────────┐
│ Management                                  │
│  - Antibiotics                              │
│  - Tube thoracostomy                        │
│  - Pleural fluid cell count &cultures       │
│  - Surgical optimization with nutrition     │
│  - Protect remaining lung: decubitus with   │
│    lung up                                  │
│  - Intubate if indicated                    │
└─────────────────────────────────────────────┘
```

Branches:

Malnourished / Unstable → Thoracostomy window (Clagett)
- Assess Size/Stump Length
  - **< 8 mm**:
    - Pleural drainage + Endobronchial sealants
    - Sealants, chest washout and debridement, chest tube until sterilized
    - Slowly withdraw tubes
  - **≥ 8 mm +/- Long stump**:
    - Drain/window until chest sterilized
    - Revision and closure of stump
    - Vascularized Flap * vs Clagget procedure vs Eloesser Flap

Early: < 2 weeks
- Pleural Drainage
- Pleural debridement
- Bronchial stump closure with tissue flap

Late: > 2 weeks → Pleural drainage
- **Small BPF**:
  - Continue pleural drain
  - VATS debridement
  - Clagett with dressing changes
  - → BPF closed → Obliterate pleural cavity
    - Antibiotic solution
    - Rarely: thoracoplasty
- **Large BPF**:
  - Transsternal/Transpleural closure with tissue flap * vs Clagett procedure (until able to close BPF)
  - → Doesn't improve → Eloesser Flap

* Intercostal muscle, latissimus, serratus, pectoralis, diaphragm, pericardial, omental pedicle flap

Chylothorax
Smarika Shrestha, Michael F. Reed

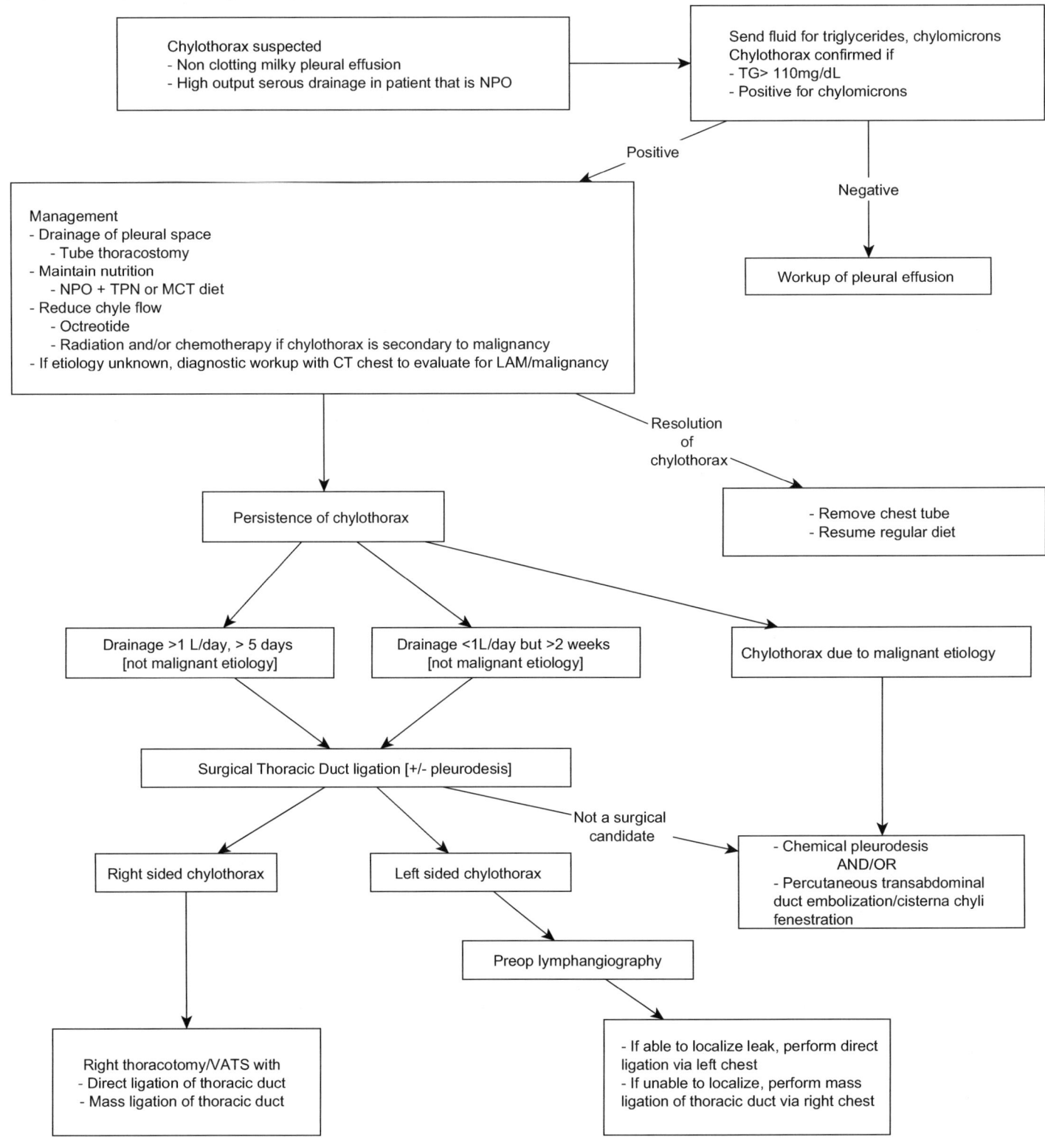

```
┌─────────────────────────────────────────────────┐         ┌─────────────────────────────────────────┐
│ Chylothorax suspected                           │         │ Send fluid for triglycerides, chylomicrons│
│  - Non clotting milky pleural effusion          │────────▶│ Chylothorax confirmed if                │
│  - High output serous drainage in patient that  │         │  - TG> 110mg/dL                         │
│    is NPO                                       │         │  - Positive for chylomicrons            │
└─────────────────────────────────────────────────┘         └─────────────────────────────────────────┘
                                                      Positive │                    │ Negative
                                                               ▼                    ▼
┌──────────────────────────────────────────────────────────────┐            ┌──────────────────────────┐
│ Management                                                   │            │ Workup of pleural effusion│
│  - Drainage of pleural space                                 │            └──────────────────────────┘
│     - Tube thoracostomy                                      │
│  - Maintain nutrition                                        │
│     - NPO + TPN or MCT diet                                  │
│  - Reduce chyle flow                                         │
│     - Octreotide                                             │
│     - Radiation and/or chemotherapy if chylothorax is        │
│       secondary to malignancy                                │
│  - If etiology unknown, diagnostic workup with CT chest to   │
│    evaluate for LAM/malignancy                               │
└──────────────────────────────────────────────────────────────┘
                            │                       Resolution of chylothorax
                            ▼                              ▼
              ┌──────────────────────────┐       ┌──────────────────────────┐
              │ Persistence of chylothorax│       │ - Remove chest tube       │
              └──────────────────────────┘       │ - Resume regular diet     │
                 │              │                └──────────────────────────┘
                 ▼              ▼                          
┌────────────────────────┐ ┌────────────────────────┐ ┌──────────────────────────────┐
│ Drainage >1 L/day,     │ │ Drainage <1L/day but   │ │ Chylothorax due to malignant │
│ > 5 days               │ │ >2 weeks               │ │ etiology                     │
│ [not malignant etiology]│ │ [not malignant etiology]│ └──────────────────────────────┘
└────────────────────────┘ └────────────────────────┘
                 │              │
                 ▼              ▼
        ┌──────────────────────────────────────┐     Not a surgical candidate
        │ Surgical Thoracic Duct ligation      │─────────────────┐
        │ [+/- pleurodesis]                    │                 │
        └──────────────────────────────────────┘                 ▼
              │                    │               ┌──────────────────────────────┐
              ▼                    ▼               │ - Chemical pleurodesis       │
    ┌──────────────────┐  ┌──────────────────┐    │   AND/OR                     │
    │ Right sided      │  │ Left sided       │    │ - Percutaneous transabdominal│
    │ chylothorax      │  │ chylothorax      │    │   duct embolization/cisterna │
    └──────────────────┘  └──────────────────┘    │   chyli fenestration         │
              │                    │               └──────────────────────────────┘
              │                    ▼
              │           ┌──────────────────────┐
              │           │ Preop lymphangiography│
              │           └──────────────────────┘
              ▼                    ▼
┌──────────────────────────┐  ┌────────────────────────────────────────────┐
│ Right thoracotomy/VATS   │  │ - If able to localize leak, perform direct │
│ with                     │  │   ligation via left chest                  │
│ - Direct ligation of     │  │ - If unable to localize, perform mass      │
│   thoracic duct          │  │   ligation of thoracic duct via right chest│
│ - Mass ligation of       │  └────────────────────────────────────────────┘
│   thoracic duct          │
└──────────────────────────┘
```

NPO, nothing by mouth; TG, triglycerides; TPN, total parenteral nutrition; MCT, medium chain triglycerides; LAM, lymphangioleiomyomatosis; VATS; video assisted thoracoscopic surgery

Pleural Mesothelioma
Panos Vardas, Jennifer Dixon, Parth Amin

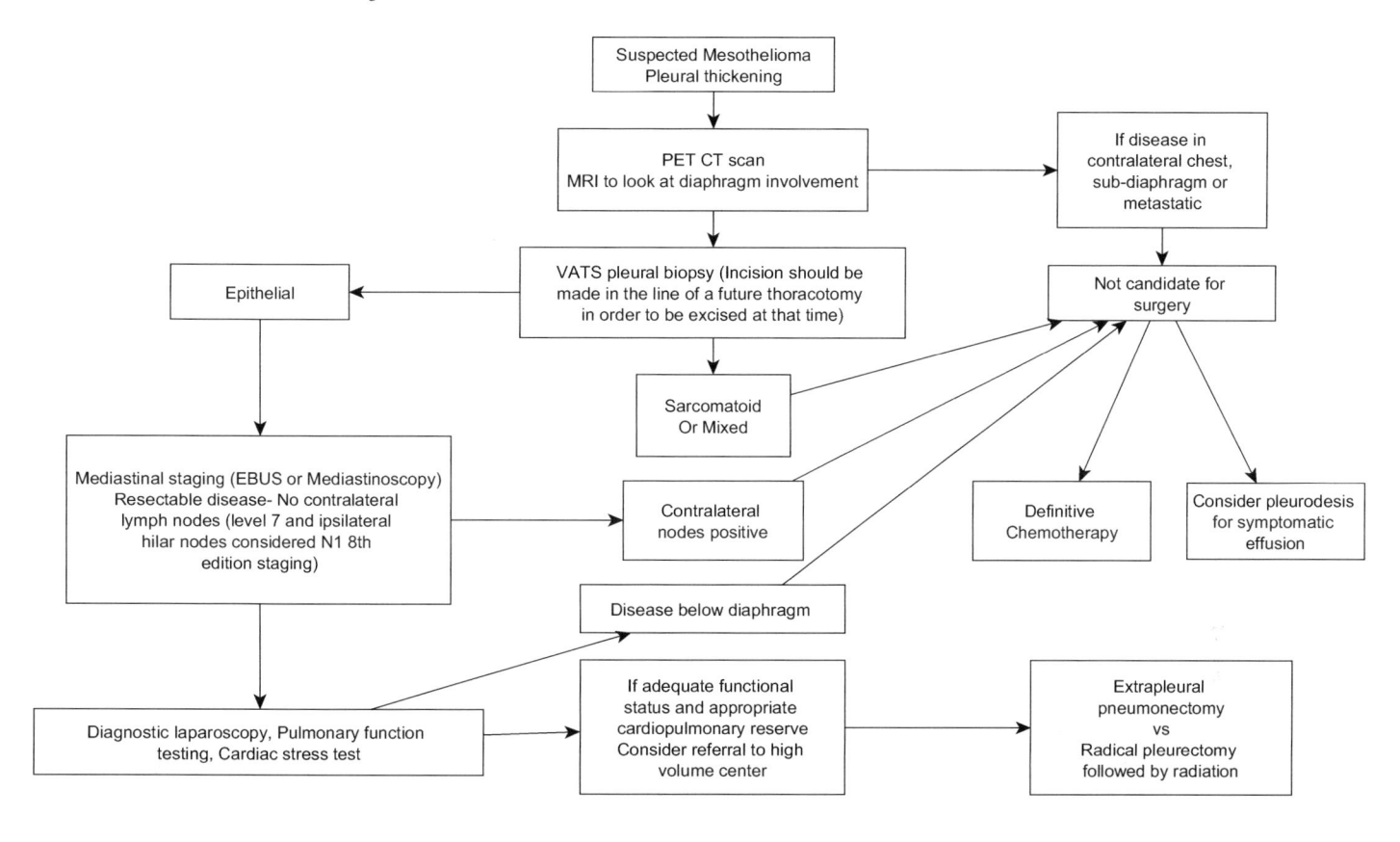

```
┌─────────────────────────┐
│ Suspected Mesothelioma  │
│   Pleural thickening    │
└───────────┬─────────────┘
            ▼
┌─────────────────────────────────────┐      ┌──────────────────────┐
│         PET CT scan                 │─────▶│  If disease in       │
│ MRI to look at diaphragm involvement│      │ contralateral chest, │
└───────────┬─────────────────────────┘      │ sub-diaphragm or     │
            │                                │    metastatic        │
            ▼                                └──────────┬───────────┘
┌──────────────┐   ┌──────────────────────────────┐     ▼
│  Epithelial  │◀──│ VATS pleural biopsy (Incision│   ┌──────────────────┐
└──────┬───────┘   │ should be made in the line of│   │ Not candidate for│
       │           │ a future thoracotomy in order│──▶│     surgery      │
       │           │     to be excised at that    │   └────┬─────┬───────┘
       │           │          time)               │        │     │
       │           └──────────┬───────────────────┘        ▼     ▼
       │                      ▼                        Definitive  Consider
       │              ┌─────────────┐                  Chemotherapy pleurodesis
       │              │ Sarcomatoid │                               for symptomatic
       │              │  Or Mixed   │                               effusion
       │              └─────────────┘
       ▼
┌─────────────────────────────┐       ┌──────────────────┐
│ Mediastinal staging (EBUS   │       │  Contralateral   │
│ or Mediastinoscopy)         │──────▶│ nodes positive   │
│ Resectable disease- No      │       └──────────────────┘
│ contralateral lymph nodes   │
│ (level 7 and ipsilateral    │
│ hilar nodes considered N1   │
│ 8th edition staging)        │
└──────────────┬──────────────┘
               │                  ┌──────────────────────┐
               │                  │ Disease below        │
               │                  │    diaphragm         │
               ▼                  └──────────┬───────────┘
┌──────────────────────────┐                 │
│ Diagnostic laparoscopy,  │      ┌──────────────────────┐    ┌─────────────────┐
│ Pulmonary function       │─────▶│ If adequate functional│───▶│ Extrapleural    │
│ testing, Cardiac stress  │      │ status and appropriate│    │ pneumonectomy   │
│ test                     │      │ cardiopulmonary reserve│   │       vs        │
└──────────────────────────┘      │ Consider referral to  │   │ Radical         │
                                  │ high volume center    │   │ pleurectomy     │
                                  └──────────────────────┘    │ followed by     │
                                                              │ radiation       │
                                                              └─────────────────┘
```

Caustic Injury
Barry Gibney, Daniel Wiener

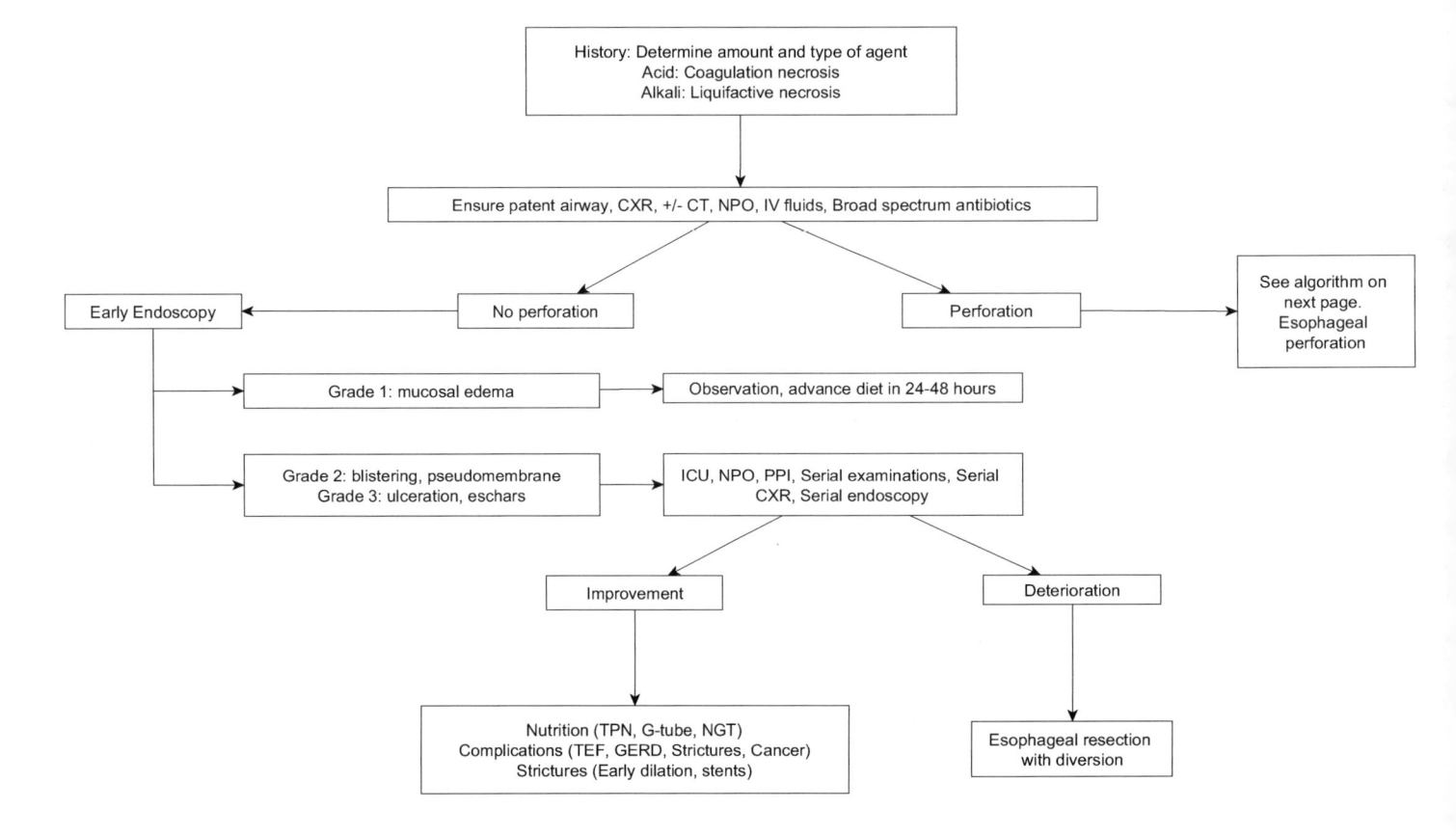

```
┌─────────────────────────────────────────┐
│ History: Determine amount and type of   │
│ agent                                   │
│    Acid: Coagulation necrosis           │
│    Alkali: Liquifactive necrosis        │
└────────────────────┬────────────────────┘
                     │
                     ▼
┌─────────────────────────────────────────────────────────┐
│ Ensure patent airway, CXR, +/- CT, NPO, IV fluids,      │
│ Broad spectrum antibiotics                              │
└──────────┬──────────────────────────────┬───────────────┘
           │                              │
           ▼                              ▼
    ┌──────────────┐              ┌──────────────┐      ┌──────────────────┐
    │ No perforation│              │ Perforation  │─────▶│ See algorithm on │
    └──────┬───────┘              └──────────────┘      │ next page.       │
           │                                            │ Esophageal       │
           ▼                                            │ perforation      │
┌──────────────────┐                                    └──────────────────┘
│ Early Endoscopy  │
└──┬───────────────┘
   │
   ├──▶ Grade 1: mucosal edema ──▶ Observation, advance diet in 24-48 hours
   │
   └──▶ Grade 2: blistering, pseudomembrane ──▶ ICU, NPO, PPI, Serial
        Grade 3: ulceration, eschars            examinations, Serial
                                                CXR, Serial endoscopy
                                                      │
                                       ┌──────────────┴──────────────┐
                                       ▼                             ▼
                                 ┌───────────┐              ┌──────────────┐
                                 │Improvement│              │Deterioration │
                                 └─────┬─────┘              └──────┬───────┘
                                       ▼                           ▼
                         Nutrition (TPN, G-tube, NGT)     Esophageal resection
                         Complications (TEF, GERD,        with diversion
                         Strictures, Cancer)
                         Strictures (Early dilation, stents)
```

Esophageal Perforation
Stevan Pupovac, Paul C. Lee

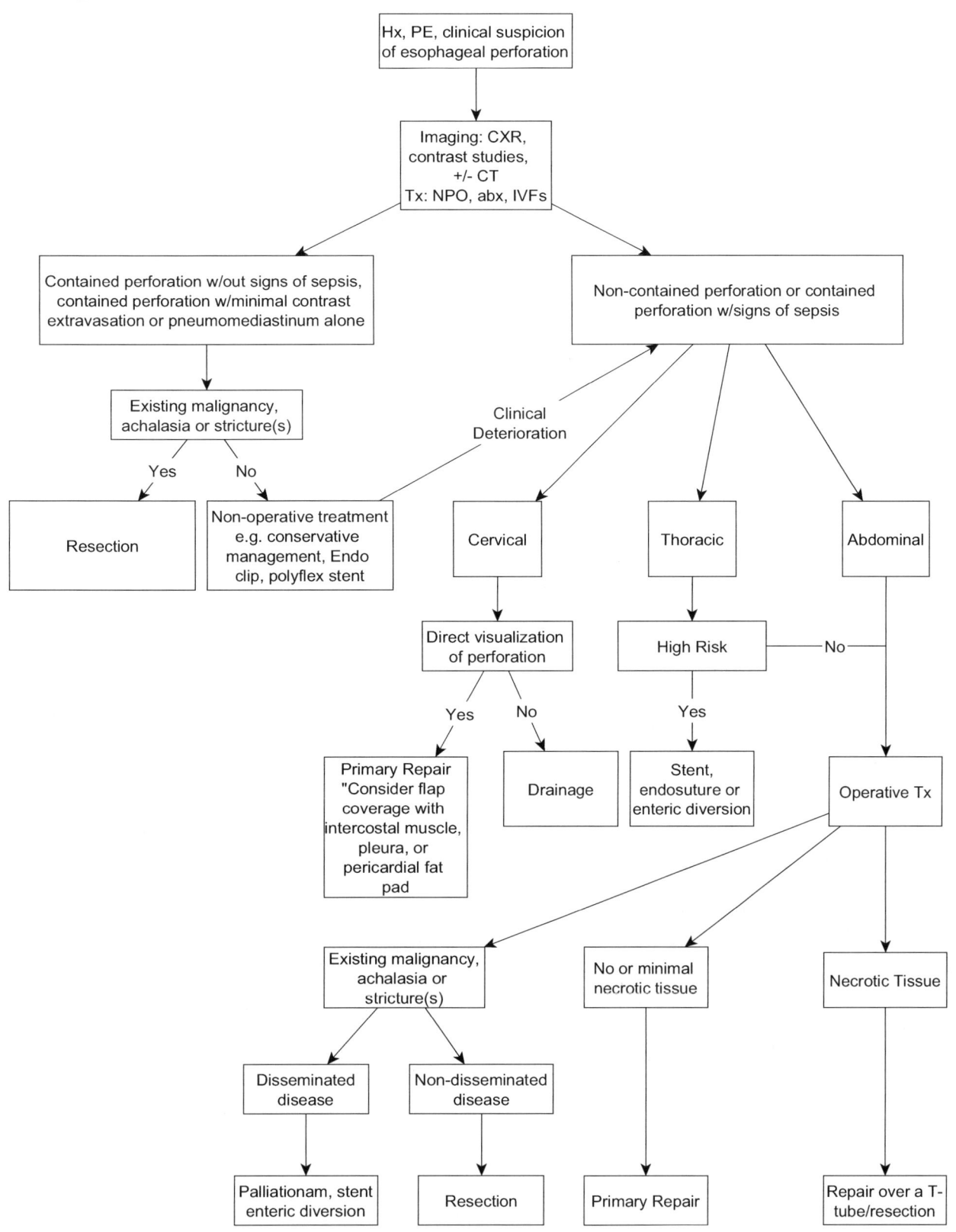

```
                    ┌─────────────────────────┐
                    │ Hx, PE, clinical        │
                    │ suspicion of            │
                    │ esophageal perforation  │
                    └───────────┬─────────────┘
                                ▼
                    ┌─────────────────────────┐
                    │ Imaging: CXR,           │
                    │ contrast studies,       │
                    │ +/- CT                  │
                    │ Tx: NPO, abx, IVFs      │
                    └───────────┬─────────────┘
                   ┌────────────┴────────────┐
                   ▼                         ▼
    ┌──────────────────────────┐   ┌──────────────────────────┐
    │ Contained perforation    │   │ Non-contained perforation│
    │ w/out signs of sepsis,   │   │ or contained perforation │
    │ contained perforation    │   │ w/signs of sepsis        │
    │ w/minimal contrast       │   └──────────────────────────┘
    │ extravasation or         │
    │ pneumomediastinum alone  │
    └────────────┬─────────────┘
                 ▼
    ┌──────────────────────────┐
    │ Existing malignancy,     │
    │ achalasia or stricture(s)│
    └──┬──────────────────┬────┘
    Yes│                No│
       ▼                  ▼
  ┌─────────┐   ┌──────────────────────┐
  │Resection│   │ Non-operative        │
  └─────────┘   │ treatment e.g.       │
                │ conservative         │
                │ management, Endo     │
                │ clip, polyflex stent │
                └──────────────────────┘
```

Clinical Deterioration → Non-contained perforation or contained perforation w/signs of sepsis → Cervical / Thoracic / Abdominal

- **Cervical** → Direct visualization of perforation
  - Yes → Primary Repair "Consider flap coverage with intercostal muscle, pleura, or pericardial fat pad
  - No → Drainage
- **Thoracic** → High Risk
  - Yes → Stent, endosuture or enteric diversion
  - No → Operative Tx
- **Abdominal** → Operative Tx

Operative Tx branches:
- Existing malignancy, achalasia or stricture(s)
  - Disseminated disease → Palliationam, stent enteric diversion
  - Non-disseminated disease → Resection
- No or minimal necrotic tissue → Primary Repair
- Necrotic Tissue → Repair over a T-tube/resection

Hx, history; CXR, chest x-ray; Abx, antibiotics; CT, computed tomography; NPO, nothing by mouth; IVFs, intravenous fluids

Acquired Trachea-esophageal Fistula
Justin Watson, Paul Schipper

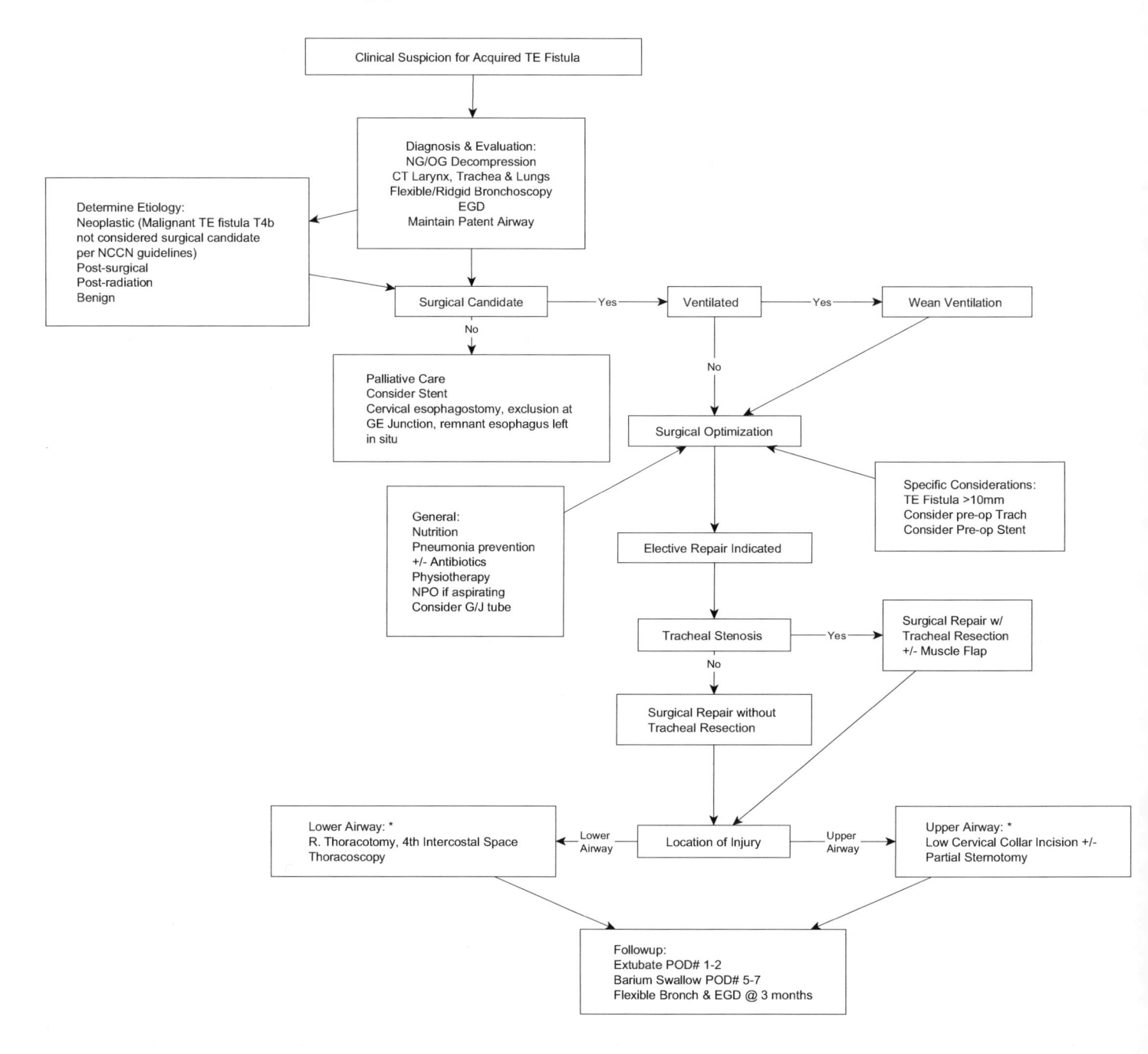

```
                          ┌─────────────────────────────────────┐
                          │ Clinical Suspicion for Acquired TE Fistula │
                          └─────────────────────────────────────┘
                                           │
                                           ▼
                          ┌─────────────────────────────────────┐
                          │ Diagnosis & Evaluation:             │
                          │ NG/OG Decompression                 │
┌──────────────────────┐  │ CT Larynx, Trachea & Lungs          │
│ Determine Etiology:  │  │ Flexible/Ridgid Bronchoscopy        │
│ Neoplastic (Malignant│◄─│ EGD                                 │
│ TE fistula T4b not   │  │ Maintain Patent Airway              │
│ considered surgical  │  └─────────────────────────────────────┘
│ candidate per NCCN   │                    │
│ guidelines)          │                    ▼
│ Post-surgical        │  ┌───────────────┐      ┌──────────┐      ┌──────────────┐
│ Post-radiation       │──│ Surgical      │─Yes─►│ Ventilated│─Yes─►│ Wean         │
│ Benign               │  │ Candidate     │      │          │      │ Ventilation  │
└──────────────────────┘  └───────────────┘      └──────────┘      └──────────────┘
                                  │No                 │No                 │
                                  ▼                   ▼                   │
                          ┌──────────────────┐  ┌──────────────────┐◄─────┘
                          │ Palliative Care  │  │ Surgical         │
                          │ Consider Stent   │  │ Optimization     │
                          │ Cervical         │  └──────────────────┘
                          │ esophagostomy,   │       ▲
                          │ exclusion at GE  │       │    ┌──────────────────────┐
                          │ Junction,        │       │    │ Specific             │
                          │ remnant esophagus│       │    │ Considerations:      │
                          │ left in situ     │       ├────│ TE Fistula >10mm     │
                          └──────────────────┘       │    │ Consider pre-op Trach│
                                                     │    │ Consider Pre-op Stent│
                          ┌─────────────────┐        │    └──────────────────────┘
                          │ General:        │        ▼
                          │ Nutrition       │   ┌──────────────────┐
                          │ Pneumonia       │   │ Elective Repair  │
                          │ prevention      │   │ Indicated        │
                          │ +/- Antibiotics │   └──────────────────┘
                          │ Physiotherapy   │        │
                          │ NPO if aspirating│       ▼
                          │ Consider G/J tube│  ┌──────────────┐       ┌──────────────────┐
                          └─────────────────┘   │ Tracheal     │─Yes──►│ Surgical Repair w/│
                                                │ Stenosis     │       │ Tracheal Resection│
                                                └──────────────┘       │ +/- Muscle Flap   │
                                                       │No             └──────────────────┘
                                                       ▼
                                                ┌──────────────────────┐
                                                │ Surgical Repair      │
                                                │ without Tracheal     │
                                                │ Resection            │
                                                └──────────────────────┘
                                                           │
 ┌────────────────────────────┐                            ▼                     ┌───────────────────────────┐
 │ Lower Airway: *            │◄──Lower Airway──┌──────────────────┐──Upper Airway►│ Upper Airway: *           │
 │ R. Thoracotomy, 4th        │                 │ Location of      │              │ Low Cervical Collar       │
 │ Intercostal Space          │                 │ Injury           │              │ Incision +/- Partial      │
 │ Thoracoscopy               │                 └──────────────────┘              │ Sternotomy                │
 └────────────────────────────┘                                                   └───────────────────────────┘
                │                                                                         │
                └──────────────────────────────┐       ┌────────────────────────────────┘
                                               ▼       ▼
                                    ┌─────────────────────────────┐
                                    │ Followup:                   │
                                    │ Extubate POD# 1-2           │
                                    │ Barium Swallow POD# 5-7     │
                                    │ Flexible Bronch & EGD @ 3 months│
                                    └─────────────────────────────┘
```

* Optimal surgical access
Lower airway is >5cm below vocal chords
Upper airway is <5cm below vocal chords

Management of Leiomyoma
Awais Ashfaq, Paul Schipper

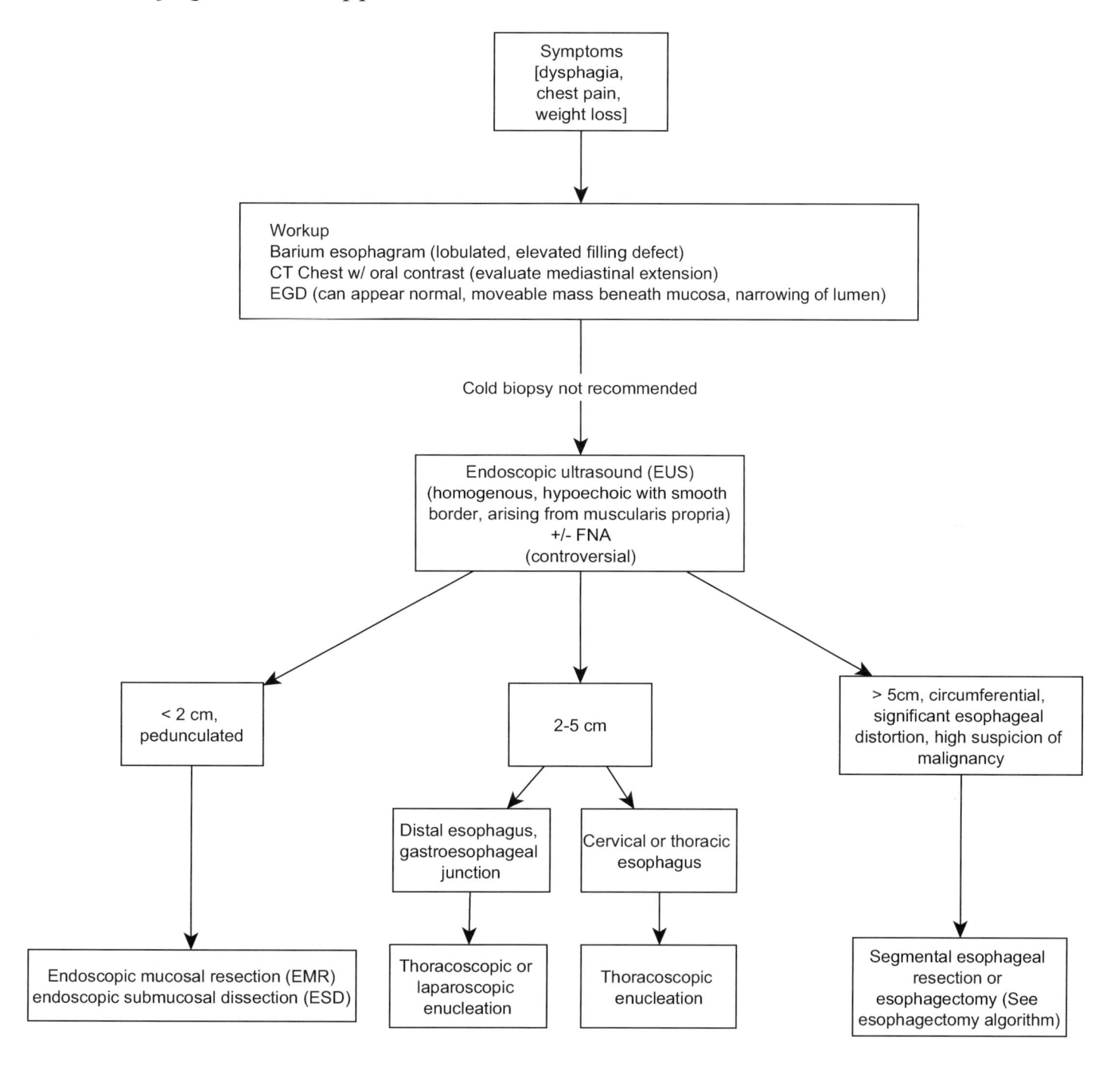

```
┌─────────────┐
│  Symptoms   │
│ [dysphagia, │
│ chest pain, │
│ weight loss]│
└──────┬──────┘
       │
       ▼
┌──────────────────────────────────────────────────────────────┐
│ Workup                                                       │
│ Barium esophagram (lobulated, elevated filling defect)       │
│ CT Chest w/ oral contrast (evaluate mediastinal extension)   │
│ EGD (can appear normal, moveable mass beneath mucosa,        │
│      narrowing of lumen)                                     │
└──────────────────────────┬───────────────────────────────────┘
                           │  Cold biopsy not recommended
                           ▼
           ┌───────────────────────────────────┐
           │ Endoscopic ultrasound (EUS)       │
           │ (homogenous, hypoechoic with      │
           │ smooth border, arising from       │
           │ muscularis propria)               │
           │ +/- FNA (controversial)           │
           └───┬──────────────┬────────────┬───┘
               ▼              ▼            ▼
      ┌──────────────┐  ┌──────────┐  ┌──────────────────┐
      │ < 2 cm,      │  │ 2-5 cm   │  │ > 5cm,           │
      │ pedunculated │  │          │  │ circumferential, │
      │              │  │          │  │ significant      │
      │              │  │          │  │ esophageal       │
      │              │  │          │  │ distortion, high │
      │              │  │          │  │ suspicion of     │
      │              │  │          │  │ malignancy       │
      └──────┬───────┘  └─┬──────┬─┘  └────────┬─────────┘
             │            ▼      ▼             │
             │    ┌──────────┐ ┌──────────┐    │
             │    │ Distal   │ │ Cervical │    │
             │    │ esophagus│ │ or       │    │
             │    │ gastro-  │ │ thoracic │    │
             │    │esophageal│ │esophagus │    │
             │    │ junction │ │          │    │
             │    └────┬─────┘ └────┬─────┘    │
             ▼         ▼            ▼          ▼
      ┌─────────────┐ ┌─────────┐ ┌─────────┐ ┌──────────────┐
      │ Endoscopic  │ │Thoraco- │ │Thoraco- │ │ Segmental    │
      │ mucosal     │ │scopic or│ │scopic   │ │ esophageal   │
      │ resection   │ │laparo-  │ │enucle-  │ │ resection or │
      │ (EMR)       │ │scopic   │ │ation    │ │ esophagectomy│
      │ endoscopic  │ │enucle-  │ │         │ │ (See esoph-  │
      │ submucosal  │ │ation    │ │         │ │ agectomy     │
      │ dissection  │ │         │ │         │ │ algorithm)   │
      │ (ESD)       │ │         │ │         │ │              │
      └─────────────┘ └─────────┘ └─────────┘ └──────────────┘
```

Surgical Approach to Esophageal Cancer
Shane P. Smith, Brian Louie

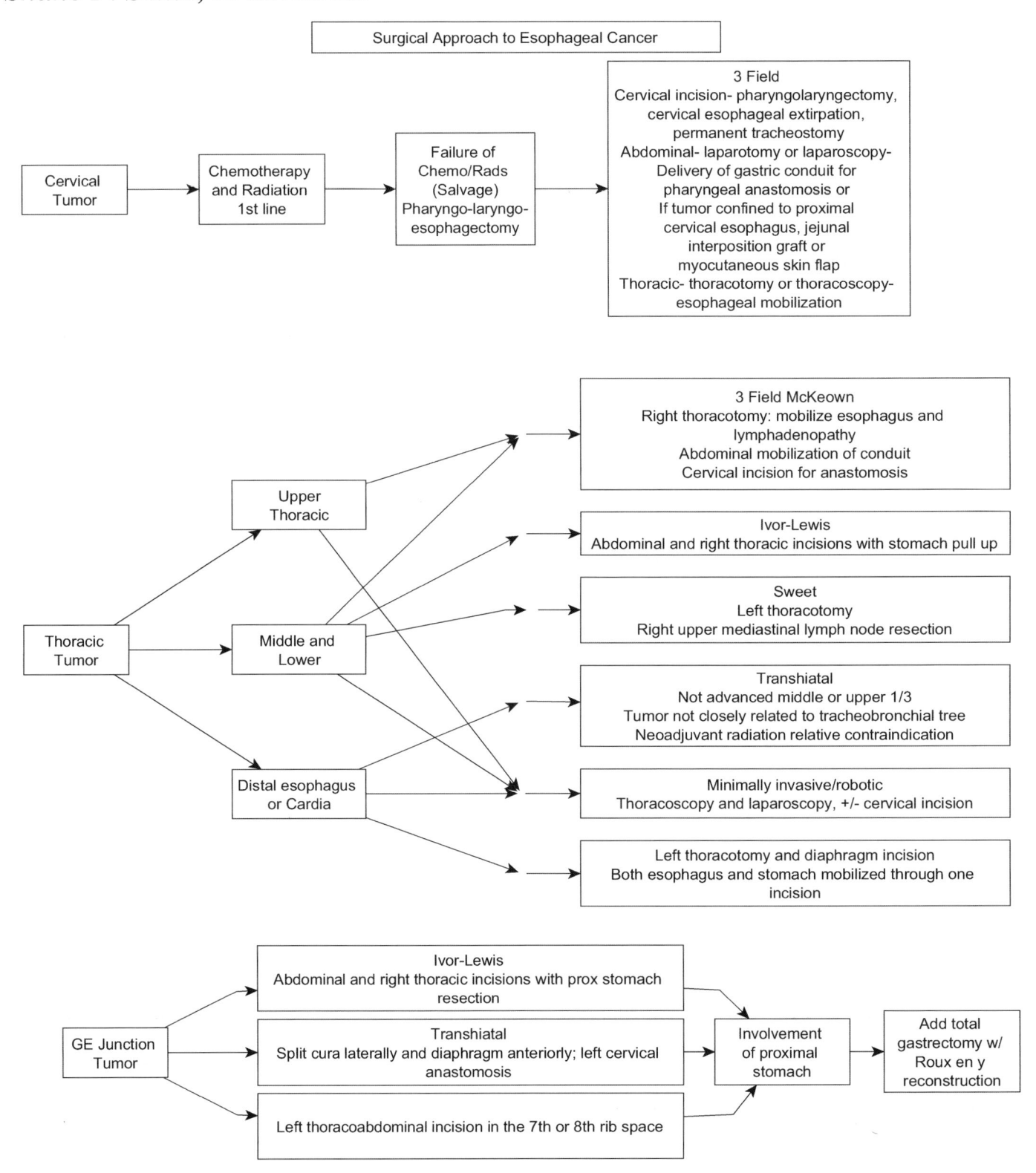

Surgical Approach to Esophageal Cancer

Cervical Tumor → Chemotherapy and Radiation 1st line → Failure of Chemo/Rads (Salvage) Pharyngo-laryngo-esophagectomy →
3 Field
Cervical incision- pharyngolaryngectomy, cervical esophageal extirpation, permanent tracheostomy
Abdominal- laparotomy or laparoscopy- Delivery of gastric conduit for pharyngeal anastomosis or
If tumor confined to proximal cervical esophagus, jejunal interposition graft or myocutaneous skin flap
Thoracic- thoracotomy or thoracoscopy- esophageal mobilization

Thoracic Tumor

- Upper Thoracic →
  - **3 Field McKeown**
    Right thoracotomy: mobilize esophagus and lymphadenopathy
    Abdominal mobilization of conduit
    Cervical incision for anastomosis
- Middle and Lower →
  - **Ivor-Lewis**
    Abdominal and right thoracic incisions with stomach pull up
  - **Sweet**
    Left thoracotomy
    Right upper mediastinal lymph node resection
  - **Transhiatal**
    Not advanced middle or upper 1/3
    Tumor not closely related to tracheobronchial tree
    Neoadjuvant radiation relative contraindication
- Distal esophagus or Cardia →
  - **Minimally invasive/robotic**
    Thoracoscopy and laparoscopy, +/- cervical incision
  - Left thoracotomy and diaphragm incision
    Both esophagus and stomach mobilized through one incision

GE Junction Tumor →
- **Ivor-Lewis**
  Abdominal and right thoracic incisions with prox stomach resection
- **Transhiatal**
  Split cura laterally and diaphragm anteriorly; left cervical anastomosis
- Left thoracoabdominal incision in the 7th or 8th rib space

→ Involvement of proximal stomach → Add total gastrectomy w/ Roux en y reconstruction

150

Choosing Esophageal Conduit
Monisha Sudarshan, Sahar Saddoughi, Dennis Wigle

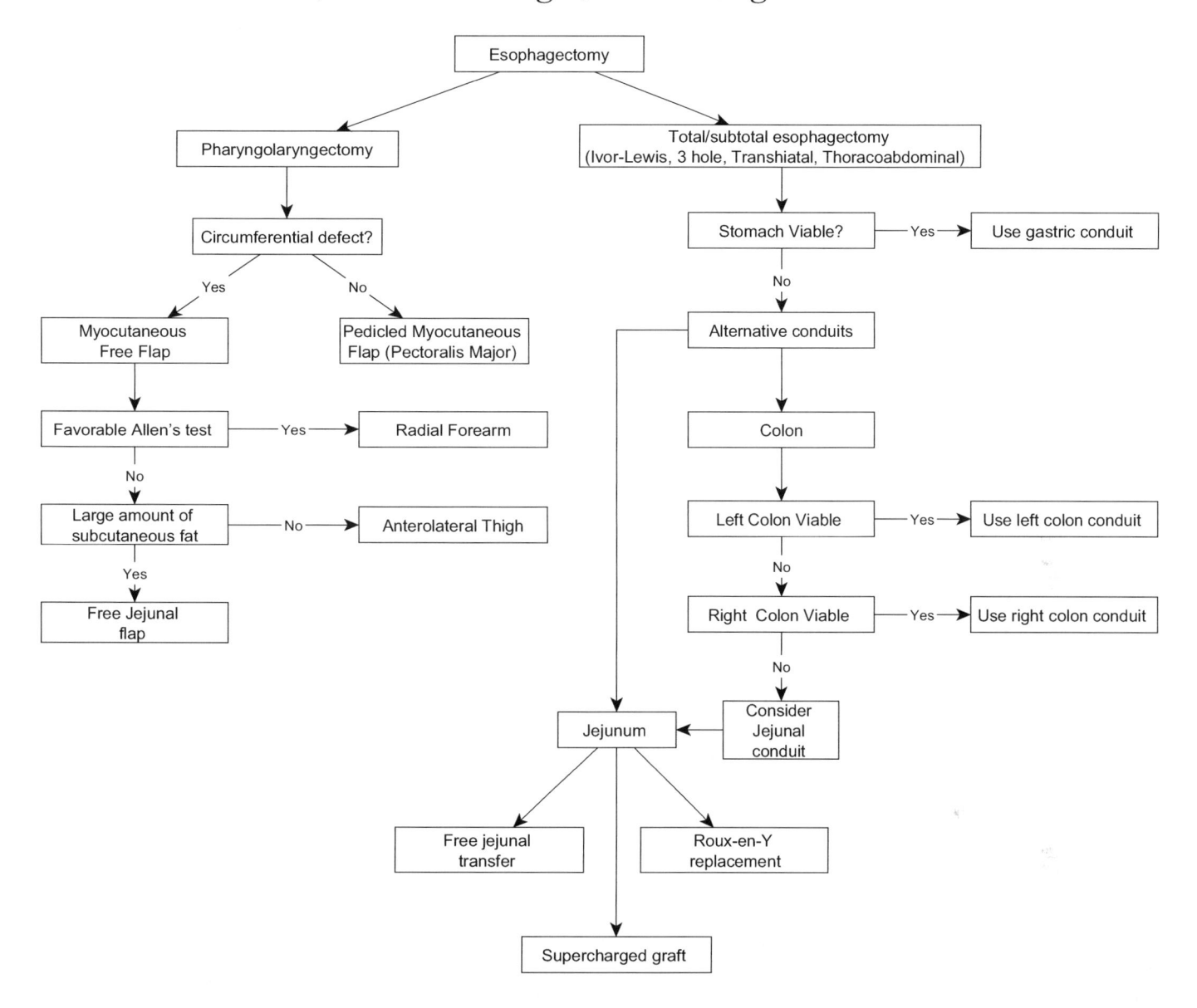

```
                            Esophagectomy
                          /              \
            Pharyngolaryngectomy        Total/subtotal esophagectomy
                    │                   (Ivor-Lewis, 3 hole, Transhiatal, Thoracoabdominal)
                    ▼                                │
            Circumferential defect?                  ▼
              /           \              Stomach Viable? ──Yes──► Use gastric conduit
           Yes            No                         │
            ▼              ▼                         No
        Myocutaneous   Pedicled Myocutaneous         ▼
        Free Flap      Flap (Pectoralis Major)   Alternative conduits
            │                                        │
            ▼                                        ▼
    Favorable Allen's test ──Yes──► Radial Forearm   Colon
            │                                        │
            No                                       ▼
            ▼                                Left Colon Viable ──Yes──► Use left colon conduit
    Large amount of                                  │
    subcutaneous fat ──No──► Anterolateral Thigh     No
            │                                        ▼
           Yes                               Right Colon Viable ──Yes──► Use right colon conduit
            ▼                                        │
        Free Jejunal                                 No
           flap                                      ▼
                                                 Consider
                                                 Jejunal
                                                 conduit
                                                     │
                                                     ▼
                                                  Jejunum
                                                 /   │   \
                                      Free jejunal   │   Roux-en-Y
                                       transfer     │   replacement
                                                     ▼
                                             Supercharged graft
```

Determining resectability of Esophageal Adenocarcinoma
Michal J. Lada, Carolyn E. Jones

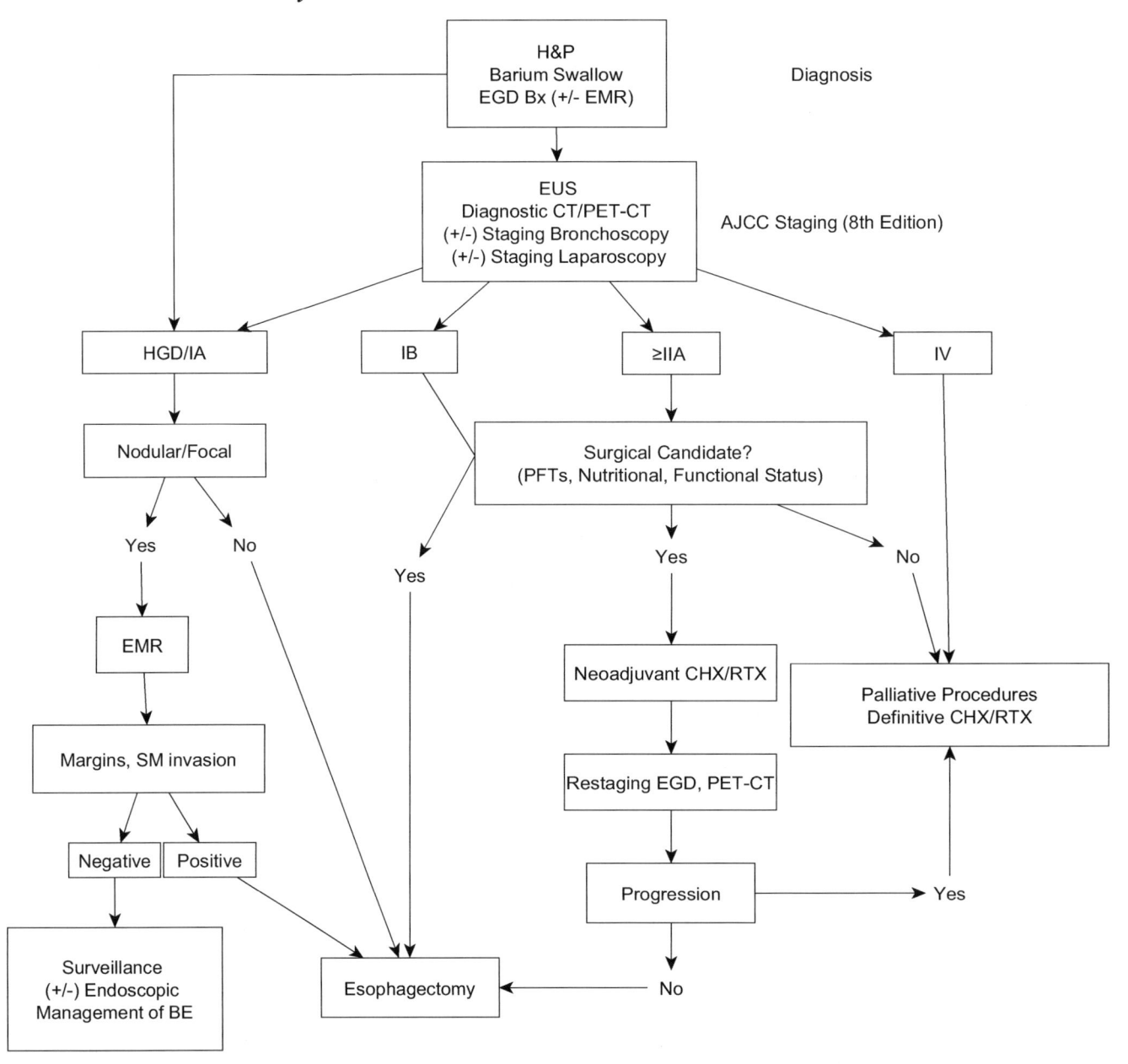

H&P, history and physical; EGD, esophagogastroduodenoscopy; Bx, biopsy; EUS, endoscopic ultrasound; PET-CT, positron emission tomography-computed tomography; AJCC, American Joint Committee on Cancer; HGD, high-grade dysplasia; PFTs, pulmonary function tests; EMR, endoscopic mucosal resection; CHX/RTX, chemotherapy/radiotherapy, BE, Barrett's Esophagus
If EMR is initial biopsy and reveals HGD or IA EAC then proceed to endoscopic therapy

Post Esophagectomy Anastomotic Leak
Mark Mankins, Thomas Birdas

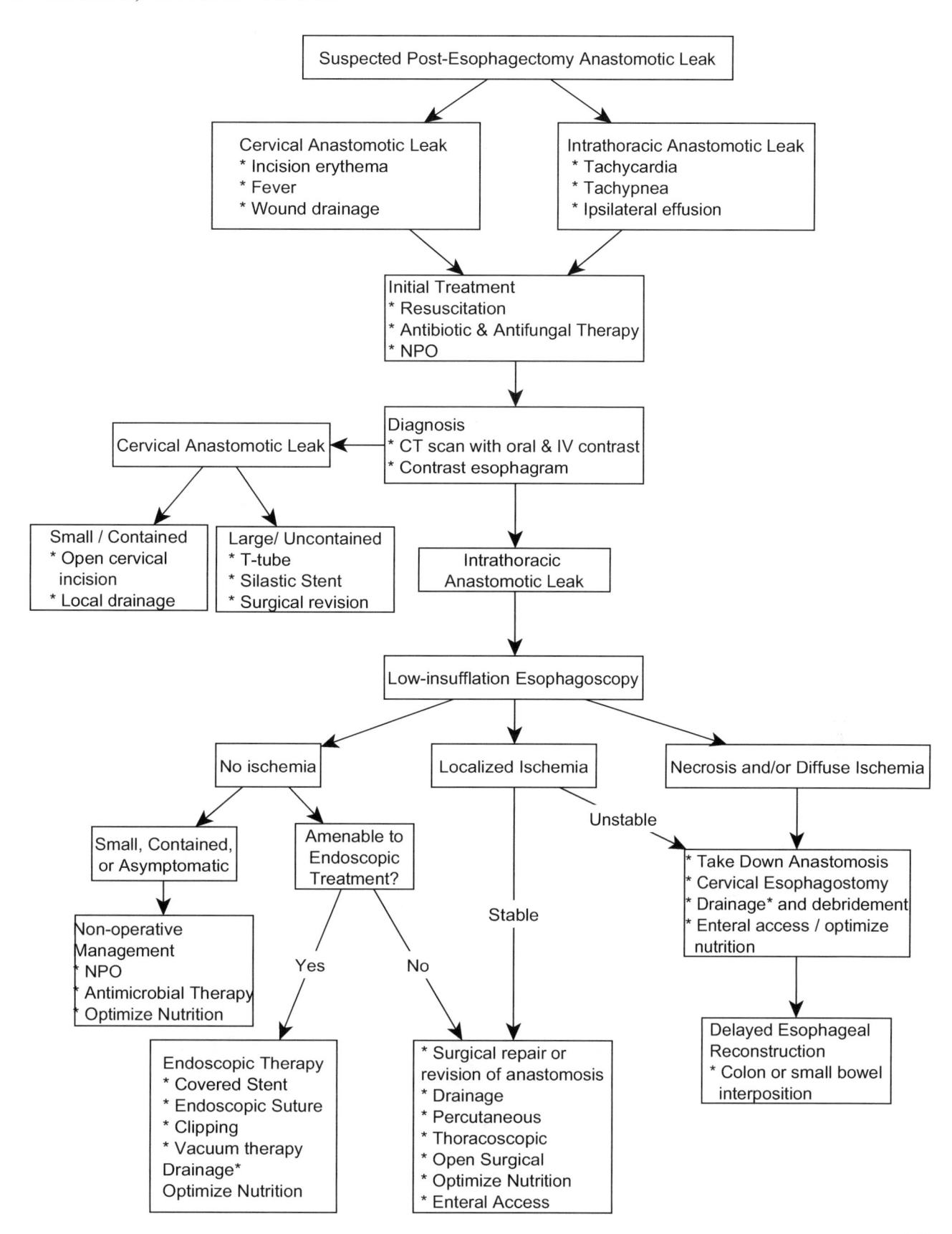

```
                    Suspected Post-Esophagectomy Anastomotic Leak
                             /                            \
          Cervical Anastomotic Leak          Intrathoracic Anastomotic Leak
          * Incision erythema                * Tachycardia
          * Fever                            * Tachypnea
          * Wound drainage                   * Ipsilateral effusion
                             \                            /
                          Initial Treatment
                          * Resuscitation
                          * Antibiotic & Antifungal Therapy
                          * NPO
                                    |
                                    v
                          Diagnosis
   Cervical Anastomotic Leak  <-- * CT scan with oral & IV contrast
         /         \              * Contrast esophagram
                                    |
  Small / Contained   Large/ Uncontained     v
  * Open cervical     * T-tube        Intrathoracic
    incision          * Silastic Stent  Anastomotic Leak
  * Local drainage    * Surgical revision    |
                                             v
                          Low-insufflation Esophagoscopy
                       /              |                \
              No ischemia      Localized Ischemia    Necrosis and/or Diffuse Ischemia
             /      \             Unstable \              |
  Small,         Amenable to                 \     * Take Down Anastomosis
  Contained,     Endoscopic                   \    * Cervical Esophagostomy
  or Asymptomatic Treatment?                   \   * Drainage* and debridement
       |         /      \                       \  * Enteral access / optimize
  Non-operative Yes      No    Stable              nutrition
  Management                                            |
  * NPO                                                 v
  * Antimicrobial Therapy                       Delayed Esophageal
  * Optimize Nutrition                          Reconstruction
                                                * Colon or small bowel
      Endoscopic Therapy    * Surgical repair or   interposition
      * Covered Stent         revision of anastomosis
      * Endoscopic Suture    * Drainage
      * Clipping             * Percutaneous
      * Vacuum therapy       * Thoracoscopic
      Drainage*              * Open Surgical
      Optimize Nutrition     * Optimize Nutrition
                             * Enteral Access
```

153

Gastroesophageal Reflux Disease
Robert Lyons, Jane Yanagawa

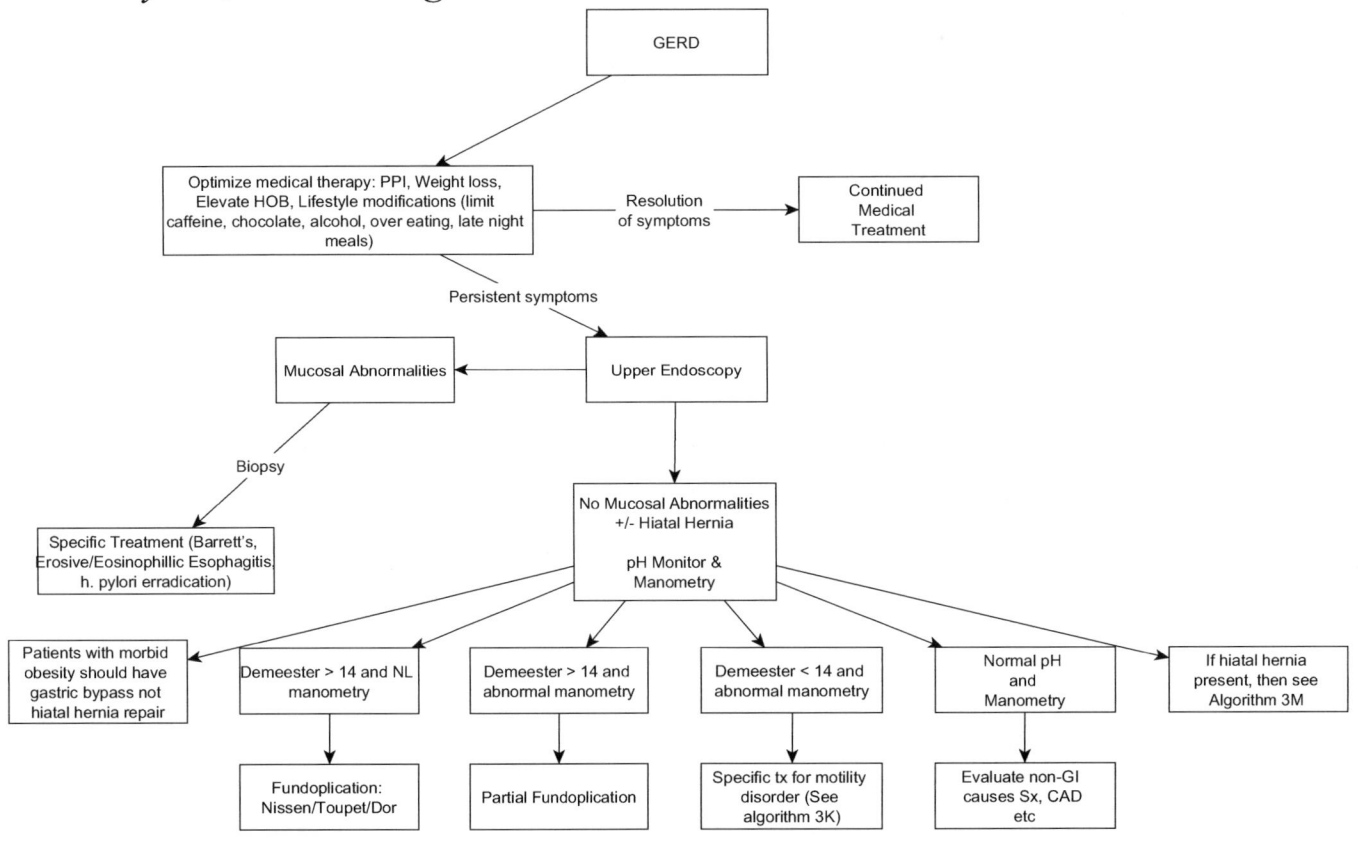

```
                          ┌──────────┐
                          │   GERD   │
                          └────┬─────┘
                               │
                               ▼
  ┌─────────────────────────────────────────────────┐    Resolution      ┌────────────┐
  │ Optimize medical therapy: PPI, Weight loss,     │ ─of symptoms──▶   │ Continued  │
  │ Elevate HOB, Lifestyle modifications (limit     │                    │  Medical   │
  │ caffeine, chocolate, alcohol, over eating,      │                    │ Treatment  │
  │ late night meals)                               │                    └────────────┘
  └─────────────────────────┬───────────────────────┘
                            │ Persistent symptoms
                            ▼
  ┌──────────────────────┐      ┌──────────────────┐
  │ Mucosal Abnormalities│◀─────│ Upper Endoscopy  │
  └──────────┬───────────┘      └────────┬─────────┘
             │ Biopsy                    │
             ▼                           ▼
  ┌──────────────────────┐      ┌─────────────────────────┐
  │ Specific Treatment   │      │ No Mucosal Abnormalities│
  │ (Barrett's,          │      │ +/- Hiatal Hernia       │
  │ Erosive/Eosinophillic│      │ pH Monitor & Manometry  │
  │ Esophagitis,         │      └─────────────────────────┘
  │ h. pylori            │
  │ erradication)        │
  └──────────────────────┘
```

- Patients with morbid obesity should have gastric bypass not hiatal hernia repair
- Demeester > 14 and NL manometry → **Fundoplication: Nissen/Toupet/Dor**
- Demeester > 14 and abnormal manometry → **Partial Fundoplication**
- Demeester < 14 and abnormal manometry → **Specific tx for motility disorder (See algorithm 3K)**
- Normal pH and Manometry → **Evaluate non-GI causes Sx, CAD etc**
- If hiatal hernia present, then see Algorithm 3M

Primary Esophageal Motility Disorders
Michal J. Lada, Carolyn E. Jones

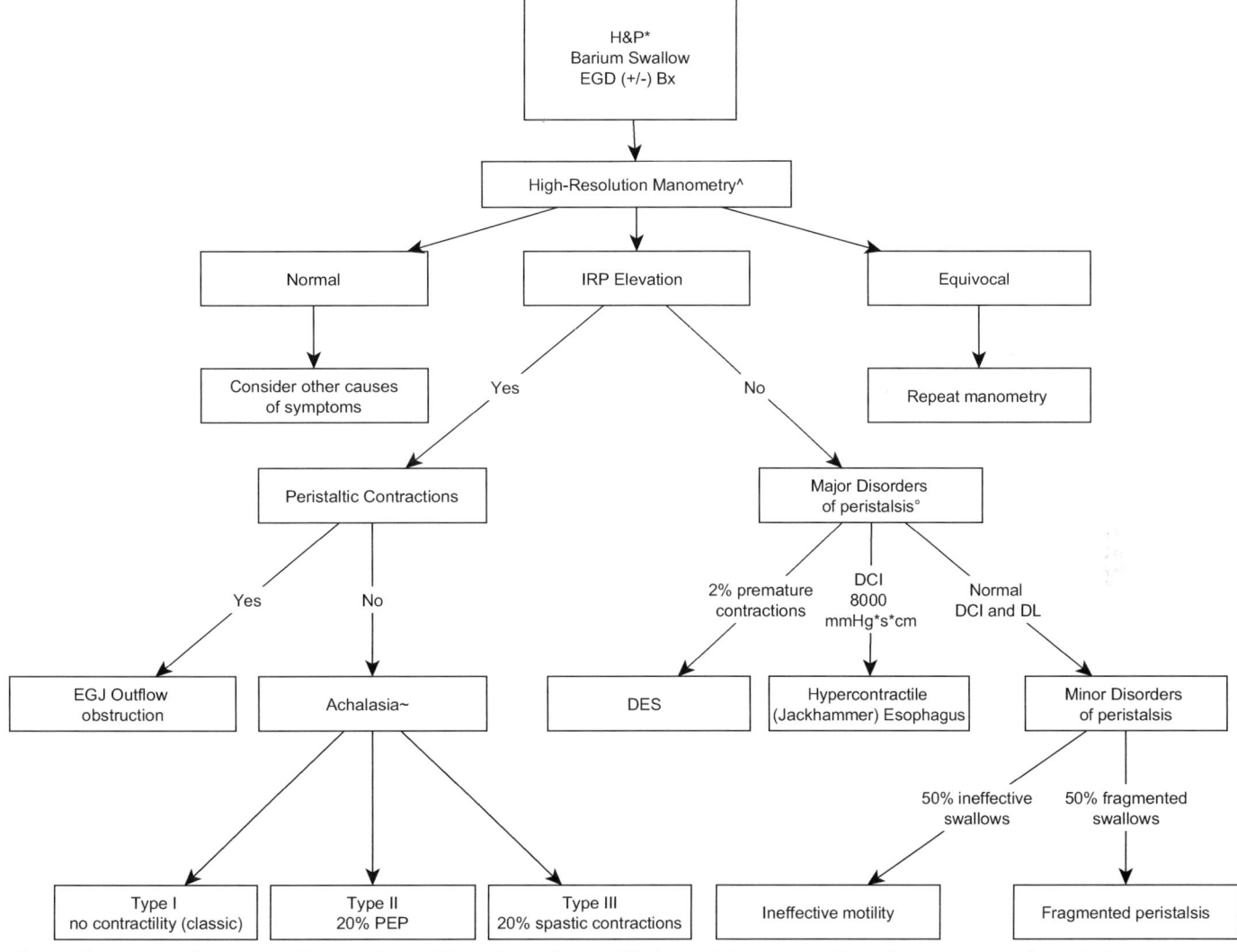

```
                    ┌─────────────────┐
                    │      H&P*       │
                    │  Barium Swallow │
                    │   EGD (+/-) Bx  │
                    └────────┬────────┘
                             ▼
                ┌──────────────────────────┐
                │ High-Resolution Manometry^│
                └──────────┬───────────────┘
         ┌─────────────────┼─────────────────┐
         ▼                 ▼                 ▼
      Normal         IRP Elevation       Equivocal
         │           ┌────┴────┐             │
         ▼          Yes        No            ▼
  Consider other    │          │       Repeat manometry
  causes of         ▼          ▼
  symptoms     Peristaltic  Major Disorders
               Contractions of peristalsis°
               ┌──┴──┐     ┌──────┼──────────┐
              Yes    No    2%    DCI       Normal
               │     │   premature 8000    DCI and DL
               ▼     ▼   contract. mmHg*s*cm    │
          EGJ      Achalasia~  ▼     ▼          ▼
          Outflow              DES  Hyper-    Minor
          obstruction               contractile Disorders
                                    (Jackhammer) of peristalsis
                                    Esophagus   ┌──┴──┐
                                              50%    50%
                                           ineffective fragmented
                                            swallows  swallows
         ┌──────┬──────┐                      ▼         ▼
         ▼      ▼      ▼                  Ineffective Fragmented
       Type I Type II Type III             motility  peristalsis
       no     20% PEP 20% spastic
       contractility  contractions
       (classic)
```

Consider secondary esophageal motility disorders: Chagas Disease, scleroderma, pseudoachalasia, chronic GERD, eosinophilic esophagitis, amyloidosis, sarcoidosis
^ Chicago Classification v3.0
° Treatment options include: calcium channel blockers (Diltiazem), Nitric oxide drugs (Sildenafil, Isosorbide), TCA, Botox injections
~ Treatment options include: dilation, Botox injection, POEM, Heller myotomy

H&P, history and physical; EGD, esophagogastroduodenoscopy; Bx, biopsy; IRP, integrated relaxation pressure; EGJ, esophagogastric junction; DCI, distal contractile integral; DL, distal latency; DES, distal esophageal spasm; PEP, panesophageal pressurization; TCA, tricyclic antidepressant; POEM, peroral endoscopic myotomy

Management of Barrett's Esophagus
Michal J. Lada, Carolyn E. Jones

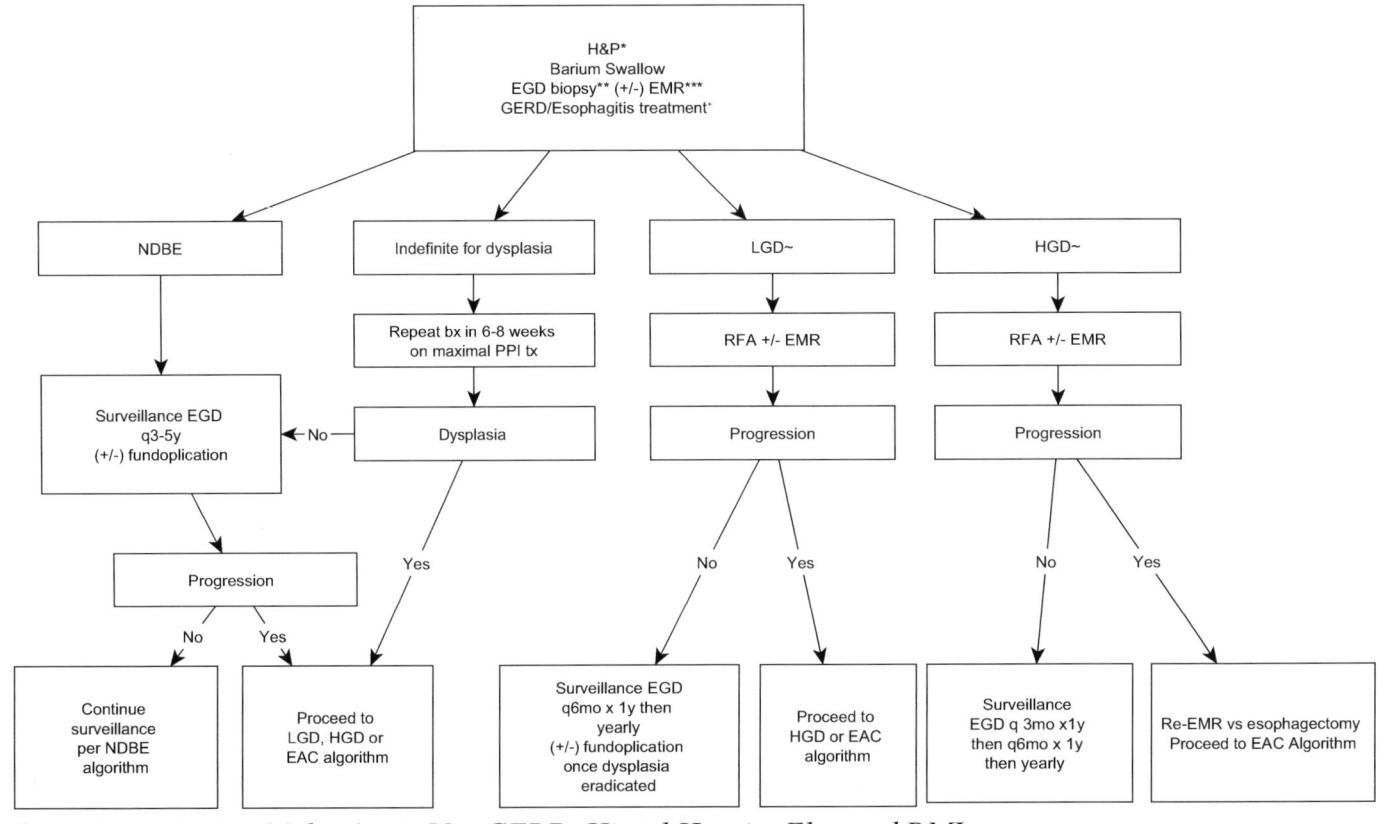

```
                    ┌─────────────────────────────┐
                    │           H&P*              │
                    │      Barium Swallow         │
                    │   EGD biopsy** (+/-) EMR*** │
                    │  GERD/Esophagitis treatment⁺│
                    └─────────────────────────────┘
                    │         │          │          │
                    ▼         ▼          ▼          ▼
                  NDBE    Indefinite    LGD~       HGD~
                          for dysplasia
```

Flow chart outline:

- **NDBE** → Surveillance EGD q3-5y (+/-) fundoplication → Progression?
  - No → Continue surveillance per NDBE algorithm
  - Yes → Proceed to LGD, HGD or EAC algorithm

- **Indefinite for dysplasia** → Repeat bx in 6-8 weeks on maximal PPI tx → Dysplasia?
  - No → Surveillance EGD q3-5y (+/-) fundoplication
  - Yes → Proceed to LGD, HGD or EAC algorithm

- **LGD~** → RFA +/- EMR → Progression?
  - No → Surveillance EGD q6mo x 1y then yearly (+/-) fundoplication once dysplasia eradicated
  - Yes → Proceed to HGD or EAC algorithm

- **HGD~** → RFA +/- EMR → Progression?
  - No → Surveillance EGD q 3mo x1y then q6mo x 1y then yearly
  - Yes → Re-EMR vs esophagectomy Proceed to EAC Algorithm

Screening criteria: Male, Age >50y, GERD, Hiatal Hernia, Elevated BMI
° *Seattle Protocol: Four-quadrant biopsies every 1cm for length of BE*
^ *If EMR is initial biopsy*
⁺ *See Management of GERD Algorithm*
~ *Confirmed by a second experienced esophageal histopathologist. Some societal guidelines support either surveillance or ablation of low-grade dysplasia*

H&P, history and physical; GERD, gastroesophageal reflux disease; EGD, esophagogastroduodenoscopy; Bx, biopsy; EMR, endoscopic mucosal resection; BE, Barrett's Esophagus; NDBE, non-dysplastic Barrett's Esophagus; LGD, low-grade dysplasia; HGD, high-grade dysplasia; PPI, proton-pump inhibitor; RFA, radiofrequency ablation; EAC, esophageal adenocarcinoma; Tx, therapy

Management of Paraesophageal Hernia
Jennifer Dixon, Parth Amin

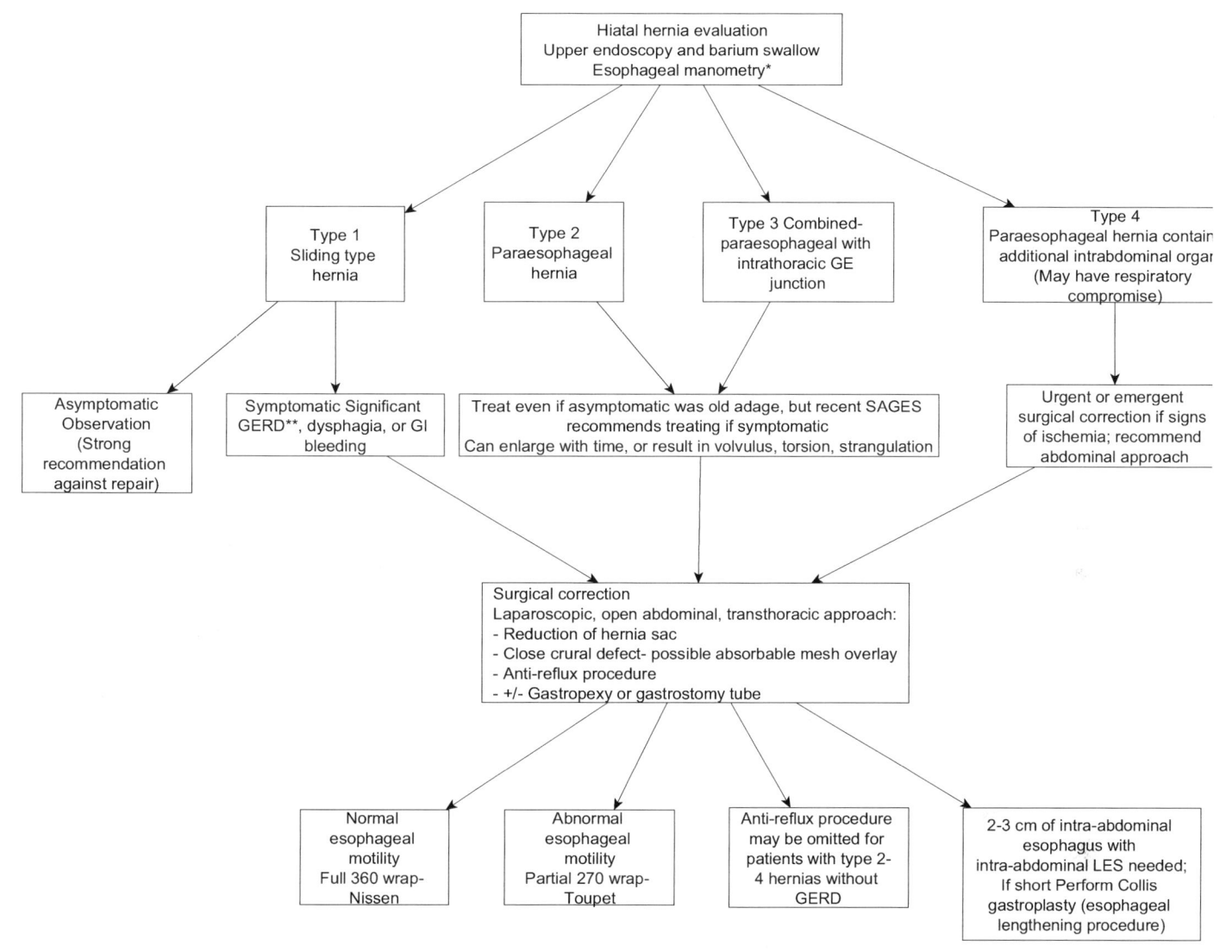

```
                    ┌─────────────────────────────────┐
                    │   Hiatal hernia evaluation      │
                    │ Upper endoscopy and barium swallow │
                    │     Esophageal manometry*       │
                    └─────────────────────────────────┘
              ┌───────────┬──────────┴──────────┬────────────┐
              ▼           ▼                     ▼            ▼
       ┌──────────┐  ┌──────────┐      ┌──────────────┐  ┌──────────────┐
       │  Type 1  │  │  Type 2  │      │Type 3 Combined-│  │   Type 4    │
       │ Sliding  │  │Paraesoph.│      │paraesophageal │  │Paraesophageal│
       │  type    │  │ hernia   │      │ with intra-   │  │hernia contain│
       │ hernia   │  │          │      │thoracic GE jxn│  │additional    │
       └──────────┘  └──────────┘      └──────────────┘  │intrabdominal │
                                                          │organ (May    │
                                                          │have respir.  │
                                                          │compromise)   │
                                                          └──────────────┘
```

- **Type 1 → Asymptomatic**: Observation (Strong recommendation against repair)
- **Type 1 → Symptomatic** Significant GERD**, dysphagia, or GI bleeding
- **Type 2, 3**: Treat even if asymptomatic was old adage, but recent SAGES recommends treating if symptomatic. Can enlarge with time, or result in volvulus, torsion, strangulation
- **Type 4**: Urgent or emergent surgical correction if signs of ischemia; recommend abdominal approach

Surgical correction
Laparoscopic, open abdominal, transthoracic approach:
- Reduction of hernia sac
- Close crural defect- possible absorbable mesh overlay
- Anti-reflux procedure
- +/- Gastropexy or gastrostomy tube

Branches from Surgical correction:
- Normal esophageal motility — Full 360 wrap- Nissen
- Abnormal esophageal motility — Partial 270 wrap- Toupet
- Anti-reflux procedure may be omitted for patients with type 2-4 hernias without GERD
- 2-3 cm of intra-abdominal esophagus with intra-abdominal LES needed; If short Perform Collis gastroplasty (esophageal lengthening procedure)

All patients should have esophageal manometry unless type 2 paraesophageal hernia with normal contrast swallow- SAGES expert consensus
** Significant GERD diagnosed by pH probe, or EGD signs of erosive esophagitis or Barrett's esophagus

Spontaneous Pneumomediastinum
Velu Balasubramanian, Kalpaj Parekh

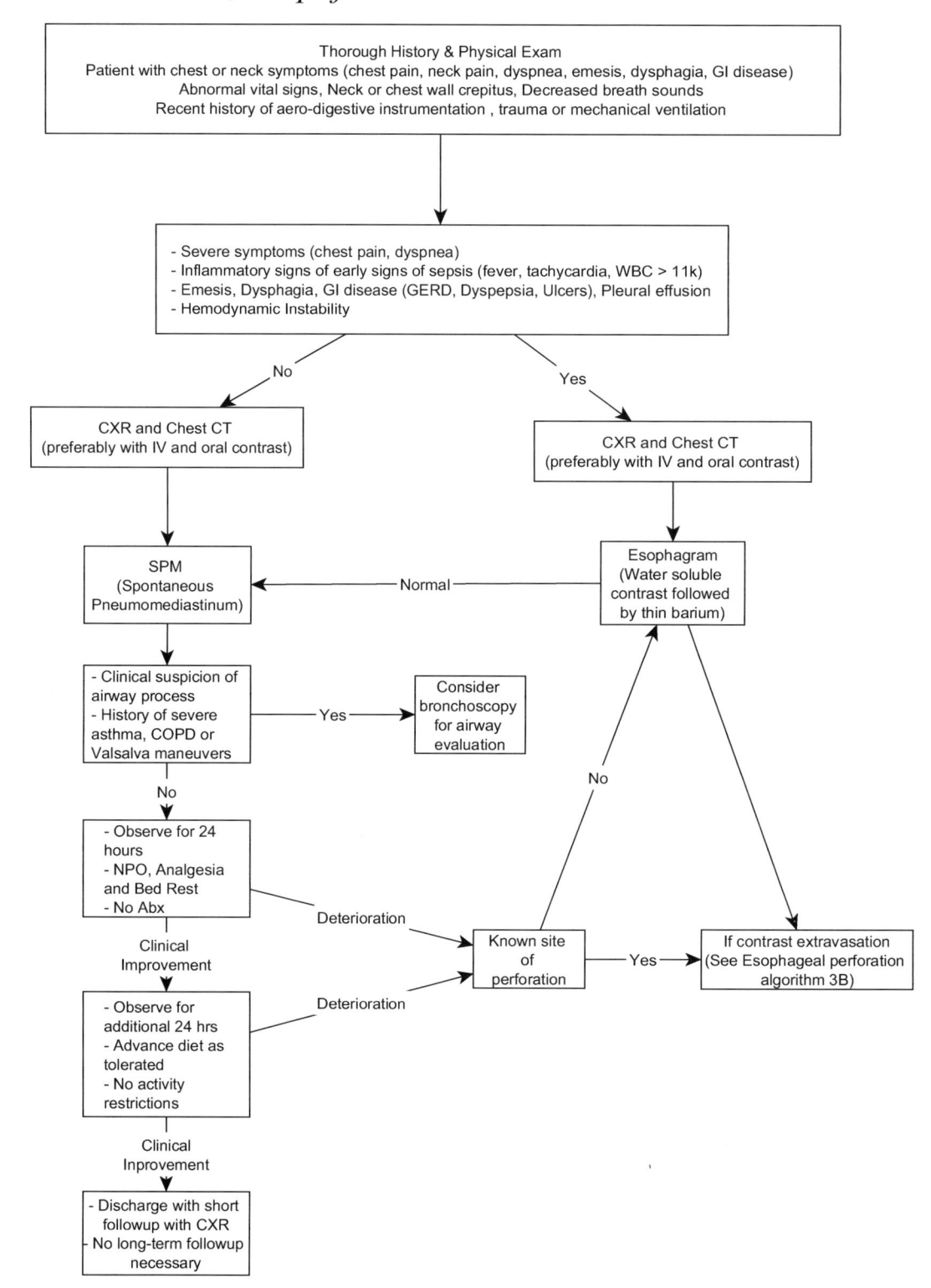

```
┌─────────────────────────────────────────────────────────────────────┐
│                    Thorough History & Physical Exam                 │
│ Patient with chest or neck symptoms (chest pain, neck pain,         │
│   dyspnea, emesis, dysphagia, GI disease)                           │
│ Abnormal vital signs, Neck or chest wall crepitus,                  │
│   Decreased breath sounds                                           │
│ Recent history of aero-digestive instrumentation, trauma            │
│   or mechanical ventilation                                         │
└─────────────────────────────────────────────────────────────────────┘
                                  │
                                  ▼
┌─────────────────────────────────────────────────────────────────────┐
│ - Severe symptoms (chest pain, dyspnea)                             │
│ - Inflammatory signs of early signs of sepsis (fever,               │
│   tachycardia, WBC > 11k)                                           │
│ - Emesis, Dysphagia, GI disease (GERD, Dyspepsia, Ulcers),          │
│   Pleural effusion                                                  │
│ - Hemodynamic Instability                                           │
└─────────────────────────────────────────────────────────────────────┘
              │ No                                  │ Yes
              ▼                                     ▼
    ┌──────────────────────┐            ┌──────────────────────┐
    │ CXR and Chest CT     │            │ CXR and Chest CT     │
    │ (preferably with IV  │            │ (preferably with IV  │
    │ and oral contrast)   │            │ and oral contrast)   │
    └──────────────────────┘            └──────────────────────┘
              │                                     │
              ▼                                     ▼
    ┌──────────────────┐                  ┌──────────────────┐
    │ SPM              │◄──── Normal ─────│ Esophagram       │
    │ (Spontaneous     │                  │ (Water soluble   │
    │ Pneumomediastinum)│                 │ contrast followed│
    └──────────────────┘                  │ by thin barium)  │
              │                           └──────────────────┘
              ▼
    ┌──────────────────┐    ┌──────────────┐
    │ - Clinical       │    │ Consider     │
    │   suspicion of   │───▶│ bronchoscopy │
    │   airway process │ Yes│ for airway   │
    │ - History of     │    │ evaluation   │
    │   severe asthma, │    └──────────────┘
    │   COPD or        │
    │   Valsalva       │
    │   maneuvers      │
    └──────────────────┘
              │ No
              ▼
    ┌──────────────────┐
    │ - Observe for 24 │
    │   hours          │
    │ - NPO, Analgesia │
    │   and Bed Rest   │       Deterioration
    │ - No Abx         │────────────────────┐
    └──────────────────┘                    │
         Clinical                           ▼
         Improvement              ┌──────────────────┐        ┌──────────────────────┐
              │                   │ Known site       │        │ If contrast          │
              ▼                   │ of           Yes │───────▶│ extravasation        │
    ┌──────────────────┐          │ perforation      │        │ (See Esophageal      │
    │ - Observe for    │          └──────────────────┘        │ perforation          │
    │   additional     │                   ▲                  │ algorithm 3B)        │
    │   24 hrs         │ Deterioration     │ No               └──────────────────────┘
    │ - Advance diet   │───────────────────┘                           ▲
    │   as tolerated   │                                               │
    │ - No activity    │                                               │
    │   restrictions   │                                               │
    └──────────────────┘                                               │
         Clinical                                                      │
         Inprovement                                                   │
              ▼
    ┌──────────────────┐
    │ - Discharge with │
    │   short followup │
    │   with CXR       │
    │ - No long-term   │
    │   followup       │
    │   necessary      │
    └──────────────────┘
```

*** - See the TSRA algorithm for Esophageal Perforation for more details
SPM – Spontaneous Pneumomediastinum; Defined as pneumomediastinum that is not caused by trauma, mechanical ventilation or recent instrumentation of the aero-digestive tract, CXR – Chest X-ray; CT – Computed Tomography; Abx – Antibiotics; NPO – Nil Per Os

Diaphragmatic Injury
Shane P. Smith, Alexander S. Farivar

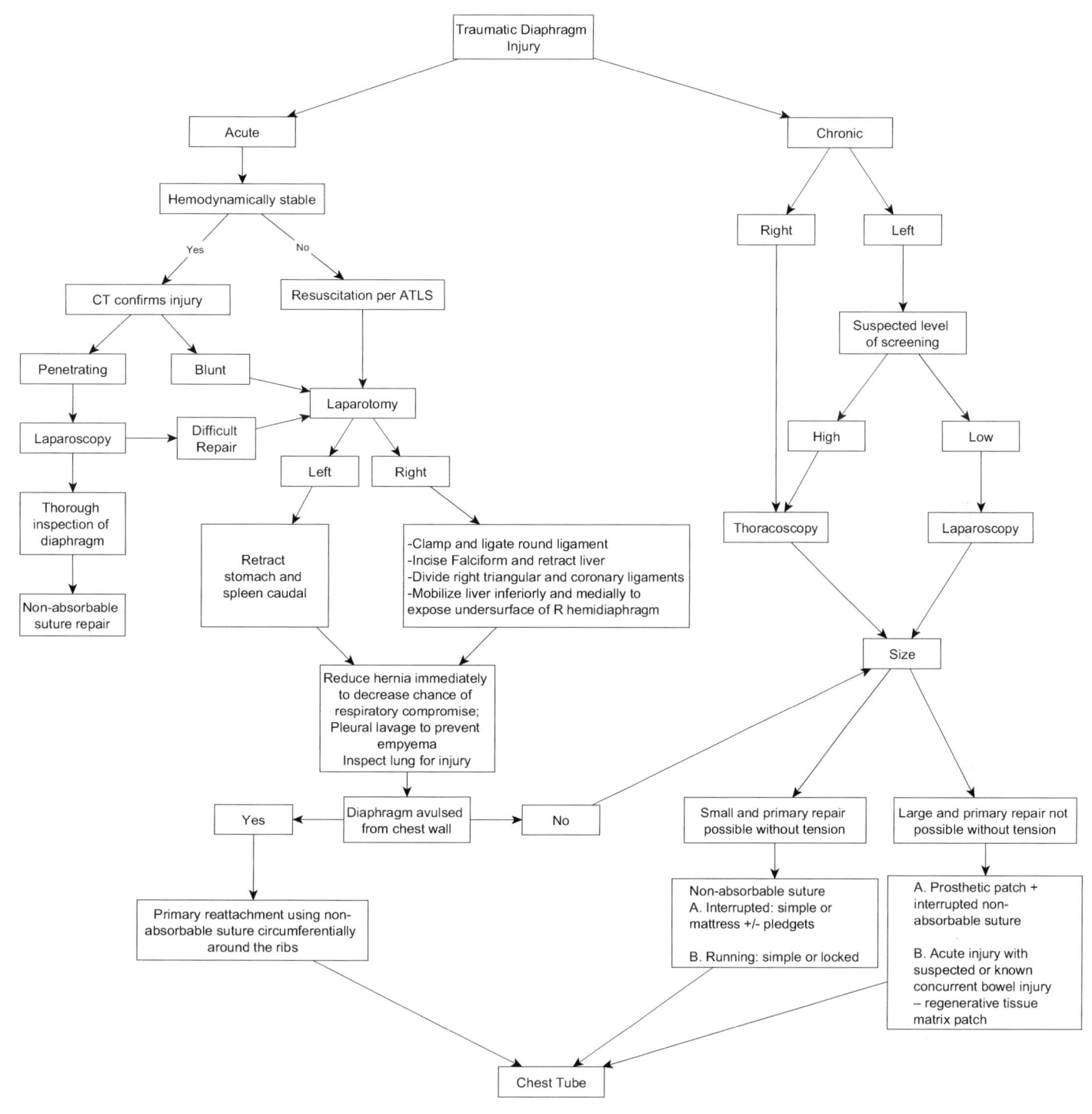

```
                          Traumatic Diaphragm
                                Injury
                         /                  \
                       Acute              Chronic
                        |                /      \
              Hemodynamically stable   Right    Left
                  /        \             \       |
                Yes         No            \   Suspected level
                 |           |             \   of screening
          CT confirms    Resuscitation      \   /      \
             injury      per ATLS          High       Low
            /      \          |             |           |
      Penetrating Blunt      Laparotomy  Thoracoscopy Laparoscopy
          |         \         /    \
      Laparoscopy  Difficult Left  Right
          |         Repair    |      |
      Thorough                |   -Clamp and ligate round ligament
      inspection              |   -Incise Falciform and retract liver
      of diaphragm            |   -Divide right triangular and coronary ligaments
          |               Retract  -Mobilize liver inferiorly and medially to
      Non-absorbable      stomach   expose undersurface of R hemidiaphragm
      suture repair       and spleen
                          caudal
                            \       /
                        Reduce hernia immediately
                        to decrease chance of
                        respiratory compromise;
                        Pleural lavage to prevent
                        empyema
                        Inspect lung for injury
                                 |
                        Diaphragm avulsed
              Yes  <--  from chest wall  -->  No
               |                                            Size
      Primary reattachment using non-            /                      \
      absorbable suture circumferentially    Small and primary    Large and primary repair
      around the ribs                        repair possible      not possible without tension
               |                              without tension            |
               |                                    |             A. Prosthetic patch +
               |                          Non-absorbable suture      interrupted non-
               |                          A. Interrupted: simple     absorbable suture
               |                             or mattress +/- pledgets
               |                          B. Running: simple         B. Acute injury with
               |                             or locked                  suspected or known
               |                                                        concurrent bowel injury
               |                                                        – regenerative tissue
               |                                                        matrix patch
               _____   Chest Tube  _____/
```

159

Anterior Mediastinal Mass
Carlo Rosati, Kenneth Kesler

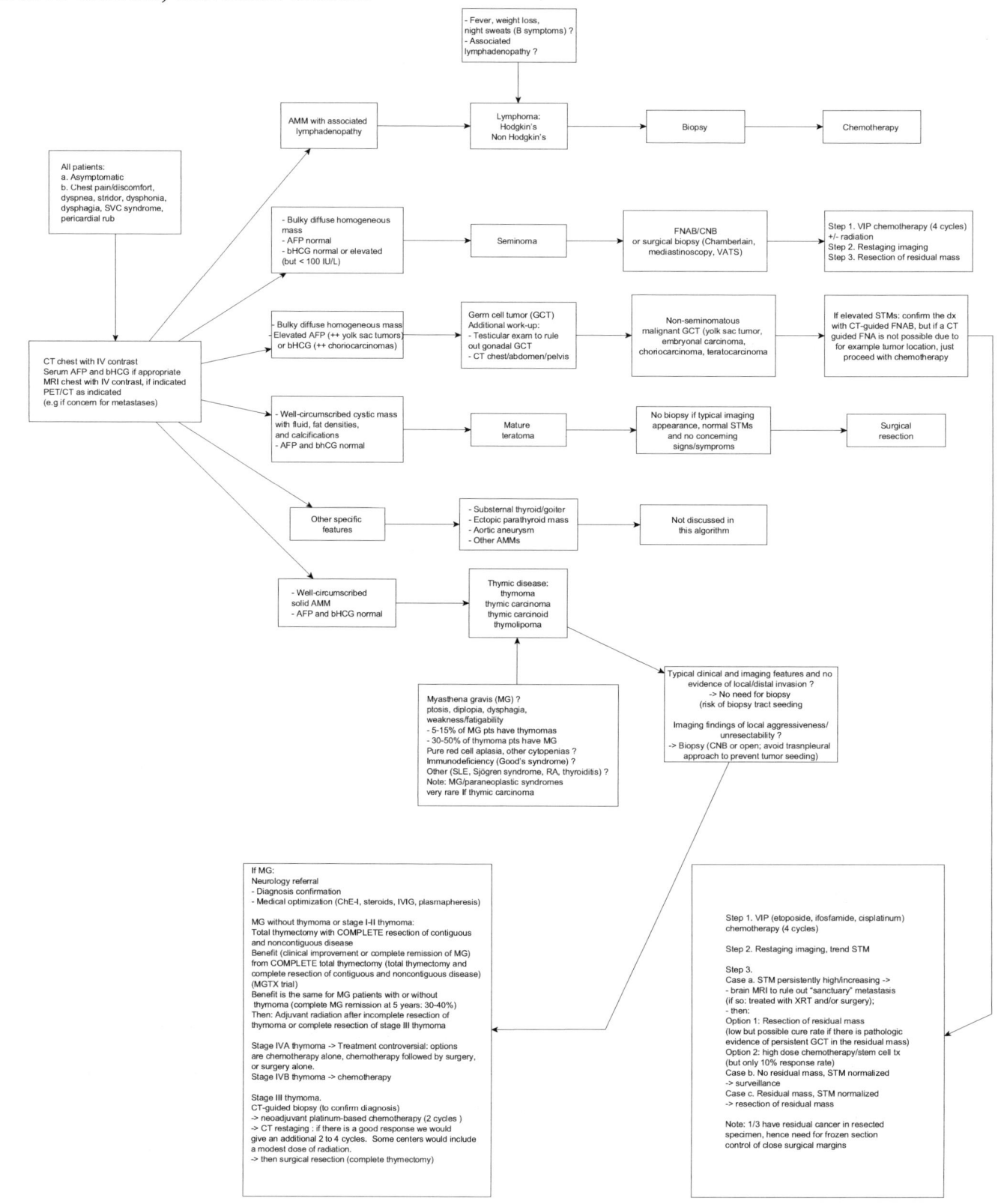

```
                                           ┌─────────────────────────┐
                                           │ - Fever, weight loss,   │
                                           │ night sweats (B symptoms)?│
                                           │ - Associated            │
                                           │ lymphadenopathy?        │
                                           └───────────┬─────────────┘
                                                       ↓
                      ┌──────────────────┐   ┌──────────────────┐   ┌──────────┐   ┌──────────────┐
                      │ AMM with associated├──▶│ Lymphoma:        │──▶│ Biopsy   │──▶│ Chemotherapy │
                      │ lymphadenopathy   │   │ Hodgkin's        │   └──────────┘   └──────────────┘
                      └──────────────────┘   │ Non Hodgkin's    │
                                             └──────────────────┘
```

All patients:
a. Asymptomatic
b. Chest pain/discomfort, dyspnea, stridor, dysphonia, dysphagia, SVC syndrome, pericardial rub

CT chest with IV contrast
Serum AFP and bHCG if appropriate
MRI chest with IV contrast, if indicated
PET/CT as indicated
(e.g if concern for metastases)

Branches:

- Bulky diffuse homogeneous mass
  - AFP normal
  - bHCG normal or elevated (but < 100 IU/L)
  → **Seminoma** → FNAB/CNB or surgical biopsy (Chamberlain, mediastinoscopy, VATS) →
  Step 1. VIP chemotherapy (4 cycles) +/- radiation
  Step 2. Restaging imaging
  Step 3. Resection of residual mass

- Bulky diffuse homogeneous mass
  - Elevated AFP (++ yolk sac tumors) or bHCG (++ choriocarcinomas)
  → **Germ cell tumor (GCT)** Additional work-up:
  - Testicular exam to rule out gonadal GCT
  - CT chest/abdomen/pelvis
  → **Non-seminomatous malignant GCT** (yolk sac tumor, embryonal carcinoma, choriocarcinoma, teratocarcinoma)
  → If elevated STMs: confirm the dx with CT-guided FNAB, but if a CT guided FNA is not possible due to for example tumor location, just proceed with chemotherapy

- Well-circumscribed cystic mass with fluid, fat densities, and calcifications
  - AFP and bhCG normal
  → **Mature teratoma** → No biopsy if typical imaging appearance, normal STMs and no concerning signs/symproms → **Surgical resection**

- **Other specific features:**
  - Substernal thyroid/goiter
  - Ectopic parathyroid mass
  - Aortic aneurysm
  - Other AMMs
  → Not discussed in this algorithm

- Well-circumscribed solid AMM
  - AFP and bHCG normal
  → **Thymic disease:** thymoma, thymic carcinoma, thymic carcinoid, thymolipoma

Myasthena gravis (MG)?
ptosis, diplopia, dysphagia, weakness/fatigability
- 5-15% of MG pts have thymomas
- 30-50% of thymoma pts have MG
Pure red cell aplasia, other cytopenias?
Immunodeficiency (Good's syndrome)?
Other (SLE, Sjögren syndrome, RA, thyroiditis)?
Note: MG/paraneoplastic syndromes very rare If thymic carcinoma

Typical clinical and imaging features and no evidence of local/distal invasion?
→ No need for biopsy (risk of biopsy tract seeding)

Imaging findings of local aggressiveness/ unresectability?
→ Biopsy (CNB or open; avoid trasnpleural approach to prevent tumor seeding)

If MG:
Neurology referral
- Diagnosis confirmation
- Medical optimization (ChE-I, steroids, IVIG, plasmapheresis)

MG without thymoma or stage I-II thymoma:
Total thymectomy with COMPLETE resection of contiguous and noncontiguous disease
Benefit (clinical improvement or complete remission of MG) from COMPLETE total thymectomy (total thymectomy and complete resection of contiguous and noncontiguous disease) (MGTX trial)
Benefit is the same for MG patients with or without thymoma (complete MG remission at 5 years: 30-40%)
Then: Adjuvant radiation after incomplete resection of thymoma or complete resection of stage III thymoma

Stage IVA thymoma → Treatment controversial: options are chemotherapy alone, chemotherapy followed by surgery, or surgery alone.
Stage IVB thymoma → chemotherapy

Stage III thymoma.
CT-guided biopsy (to confirm diagnosis)
→ neoadjuvant platinum-based chemotherapy (2 cycles)
→ CT restaging ; if there is a good response we would give an additional 2 to 4 cycles. Some centers would include a modest dose of radiation.
→ then surgical resection (complete thymectomy)

Step 1. VIP (etoposide, ifosfamide, cisplatinum) chemotherapy (4 cycles)

Step 2. Restaging imaging, trend STM

Step 3.
Case a. STM persistently high/increasing →
- brain MRI to rule out "sanctuary" metastasis (if so: treated with XRT and/or surgery);
- then:
Option 1: Resection of residual mass (low but possible cure rate if there is pathologic evidence of persistent GCT in the residual mass)
Option 2: high dose chemotherapy/stem cell tx (but only 10% response rate)
Case b. No residual mass, STM normalized
→ surveillance
Case c. Residual mass, STM normalized
→ resection of residual mass

Note: 1/3 have residual cancer in resected specimen, hence need for frozen section control of close surgical margins

Surgical approach
Fairly localized-> Sternotomy
Larger masses extending into pleural space or pulmonary hilum -> Clamshell thoracotomy
Consider VATS/robotic, without compromising oncologic principles

AMM- anterior mediastinal mass; AFP- alpha fetoprotein; bHCG- beta human chorionic gonadotropin; ChE-I - cholinesterase inhibitor; CNB- core needle biopsy; FNAB- fine needle aspiration biopsy; GCT- germ cell tumor; IVIG- intravenous immunoglobulin; MG- myasthenia gravis; RA- rheumatoid arthritis; SLE- systemic lupus erythematosus; STM- serum tumor markers; VIP- etoposide, ifosfamide, cisplatinum

Thoracic Outlet Syndrome
Shane P. Smith, Kaj H. Johansen

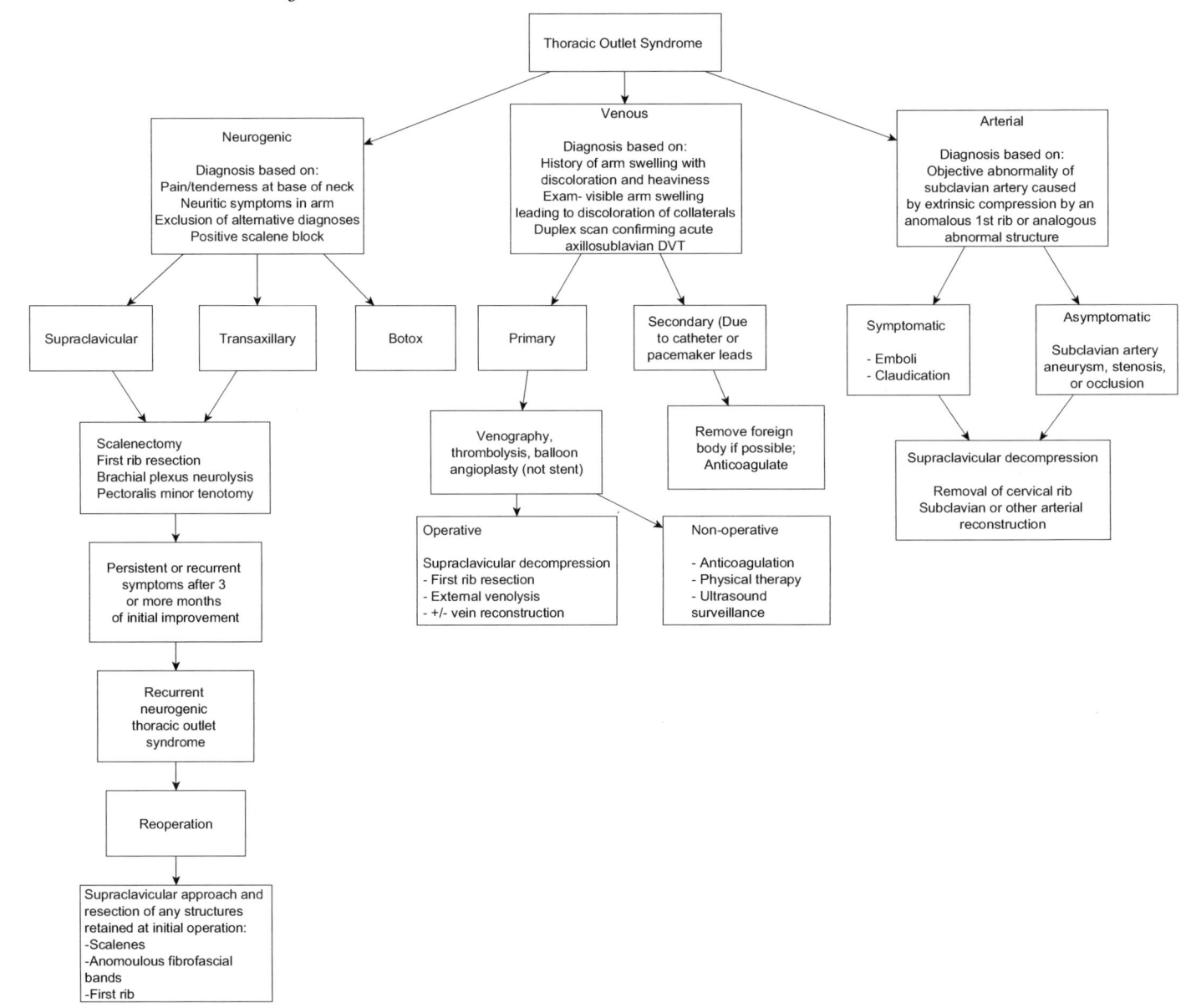

```
                          ┌─────────────────────────┐
                          │ Thoracic Outlet Syndrome│
                          └───────────┬─────────────┘
        ┌─────────────────────────────┼─────────────────────────────┐
        ▼                             ▼                             ▼
┌──────────────────┐         ┌──────────────────┐         ┌──────────────────┐
│   Neurogenic     │         │      Venous      │         │     Arterial     │
│                  │         │                  │         │                  │
│ Diagnosis based  │         │ Diagnosis based  │         │ Diagnosis based  │
│ on:              │         │ on:              │         │ on:              │
│ Pain/tenderness  │         │ History of arm   │         │ Objective        │
│ at base of neck  │         │ swelling with    │         │ abnormality of   │
│ Neuritic         │         │ discoloration    │         │ subclavian       │
│ symptoms in arm  │         │ and heaviness    │         │ artery caused    │
│ Exclusion of     │         │ Exam- visible    │         │ by extrinsic     │
│ alternative      │         │ arm swelling     │         │ compression by   │
│ diagnoses        │         │ leading to       │         │ an anomalous 1st │
│ Positive scalene │         │ discoloration of │         │ rib or analogous │
│ block            │         │ collaterals      │         │ abnormal         │
│                  │         │ Duplex scan      │         │ structure        │
│                  │         │ confirming acute │         │                  │
│                  │         │ axillosubclavian │         │                  │
│                  │         │ DVT              │         │                  │
└──────────────────┘         └──────────────────┘         └──────────────────┘
```

Neurogenic branch:
- Supraclavicular
- Transaxillary
- Botox

Scalenectomy
First rib resection
Brachial plexus neurolysis
Pectoralis minor tenotomy

↓

Persistent or recurrent symptoms after 3 or more months of initial improvement

↓

Recurrent neurogenic thoracic outlet syndrome

↓

Reoperation

↓

Supraclavicular approach and resection of any structures retained at initial operation:
- Scalenes
- Anomoulous fibrofascial bands
- First rib

Venous branch:
- **Primary** → Venography, thrombolysis, balloon angioplasty (not stent)
  - Operative: Supraclavicular decompression
    - First rib resection
    - External venolysis
    - +/- vein reconstruction
  - Non-operative:
    - Anticoagulation
    - Physical therapy
    - Ultrasound surveillance
- **Secondary** (Due to catheter or pacemaker leads) → Remove foreign body if possible; Anticoagulate

Arterial branch:
- **Symptomatic**
  - Emboli
  - Claudication
- **Asymptomatic**
  - Subclavian artery aneurysm, stenosis, or occlusion

Supraclavicular decompression
Removal of cervical rib
Subclavian or other arterial reconstruction

Chest Wall Tumors
Panos Vardas, Jennifer Dixon

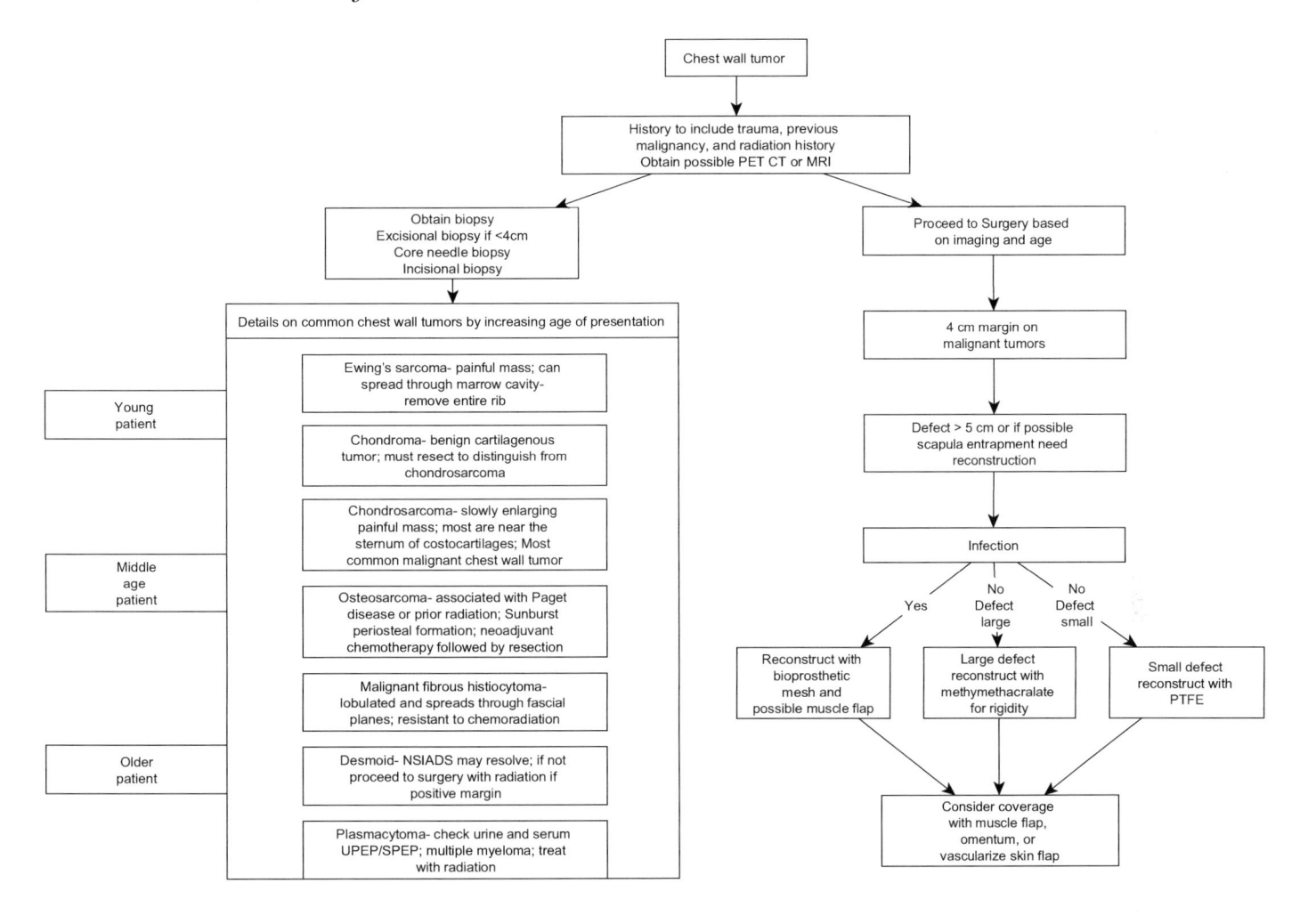

```
                    ┌─────────────────────┐
                    │  Chest wall tumor   │
                    └──────────┬──────────┘
                               ▼
            ┌──────────────────────────────────────┐
            │ History to include trauma, previous  │
            │ malignancy, and radiation history    │
            │ Obtain possible PET CT or MRI        │
            └──────────────────────────────────────┘
                   │                           │
                   ▼                           ▼
     ┌──────────────────────────┐   ┌──────────────────────────┐
     │ Obtain biopsy            │   │ Proceed to Surgery based │
     │ Excisional biopsy if <4cm│   │ on imaging and age       │
     │ Core needle biopsy       │   └────────────┬─────────────┘
     │ Incisional biopsy        │                ▼
     └──────────────────────────┘   ┌──────────────────────────┐
                                    │ 4 cm margin on           │
                                    │ malignant tumors         │
                                    └────────────┬─────────────┘
                                                 ▼
                                    ┌──────────────────────────┐
                                    │ Defect > 5 cm or if      │
                                    │ possible scapula         │
                                    │ entrapment need          │
                                    │ reconstruction           │
                                    └────────────┬─────────────┘
                                                 ▼
                                         ┌───────────────┐
                                         │   Infection   │
                                         └───────┬───────┘
```

Details on common chest wall tumors by increasing age of presentation

Young patient
- Ewing's sarcoma- painful mass; can spread through marrow cavity- remove entire rib
- Chondroma- benign cartilagenous tumor; must resect to distinguish from chondrosarcoma

Middle age patient
- Chondrosarcoma- slowly enlarging painful mass; most are near the sternum of costocartilages; Most common malignant chest wall tumor
- Osteosarcoma- associated with Paget disease or prior radiation; Sunburst periosteal formation; neoadjuvant chemotherapy followed by resection
- Malignant fibrous histiocytoma- lobulated and spreads through fascial planes; resistant to chemoradiation

Older patient
- Desmoid- NSIADS may resolve; if not proceed to surgery with radiation if positive margin
- Plasmacytoma- check urine and serum UPEP/SPEP; multiple myeloma; treat with radiation

Infection:
- **Yes**: Reconstruct with bioprosthetic mesh and possible muscle flap
- **No Defect large**: Large defect reconstruct with methymethacralate for rigidity
- **No Defect small**: Small defect reconstruct with PTFE

Consider coverage with muscle flap, omentum, or vascularize skin flap

Patent Ductus Arteriosus
Awais Ashfaq, Ashok Muralidaran

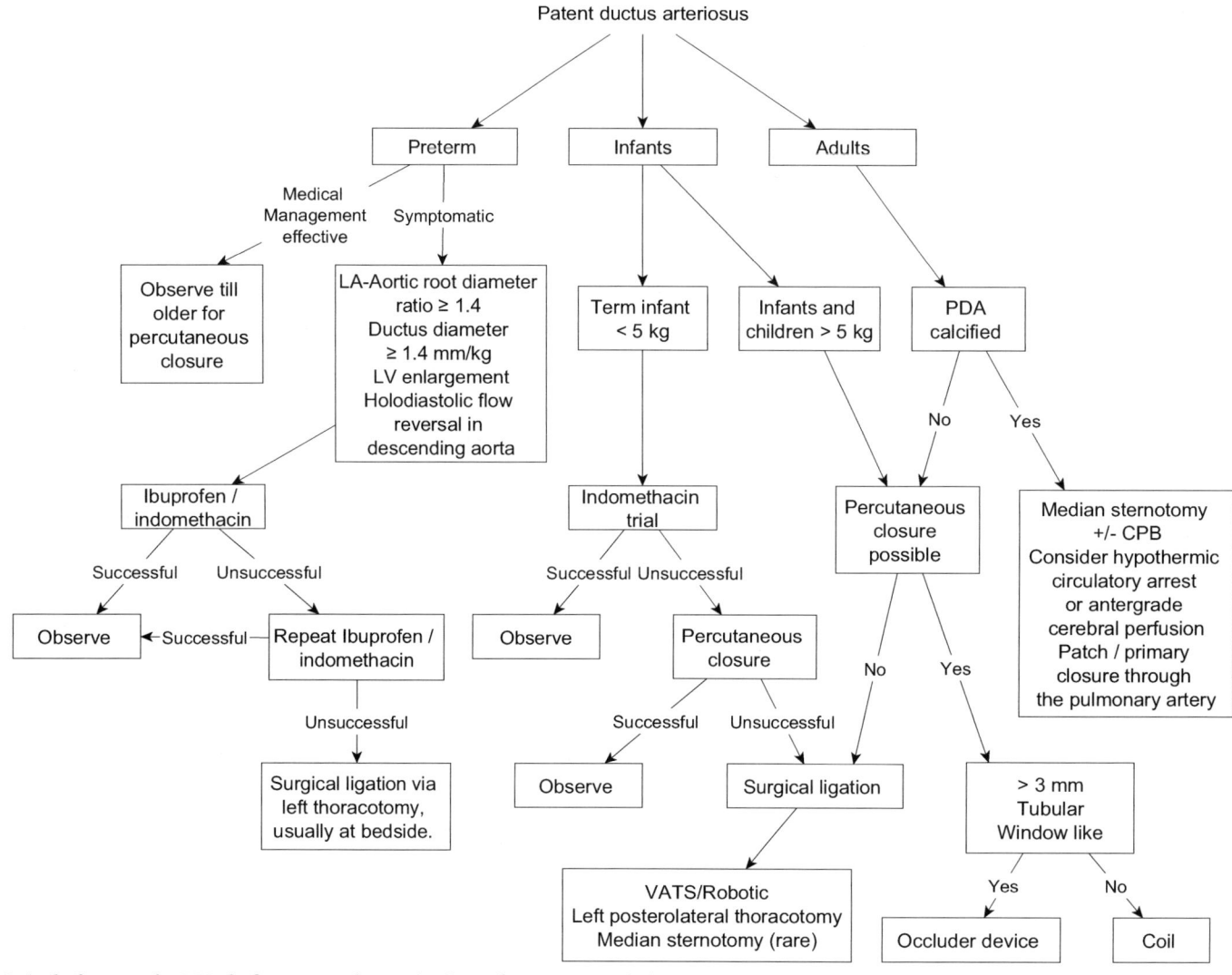

```
                        Patent ductus arteriosus
              ┌──────────────────┼──────────────────┐
           Preterm            Infants             Adults
```

Preterm:
- Medical Management effective → Observe till older for percutaneous closure
- Symptomatic → LA-Aortic root diameter ratio ≥ 1.4; Ductus diameter ≥ 1.4 mm/kg; LV enlargement; Holodiastolic flow reversal in descending aorta → Ibuprofen / indomethacin
  - Successful → Observe
  - Unsuccessful → Repeat Ibuprofen / indomethacin
    - Successful → Observe
    - Unsuccessful → Surgical ligation via left thoracotomy, usually at bedside.

Infants:
- Term infant < 5 kg → Indomethacin trial
  - Successful → Observe
  - Unsuccessful → Percutaneous closure
    - Successful → Observe
    - Unsuccessful → Surgical ligation → VATS/Robotic, Left posterolateral thoracotomy, Median sternotomy (rare)
- Infants and children > 5 kg → Percutaneous closure possible
  - No → Surgical ligation
  - Yes → > 3 mm Tubular Window like
    - Yes → Occluder device
    - No → Coil

Adults:
- PDA calcified
  - No → Percutaneous closure possible (see above)
  - Yes → Median sternotomy +/- CPB; Consider hypothermic circulatory arrest or antegrade cerebral perfusion; Patch / primary closure through the pulmonary artery

LA, left atrial; LV, left ventricle; VATS, video assisted thoracoscopic surgery

Atrial Septal Defect (ASD)
Sandeep Sainathan, Carl Backer

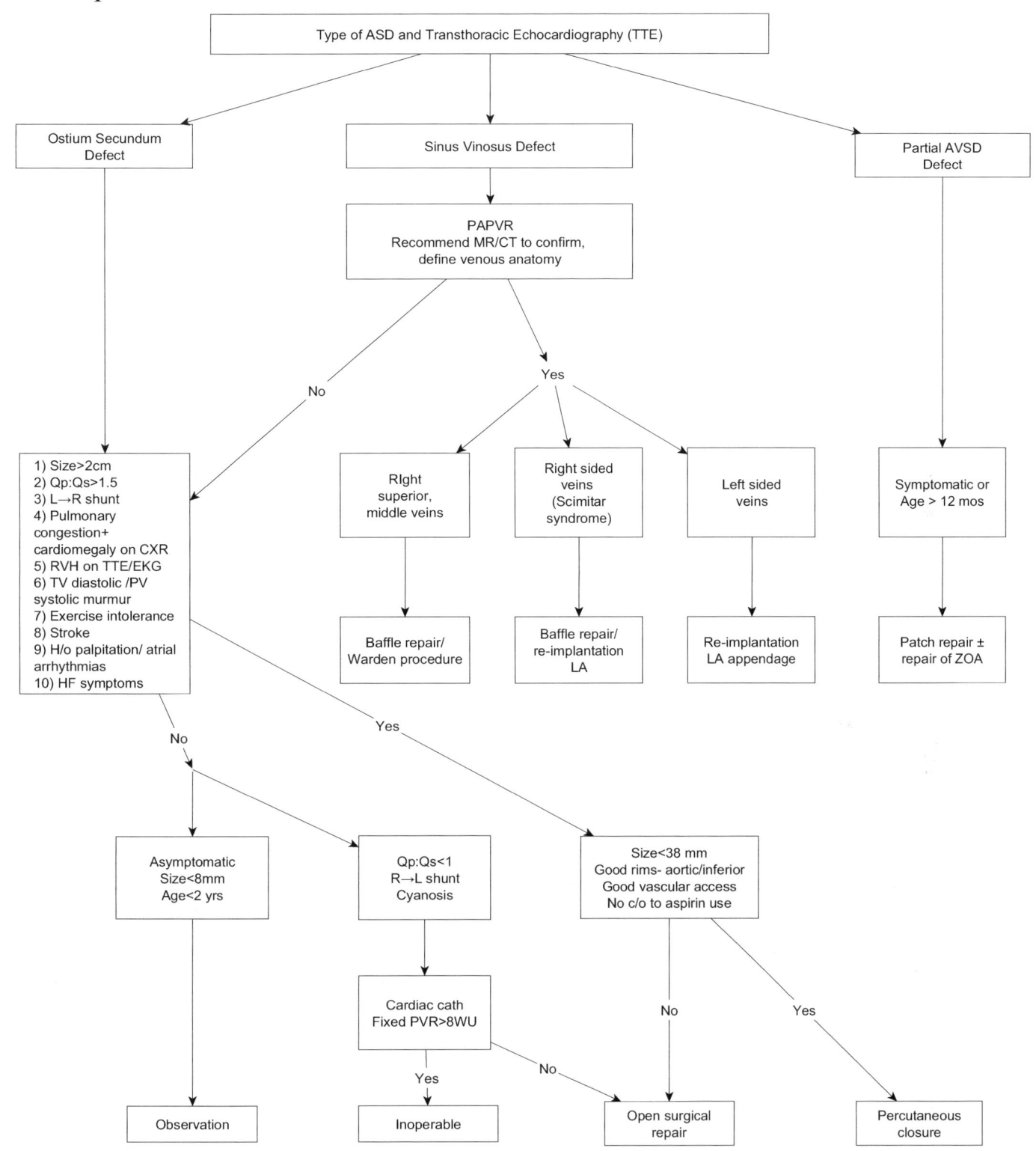

```
                    ┌─────────────────────────────────────────────────┐
                    │ Type of ASD and Transthoracic Echocardiography (TTE) │
                    └─────────────────────────────────────────────────┘
                         │              │                │
              ┌──────────┘              │                └──────────┐
              ▼                         ▼                           ▼
    ┌──────────────────┐    ┌──────────────────┐        ┌──────────────────┐
    │ Ostium Secundum  │    │  Sinus Vinosus   │        │   Partial AVSD   │
    │     Defect       │    │     Defect       │        │     Defect       │
    └──────────────────┘    └──────────────────┘        └──────────────────┘
                                     │                           │
                                     ▼                           │
                         ┌──────────────────────┐                │
                         │       PAPVR          │                │
                         │ Recommend MR/CT to   │                │
                         │ confirm, define      │                │
                         │ venous anatomy       │                │
                         └──────────────────────┘                │
                              │           │                      │
                           No │           │ Yes                  │
```

Ostium Secundum / "No PAPVR" branch — indications:
1) Size>2cm
2) Qp:Qs>1.5
3) L→R shunt
4) Pulmonary congestion+ cardiomegaly on CXR
5) RVH on TTE/EKG
6) TV diastolic /PV systolic murmur
7) Exercise intolerance
8) Stroke
9) H/o palpitation/ atrial arrhythmias
10) HF symptoms

Sinus Venosus with PAPVR — Yes branch:
- Right superior, middle veins → Baffle repair/ Warden procedure
- Right sided veins (Scimitar syndrome) → Baffle repair/ re-implantation LA
- Left sided veins → Re-implantation LA appendage

Partial AVSD:
- Symptomatic or Age > 12 mos → Patch repair ± repair of ZOA

Ostium Secundum decision outcomes:
- No (criteria not met): Asymptomatic, Size<8mm, Age<2 yrs → Observation
- Qp:Qs<1, R→L shunt, Cyanosis → Cardiac cath, Fixed PVR>8WU
  - Yes → Inoperable
  - No → Open surgical repair
- Yes (criteria met): Size<38 mm, Good rims- aortic/inferior, Good vascular access, No c/o to aspirin use
  - No → Open surgical repair
  - Yes → Percutaneous closure

WU, Wood units; PAPVR, partial anomalous pulmonary venous return; RVH, right ventricular hypertrophy; HF, heart failure; ZOA, zone of apposition; AVSD, atrioventricular septal defect; Qp, pulmonary flow; Qs, systemic flow; PVR, pulmonary vascular resistance; LA, left atrium; TV, tricuspid valve; PV, pulmonary valve; TTE, transthoracic echocardiogram; EKG, electrocardiogram

Evaluation of Aortopulmonary window
Edo Bedzra, Lester Permut

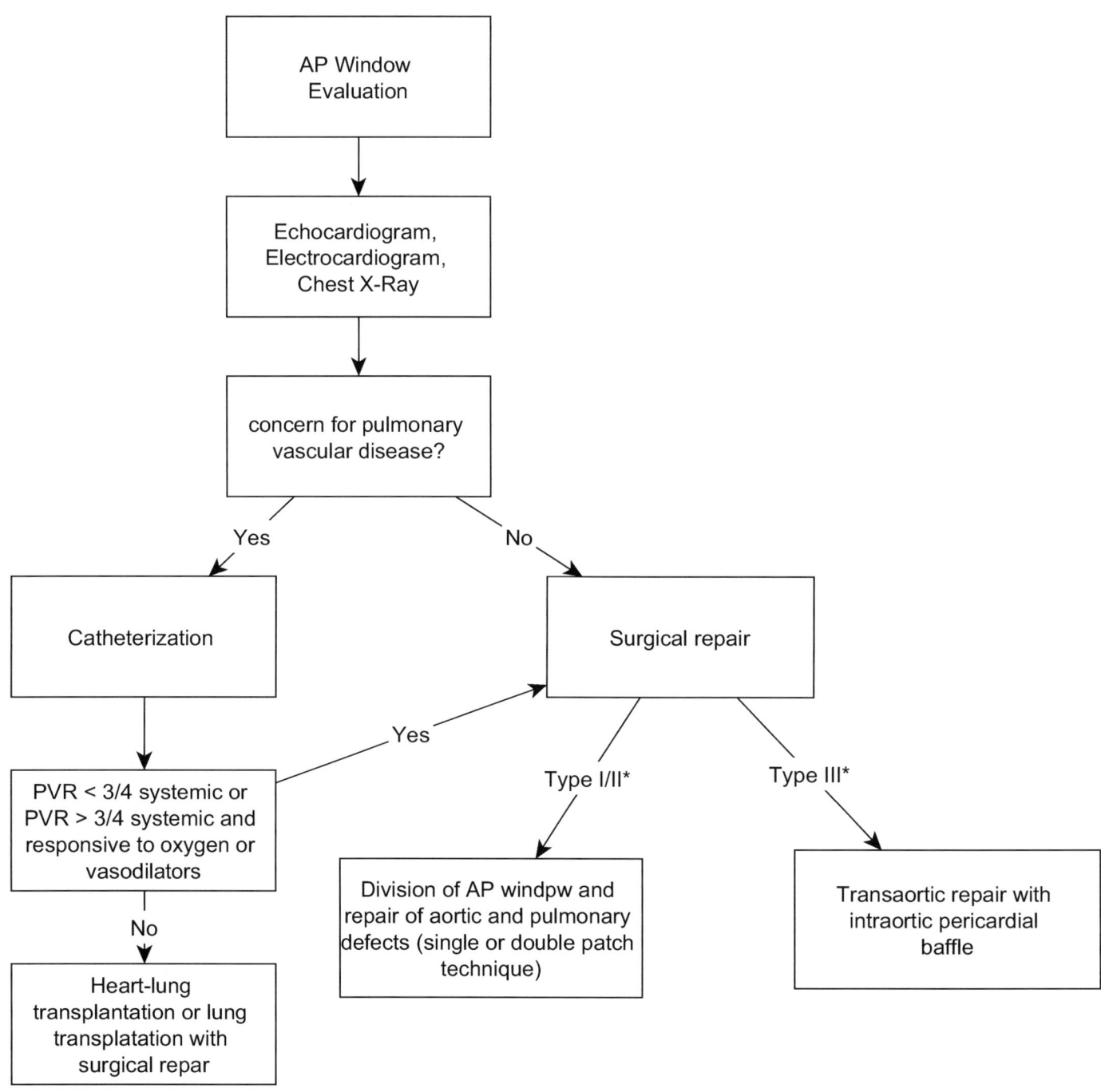

```
┌─────────────────┐
│   AP Window     │
│   Evaluation    │
└────────┬────────┘
         ▼
┌─────────────────┐
│  Echocardiogram,│
│ Electrocardiogram,│
│   Chest X-Ray   │
└────────┬────────┘
         ▼
┌─────────────────┐
│ concern for pulmonary│
│ vascular disease?│
└──┬───────────┬──┘
 Yes          No
  ▼            ▼
┌──────────┐  ┌──────────────┐
│Catheter- │  │Surgical repair│
│ ization  │  └──────────────┘
└────┬─────┘       │       │
     ▼          Type I/II* Type III*
┌──────────────┐    ▼         ▼
│PVR < 3/4 systemic│ ┌──────────┐ ┌──────────┐
│or PVR > 3/4      │ │Division  │ │Transaortic│
│systemic and      │ │of AP     │ │repair with│
│responsive to     │ │windpw and│ │intraortic │
│oxygen or         │ │repair of │ │pericardial│
│vasodilators      │ │aortic and│ │  baffle   │
└──────┬───────────┘ │pulmonary │ └──────────┘
      No             │defects   │
       ▼             │(single or│
┌──────────────┐     │double    │
│Heart-lung    │     │patch     │
│transplantation│    │technique)│
│or lung       │     └──────────┘
│transplatation│
│with surgical │
│repar         │
└──────────────┘
```

AP, Aortopulmonary; ECG, electrocardiogram; CXR, Chest X-ray; PVR, Pulmonary vascular resistance
*Surgical repair usually performed with CPB. Concomitant arch repair should be performed if interrupted arch present.

Cor Triatriatum
Corinne Tan, Carlos Mery

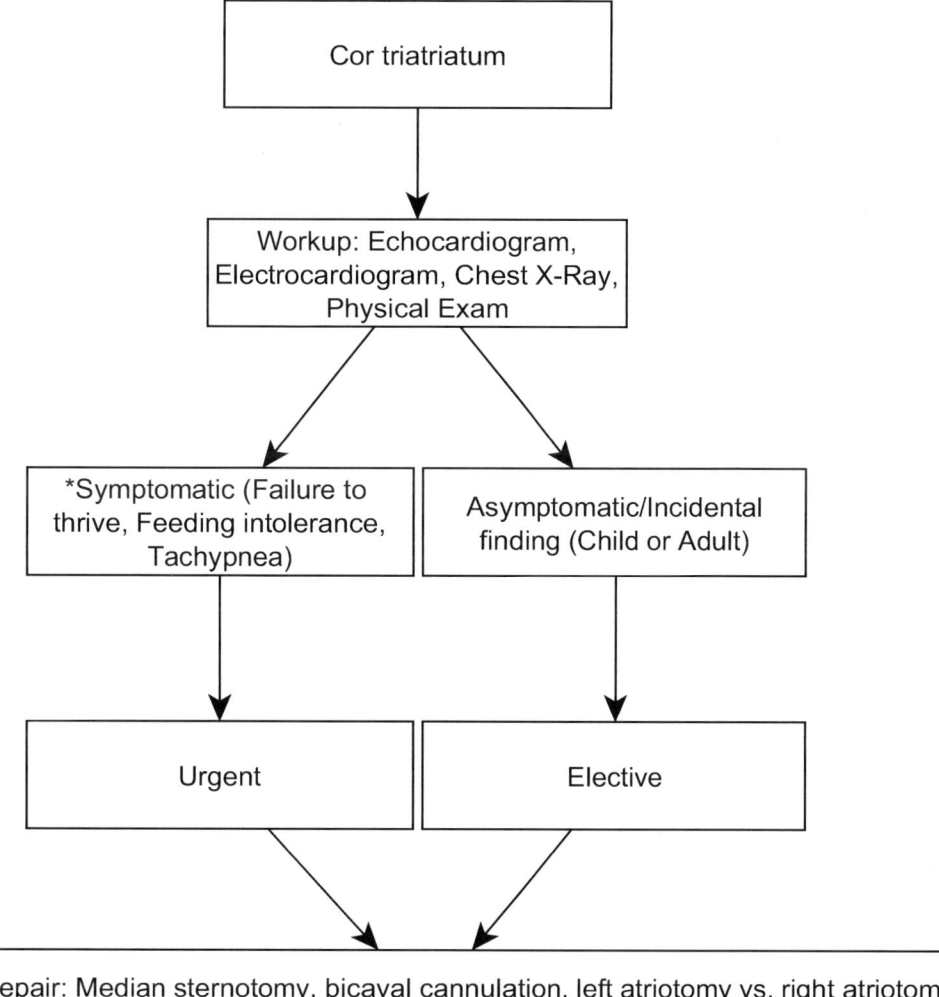

```
┌─────────────────────┐
│   Cor triatriatum   │
└──────────┬──────────┘
           ▼
┌─────────────────────────────┐
│ Workup: Echocardiogram,     │
│ Electrocardiogram, Chest X-Ray, │
│ Physical Exam               │
└──────┬───────────────┬──────┘
       ▼               ▼
┌──────────────┐  ┌──────────────┐
│ *Symptomatic │  │ Asymptomatic/│
│ (Failure to  │  │ Incidental   │
│ thrive,      │  │ finding      │
│ Feeding      │  │ (Child or    │
│ intolerance, │  │ Adult)       │
│ Tachypnea)   │  │              │
└──────┬───────┘  └──────┬───────┘
       ▼                 ▼
┌──────────────┐  ┌──────────────┐
│   Urgent     │  │   Elective   │
└──────┬───────┘  └──────┬───────┘
       └────────┬────────┘
                ▼
┌─────────────────────────────────────────────────┐
│ Surgical repair: Median sternotomy, bicaval     │
│ cannulation, left atriotomy vs. right atriotomy │
│ with trans-septal approach, resection of        │
│ fibromuscular membrane +/- ASD repair           │
└─────────────────────────────────────────────────┘
```

ASD, atrial septal defect
The more restrictive the membrane the more symptomatic the patient

Ventricular Septal Defect (VSD)
David Blitzer, John Brown

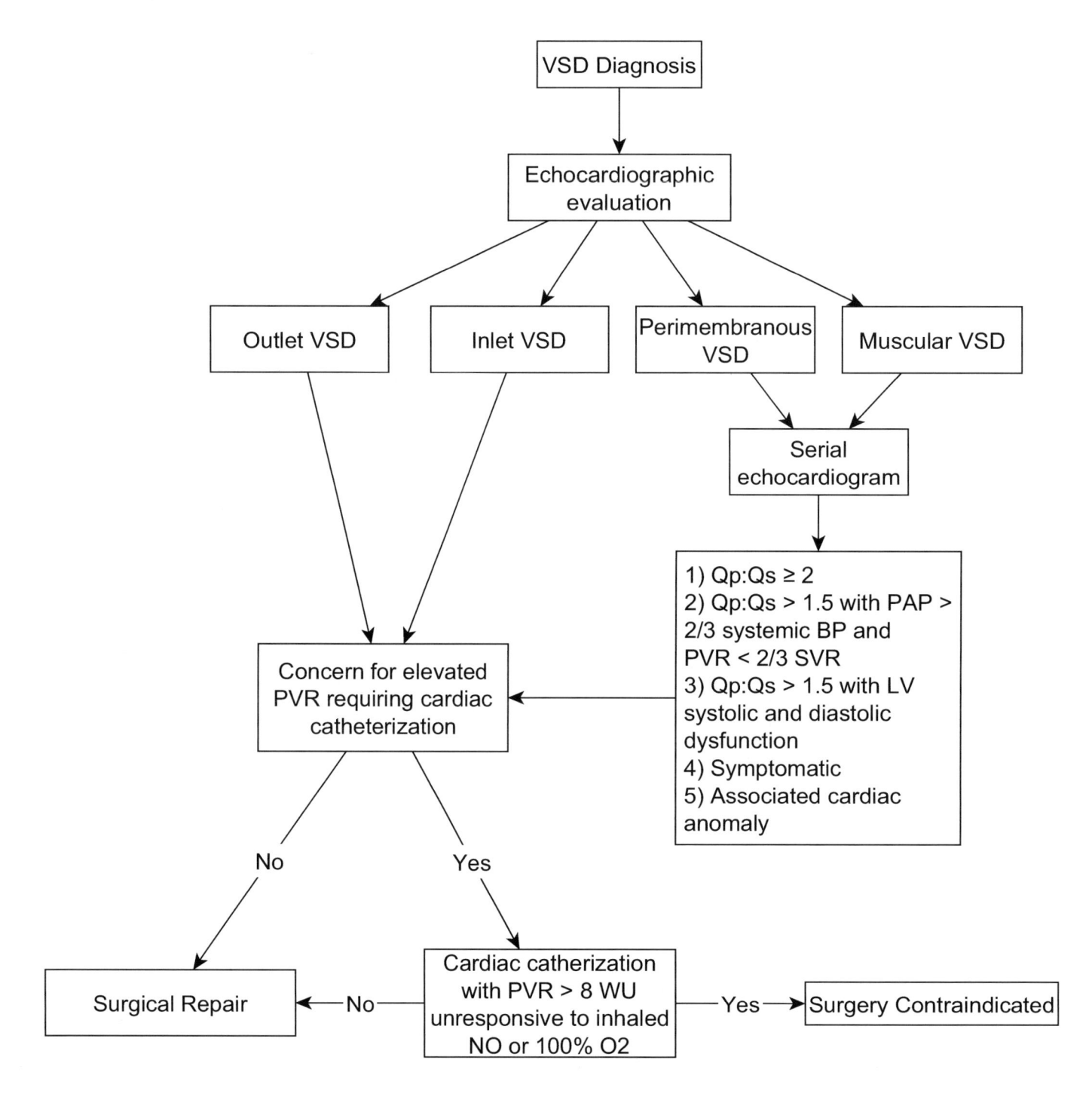

```
                    ┌─────────────────┐
                    │  VSD Diagnosis  │
                    └────────┬────────┘
                             ▼
                    ┌─────────────────┐
                    │ Echocardiographic│
                    │    evaluation   │
                    └────────┬────────┘
         ┌──────────┬────────┼────────┬──────────┐
         ▼          ▼                 ▼          ▼
    ┌─────────┐ ┌─────────┐ ┌──────────────┐ ┌─────────────┐
    │Outlet VSD│ │Inlet VSD│ │Perimembranous│ │Muscular VSD │
    │          │ │         │ │     VSD      │ │             │
    └────┬─────┘ └────┬────┘ └──────┬───────┘ └──────┬──────┘
         │            │             └────┬───────────┘
         │            │                  ▼
         │            │         ┌─────────────────┐
         │            │         │     Serial      │
         │            │         │ echocardiogram  │
         │            │         └────────┬────────┘
         │            │                  ▼
         │            │    ┌─────────────────────────────┐
         │            │    │ 1) Qp:Qs ≥ 2                │
         │            │    │ 2) Qp:Qs > 1.5 with PAP >   │
         │            │    │    2/3 systemic BP and      │
         │            │    │    PVR < 2/3 SVR            │
         ▼            ▼    │ 3) Qp:Qs > 1.5 with LV      │
    ┌──────────────────┐   │    systolic and diastolic   │
    │  Concern for     │◄──│    dysfunction              │
    │  elevated PVR    │   │ 4) Symptomatic              │
    │ requiring cardiac│   │ 5) Associated cardiac       │
    │ catheterization  │   │    anomaly                  │
    └────┬────────┬────┘   └─────────────────────────────┘
       No│        │Yes
         ▼        ▼
  ┌──────────┐  ┌──────────────────┐         ┌──────────────┐
  │ Surgical │◄─│Cardiac catherization│──Yes──►│   Surgery    │
  │  Repair  │No│ with PVR > 8 WU  │         │Contraindicated│
  └──────────┘  │unresponsive to inhaled│     └──────────────┘
                │   NO or 100% O2  │
                └──────────────────┘
```

VSD, ventricular septal defect; Qp, pulmonary flow; Qs, systemic flow; PVR, pulmonary vascular resistance; SVR, systemic vascular resistance; LV, left ventricular; NO, nitric oxide; WU, woods units

Coarctation of the Aorta
Corinne Tan, Carlos Mery

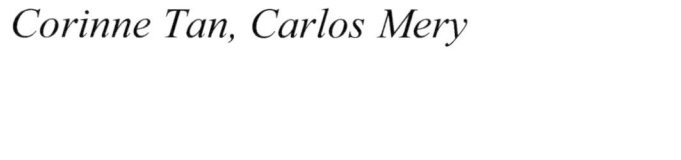

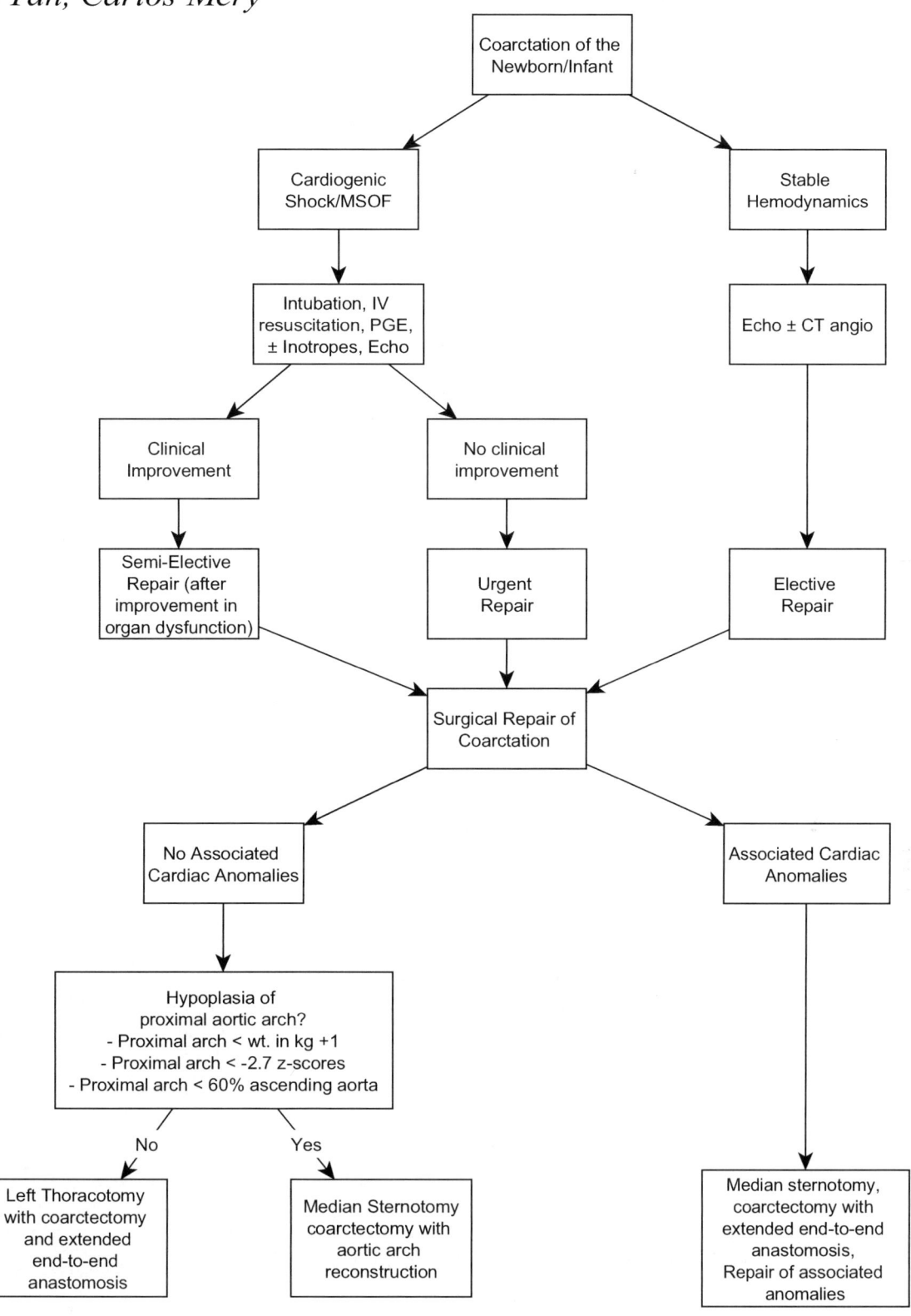

```
                    ┌─────────────────────┐
                    │ Coarctation of the  │
                    │  Newborn/Infant     │
                    └──────────┬──────────┘
                  ┌────────────┴────────────┐
                  ▼                         ▼
         ┌────────────────┐         ┌────────────────┐
         │  Cardiogenic   │         │    Stable      │
         │  Shock/MSOF    │         │  Hemodynamics  │
         └───────┬────────┘         └────────┬───────┘
                 ▼                           ▼
         ┌────────────────┐         ┌────────────────┐
         │ Intubation, IV │         │ Echo ± CT angio│
         │ resuscitation, │         └────────┬───────┘
         │ PGE, ± Inotropes│                 │
         │     , Echo     │                  │
         └───┬────────┬───┘                  │
             ▼        ▼                      │
     ┌─────────┐  ┌──────────┐               │
     │Clinical │  │No clinical│              │
     │Improve- │  │improvement│              │
     │ment     │  │           │              │
     └────┬────┘  └─────┬─────┘              │
          ▼             ▼                    ▼
   ┌──────────┐   ┌──────────┐        ┌──────────┐
   │Semi-     │   │ Urgent   │        │ Elective │
   │Elective  │   │ Repair   │        │ Repair   │
   │Repair    │   └────┬─────┘        └────┬─────┘
   │(after    │        │                   │
   │improvement│       │                   │
   │in organ  │        │                   │
   │dysfunction)│      │                   │
   └─────┬────┘        │                   │
         └─────────────┼───────────────────┘
                       ▼
              ┌─────────────────┐
              │Surgical Repair  │
              │ of Coarctation  │
              └────┬───────┬────┘
                   ▼       ▼
       ┌──────────────┐ ┌──────────────┐
       │No Associated │ │  Associated  │
       │Cardiac       │ │   Cardiac    │
       │Anomalies     │ │  Anomalies   │
       └──────┬───────┘ └──────┬───────┘
              ▼                │
   ┌────────────────────┐      │
   │ Hypoplasia of      │      │
   │ proximal aortic arch?│    │
   │ - Proximal arch    │      │
   │   < wt. in kg +1   │      │
   │ - Proximal arch    │      │
   │   < -2.7 z-scores  │      │
   │ - Proximal arch    │      │
   │   < 60% ascending  │      │
   │   aorta            │      │
   └──┬──────────────┬──┘      │
    No│              │Yes      │
      ▼              ▼         ▼
 ┌─────────┐  ┌─────────┐  ┌─────────────┐
 │Left     │  │Median   │  │Median       │
 │Thoracotomy│ │Sternotomy│ │sternotomy,  │
 │with     │  │coarctectomy│ │coarctectomy │
 │coarctectomy│ │with    │  │with extended│
 │and      │  │aortic   │  │end-to-end   │
 │extended │  │arch     │  │anastomosis, │
 │end-to-end│ │reconstruction│ │Repair of  │
 │anastomosis│ │        │  │associated   │
 │         │  │         │  │anomalies    │
 └─────────┘  └─────────┘  └─────────────┘
```

MSOF, multisystem organ failure; PGE, Prostaglandin E

Tetralogy of Fallot with Pulmonary Stenosis
Kyle Riggs, Vincent Parnell

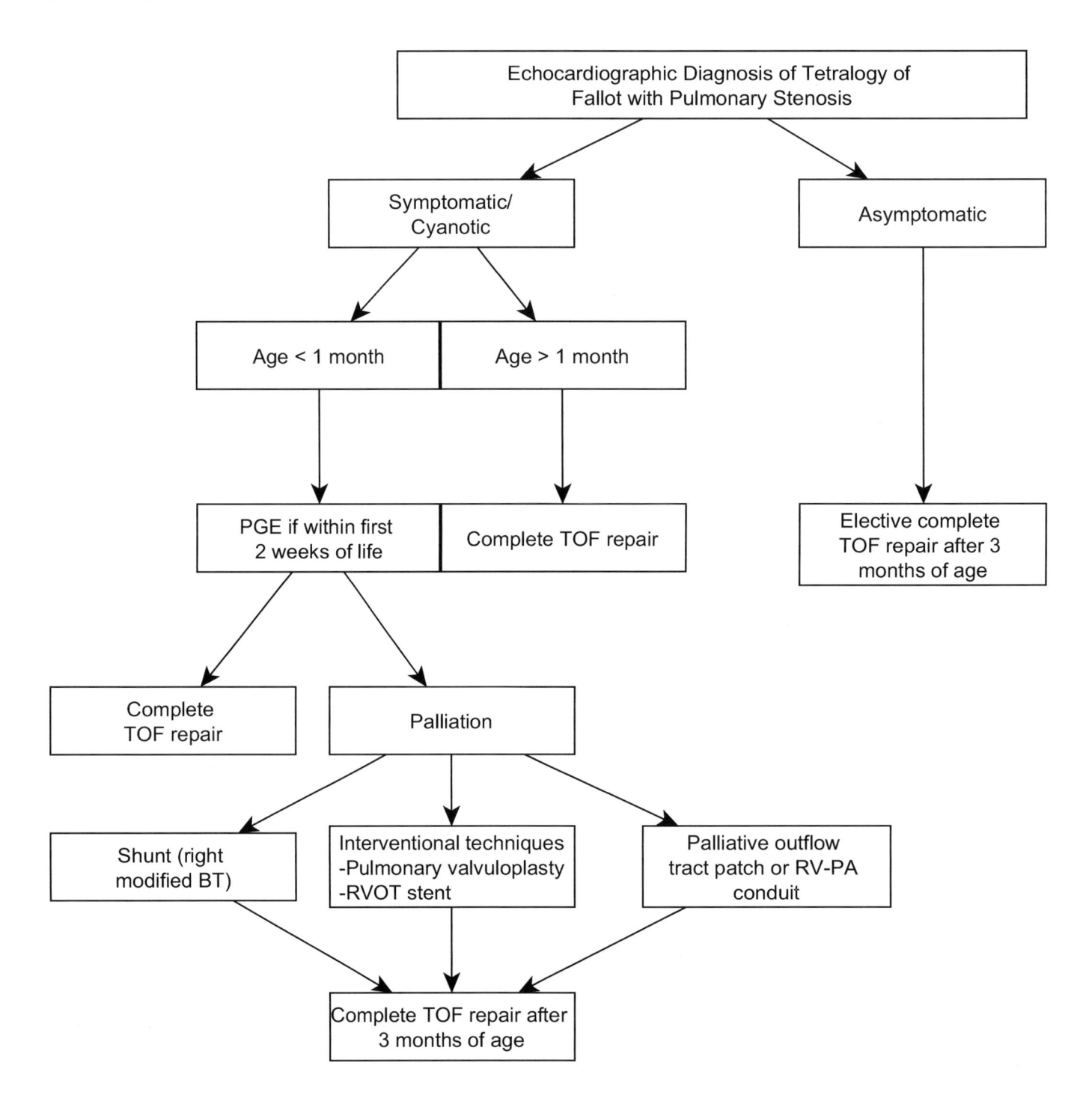

```
                    ┌─────────────────────────────────┐
                    │ Echocardiographic Diagnosis of  │
                    │ Tetralogy of Fallot with        │
                    │ Pulmonary Stenosis              │
                    └─────────────────────────────────┘
                         ↓                    ↓
              ┌──────────────────┐    ┌──────────────┐
              │ Symptomatic/     │    │ Asymptomatic │
              │ Cyanotic         │    │              │
              └──────────────────┘    └──────────────┘
                  ↓         ↓                 ↓
         ┌──────────────┐ ┌──────────────┐  ┌────────────────┐
         │ Age < 1 month│ │ Age > 1 month│  │ Elective       │
         └──────────────┘ └──────────────┘  │ complete TOF   │
                ↓                ↓          │ repair after 3 │
         ┌──────────────┐ ┌──────────────┐  │ months of age  │
         │ PGE if within│ │ Complete TOF │  └────────────────┘
         │ first 2 weeks│ │ repair       │
         │ of life      │ │              │
         └──────────────┘ └──────────────┘
              ↓       ↓
    ┌──────────┐  ┌───────────┐
    │ Complete │  │ Palliation│
    │ TOF      │  └───────────┘
    │ repair   │   ↓    ↓    ↓
    └──────────┘
```

- Shunt (right modified BT)
- Interventional techniques
  - Pulmonary valvuloplasty
  - RVOT stent
- Palliative outflow tract patch or RV-PA conduit

→ Complete TOF repair after 3 months of age

PGE, Prostaglandin; TOF, Tetralogy of Fallot; BT, Blalock-Taussig; RVOT, Right ventricular outflow tract; RV-PA, Right ventricle-pulmonary artery

Transposition of the Great Arteries
Mahim Malik, Lester Permut

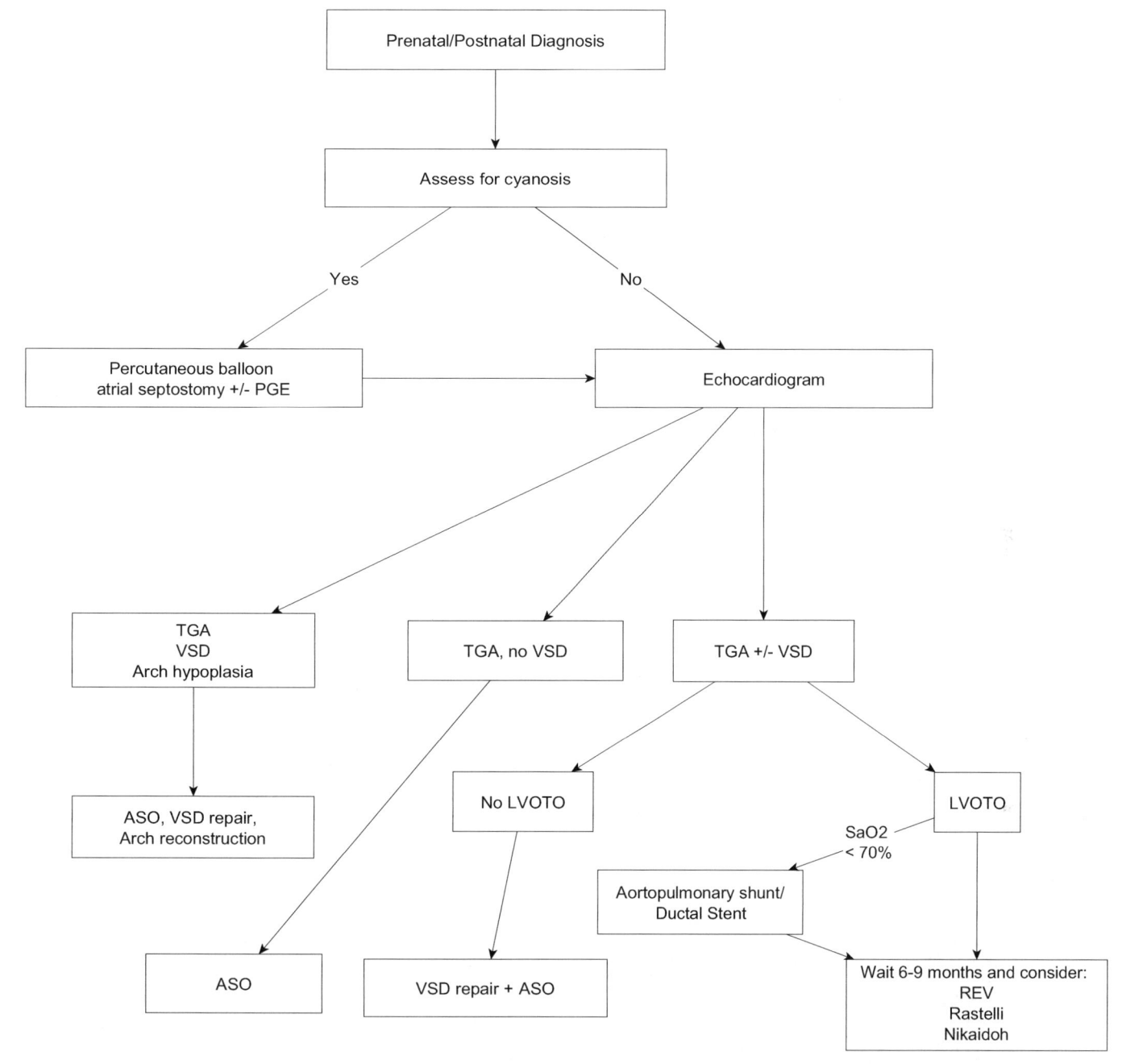

```
┌─────────────────────────────┐
│ Prenatal/Postnatal Diagnosis │
└──────────────┬──────────────┘
               ▼
┌─────────────────────────────┐
│     Assess for cyanosis     │
└──────────────┬──────────────┘
         Yes ◄─┴─► No
```

- **Yes** → Percutaneous balloon atrial septostomy +/- PGE → Echocardiogram
- **No** → Echocardiogram

Echocardiogram branches:

- **TGA, VSD, Arch hypoplasia** → ASO, VSD repair, Arch reconstruction
- **TGA, no VSD** → ASO
- **TGA +/- VSD**:
  - **No LVOTO** → VSD repair + ASO
  - **LVOTO**:
    - SaO2 < 70% → Aortopulmonary shunt/Ductal Stent → Wait 6-9 months and consider: REV, Rastelli, Nikaidoh
    - → Wait 6-9 months and consider: REV, Rastelli, Nikaidoh

PGE, Prostaglandin; TGA, transposition of great arteries; VSD, ventricular septal defect; LVOTO, left ventricular outflow tract obstruction; ASO, arterial switch operation; REV, Reparation a l'etage ventriculaire.

Pulmonary Atresia with Ventricular Septal Defect and Major Aortopulmonary Collaterals (PA/VSD/MAPCAs)
Christopher Greenleaf, Ali Dodge-Khatami

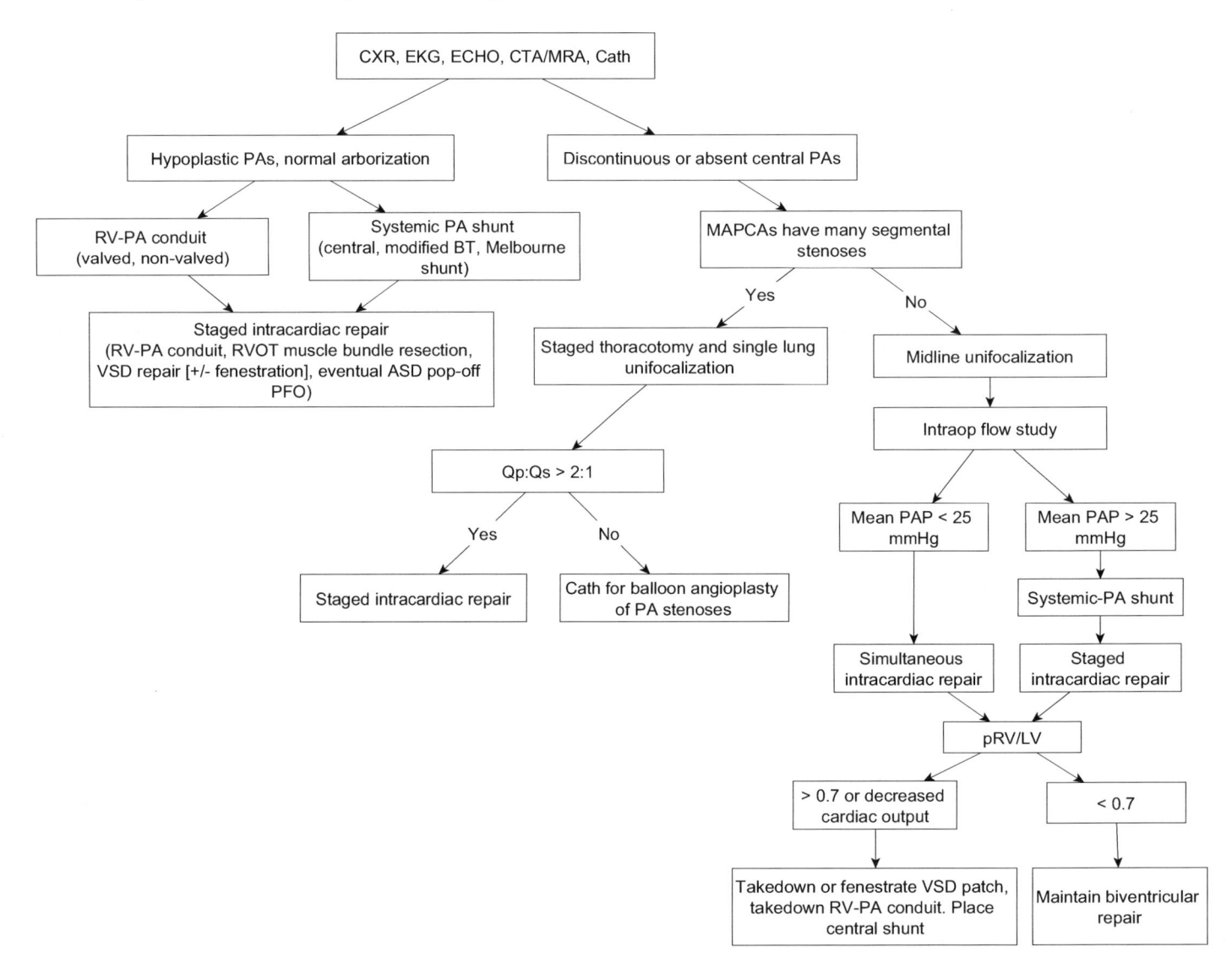

```
                        ┌─────────────────────────────────┐
                        │ CXR, EKG, ECHO, CTA/MRA, Cath   │
                        └─────────────────────────────────┘
                           │                           │
                           ▼                           ▼
         ┌──────────────────────────────┐   ┌──────────────────────────────┐
         │ Hypoplastic PAs,             │   │ Discontinuous or absent      │
         │ normal arborization          │   │ central PAs                  │
         └──────────────────────────────┘   └──────────────────────────────┘
              │               │                         │
              ▼               ▼                         ▼
     ┌──────────────┐  ┌──────────────────┐   ┌────────────────────────┐
     │ RV-PA conduit│  │ Systemic PA shunt│   │ MAPCAs have many       │
     │ (valved,     │  │ (central, mod.   │   │ segmental stenoses     │
     │ non-valved)  │  │ BT, Melbourne    │   └────────────────────────┘
     └──────────────┘  │ shunt)           │       Yes │    │ No
              │        └──────────────────┘           ▼    ▼
              ▼               ▼              ┌──────────────┐  ┌──────────────┐
     ┌─────────────────────────────────┐     │ Staged       │  │ Midline      │
     │ Staged intracardiac repair      │     │ thoracotomy  │  │ unifocal-    │
     │ (RV-PA conduit, RVOT muscle     │     │ and single   │  │ ization      │
     │ bundle resection, VSD repair    │     │ lung unifoc. │  └──────────────┘
     │ [+/- fenestration], eventual    │     └──────────────┘         │
     │ ASD pop-off PFO)                │            │                 ▼
     └─────────────────────────────────┘            ▼          ┌──────────────┐
                                            ┌──────────────┐   │ Intraop flow │
                                            │ Qp:Qs > 2:1  │   │ study        │
                                            └──────────────┘   └──────────────┘
                                             Yes │   │ No          │     │
                                                 ▼   ▼             ▼     ▼
                                    ┌───────────┐ ┌─────────────┐ ┌────────────┐ ┌────────────┐
                                    │ Staged    │ │ Cath for    │ │ Mean PAP   │ │ Mean PAP   │
                                    │ intra-    │ │ balloon     │ │ < 25 mmHg  │ │ > 25 mmHg  │
                                    │ cardiac   │ │ angioplasty │ └────────────┘ └────────────┘
                                    │ repair    │ │ of PA       │       │            │
                                    └───────────┘ │ stenoses    │       │            ▼
                                                  └─────────────┘       │     ┌──────────────┐
                                                                        │     │ Systemic-PA  │
                                                                        │     │ shunt        │
                                                                        │     └──────────────┘
                                                                        ▼            ▼
                                                                ┌──────────────┐ ┌──────────────┐
                                                                │ Simultaneous │ │ Staged       │
                                                                │ intracardiac │ │ intracardiac │
                                                                │ repair       │ │ repair       │
                                                                └──────────────┘ └──────────────┘
                                                                        │
                                                                        ▼
                                                                 ┌──────────┐
                                                                 │  pRV/LV  │
                                                                 └──────────┘
                                                                   │      │
                                                                   ▼      ▼
                                                         ┌──────────────┐ ┌────────┐
                                                         │ > 0.7 or     │ │ < 0.7  │
                                                         │ decreased    │ └────────┘
                                                         │ cardiac out. │     │
                                                         └──────────────┘     ▼
                                                                │    ┌──────────────┐
                                                                ▼    │ Maintain     │
                                                    ┌──────────────────┐│ biventricular│
                                                    │ Takedown or      ││ repair       │
                                                    │ fenestrate VSD   │└──────────────┘
                                                    │ patch, takedown  │
                                                    │ RV-PA conduit.   │
                                                    │ Place central    │
                                                    │ shunt            │
                                                    └──────────────────┘
```

CTA, CT angiogram; MRA, MR angiogram; PA, pulmonary artery; RV-PA, right ventricle-pulmonary artery; BT, Blalock Taussig; RVOT – right ventricular outflow tract; PFO, patent foramen ovale; ASD, atrial septal defect; Qp, pulmonary flow; Qs, systemic flow; PAP, pulmonary artery pressure

Pulmonary Atresia with Intact Ventricular Septum
Christopher Greenleaf, Ali Dodge-Khatami

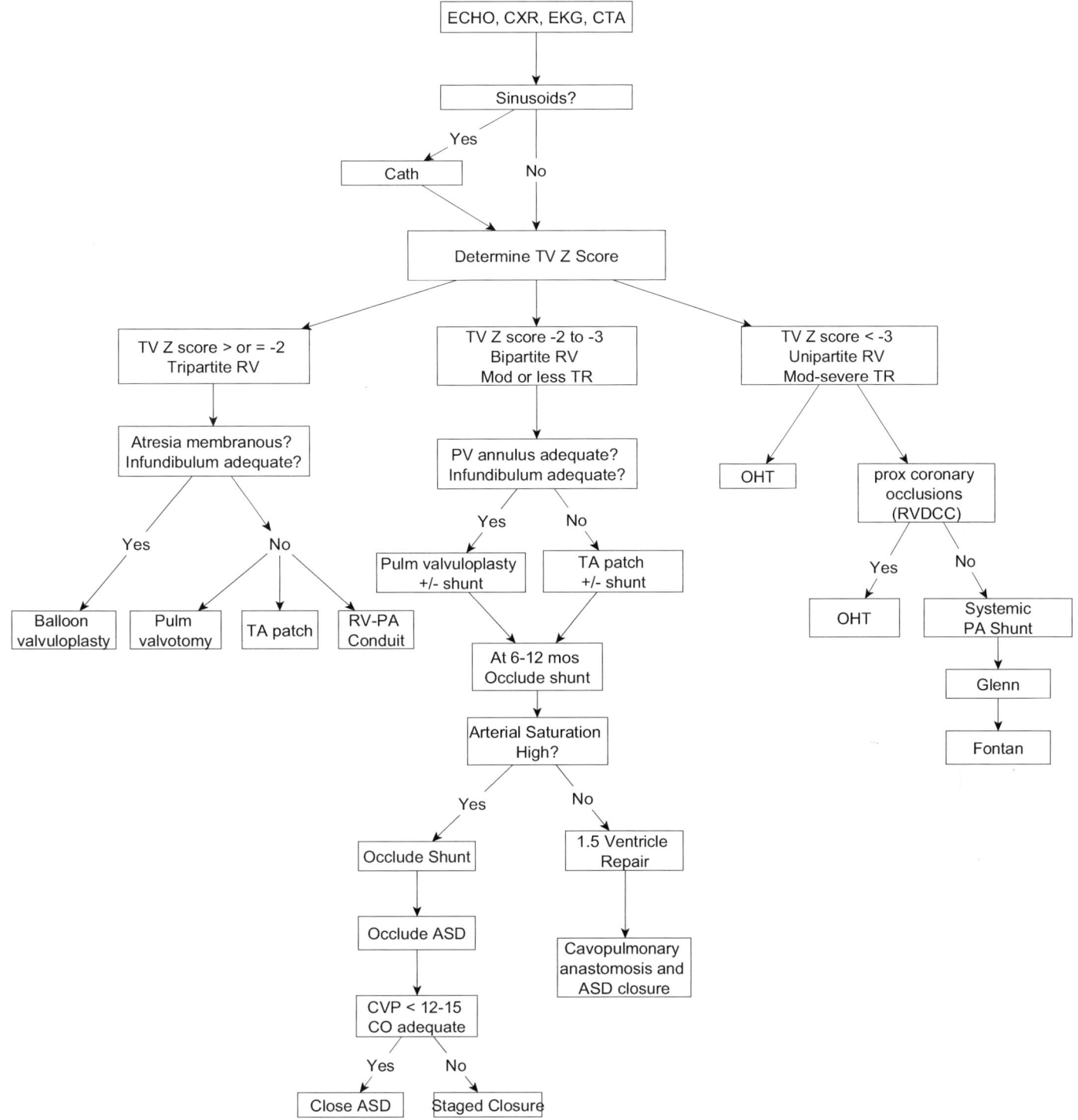

```
                         ECHO, CXR, EKG, CTA
                                 │
                                 ▼
                            Sinusoids?
                         ┌───┴───┐
                       Yes      No
                        │        │
                      Cath       │
                                 ▼
                       Determine TV Z Score
             ┌───────────────┼───────────────┐
             ▼               ▼               ▼
      TV Z score ≥ -2   TV Z score -2 to -3   TV Z score < -3
       Tripartite RV     Bipartite RV          Unipartite RV
                        Mod or less TR         Mod-severe TR
             │               │              ┌──┴──┐
             ▼               ▼              ▼     ▼
      Atresia membranous?  PV annulus      OHT   prox coronary
      Infundibulum         adequate?              occlusions
      adequate?            Infundibulum           (RVDCC)
       ┌──┴──┐             adequate?            ┌──┴──┐
      Yes   No            ┌──┴──┐              Yes    No
       │   ┌─┼─┐         Yes    No              │     │
       ▼   ▼ ▼ ▼          │     │              OHT   Systemic
   Balloon Pulm TA RV-PA  ▼     ▼                    PA Shunt
   valvulo valvo patch Conduit                        │
   plasty  tomy    Pulm    TA patch                   ▼
              valvuloplasty +/- shunt               Glenn
              +/- shunt                               │
                  └────┬────┘                         ▼
                       ▼                           Fontan
                 At 6-12 mos
                 Occlude shunt
                       │
                       ▼
                 Arterial Saturation
                      High?
                  ┌────┴────┐
                 Yes        No
                  │          │
                  ▼          ▼
             Occlude Shunt  1.5 Ventricle Repair
                  │          │
                  ▼          ▼
             Occlude ASD    Cavopulmonary
                  │         anastomosis and
                  ▼         ASD closure
             CVP < 12-15
             CO adequate
              ┌──┴──┐
             Yes    No
              │     │
              ▼     ▼
          Close  Staged
           ASD   Closure
```

TV, tricuspid valve; TA, Transannular; RV, Right Ventricle; TR, Tricuspid Regurgitation; OHT, Orthotopic Heart Transplant; ASD, atrial septal defect; CVP, central venous pressure; CO, cardiac output; RVDCC, RV dependent coronary circulation; PA, pulmonary artery

Neonatal Ebstein's Anomaly
W. Hampton Gray, S. Ram Kumar

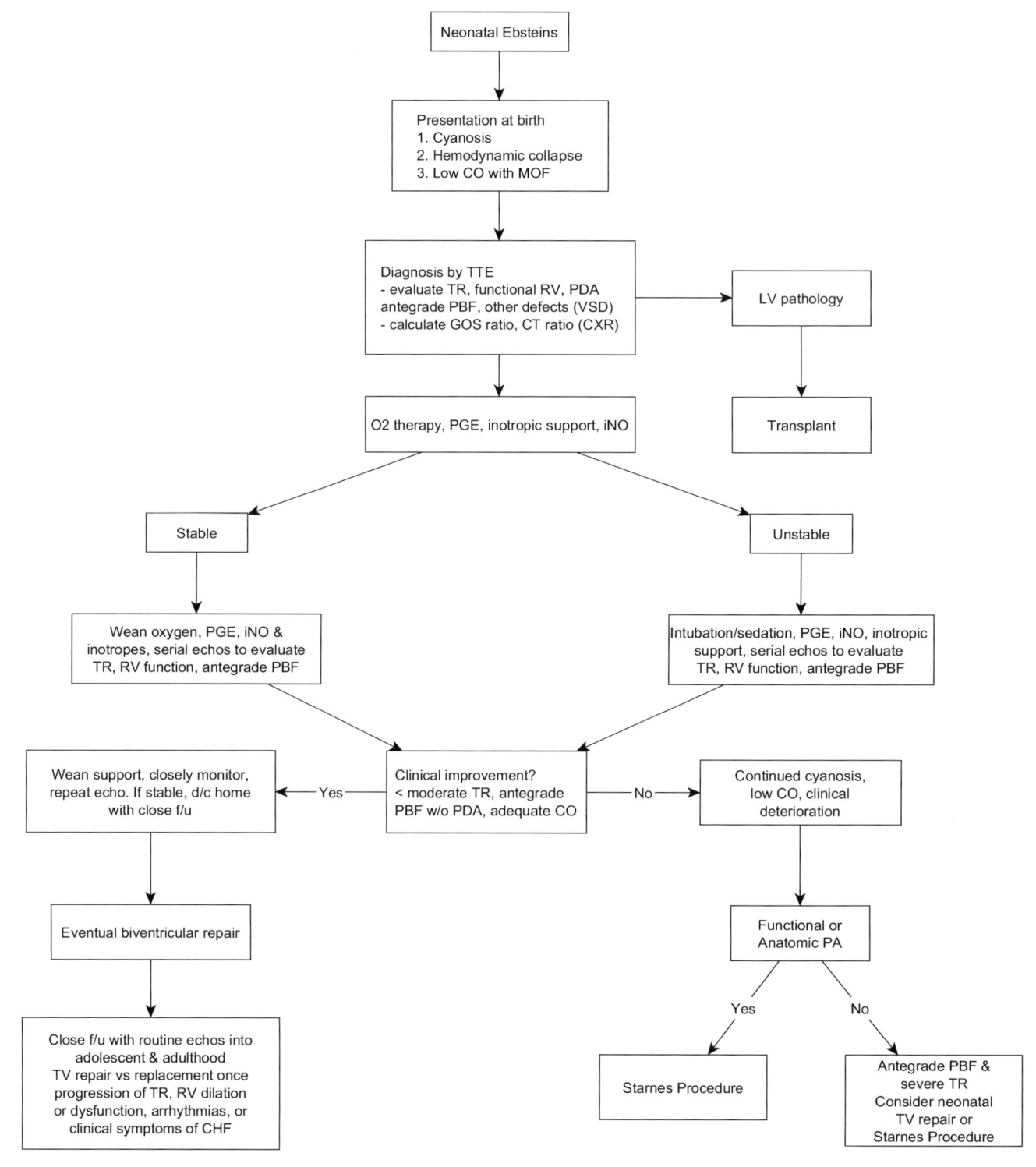

```
                    ┌──────────────────┐
                    │ Neonatal Ebsteins│
                    └────────┬─────────┘
                             ▼
                  ┌──────────────────────┐
                  │ Presentation at birth│
                  │ 1. Cyanosis          │
                  │ 2. Hemodynamic collapse│
                  │ 3. Low CO with MOF   │
                  └──────────┬───────────┘
                             ▼
          ┌─────────────────────────────────────┐       ┌──────────────┐
          │ Diagnosis by TTE                    │──────▶│ LV pathology │
          │ - evaluate TR, functional RV, PDA   │       └──────┬───────┘
          │   antegrade PBF, other defects (VSD)│              ▼
          │ - calculate GOS ratio, CT ratio(CXR)│       ┌──────────────┐
          └──────────────────┬──────────────────┘       │  Transplant  │
                             ▼                          └──────────────┘
          ┌──────────────────────────────────────┐
          │ O2 therapy, PGE, inotropic support, iNO│
          └────────┬────────────────────┬────────┘
                   ▼                    ▼
              ┌────────┐           ┌──────────┐
              │ Stable │           │ Unstable │
              └────┬───┘           └────┬─────┘
                   ▼                    ▼
      ┌──────────────────────┐  ┌──────────────────────┐
      │ Wean oxygen, PGE, iNO│  │ Intubation/sedation, │
      │ & inotropes, serial  │  │ PGE, iNO, inotropic  │
      │ echos to evaluate    │  │ support, serial echos│
      │ TR, RV function,     │  │ to evaluate TR, RV   │
      │ antegrade PBF        │  │ function,antegrade PBF│
      └──────────┬───────────┘  └───────────┬──────────┘
                 └────────┬─────────────────┘
                          ▼
   ┌──────────────┐  ┌──────────────────┐  ┌──────────────────┐
   │Wean support, │◀─│ Clinical         │─▶│ Continued cyanosis│
   │closely monitor│Yes│ improvement?    │No│ low CO, clinical │
   │repeat echo.  │  │ < moderate TR,   │  │ deterioration    │
   │If stable, d/c│  │ antegrade PBF    │  └─────────┬────────┘
   │home with     │  │ w/o PDA,adequate CO│            ▼
   │close f/u     │  └──────────────────┘  ┌──────────────────┐
   └──────┬───────┘                        │ Functional or    │
          ▼                                │ Anatomic PA      │
   ┌──────────────┐                        └────┬────────┬────┘
   │ Eventual     │                          Yes│        │No
   │ biventricular│                             ▼        ▼
   │ repair       │                      ┌────────┐ ┌─────────────┐
   └──────┬───────┘                      │Starnes │ │Antegrade PBF│
          ▼                              │Procedure│ │& severe TR │
   ┌──────────────────────┐              └────────┘ │Consider     │
   │Close f/u with routine│                         │neonatal     │
   │echos into adolescent │                         │TV repair or │
   │& adulthood TV repair │                         │Starnes      │
   │vs replacement once   │                         │Procedure    │
   │progression of TR, RV │                         └─────────────┘
   │dilation or dysfunction,│
   │arrhythmias, or       │
   │clinical symptoms of CHF│
   └──────────────────────┘
```

CO, cardiac output; MOF, multiorgan failure; TTE, transthoracic echocardiogram; TR, tricuspid regurgitation; RV, right ventricle; LV, left ventricle; PDA, patent ductus arteriosus; PBF, pulmonary blood flow; VSD, ventricular septal defect; GOS, Great Ormond Street; CT, cardiothoracic; CXR, chest X-ray; O2, oxygen; Vent, ventilation; PGE, prostaglandin E1; iNO, nitric oxide; echo, echocardiogram; CHF, congestive heart failure; PA, pulmonary atresia; BiV, biventricular

Left Ventricular Outflow Tract Obstruction
Awais Ashfaq, Ashok Muralidaran

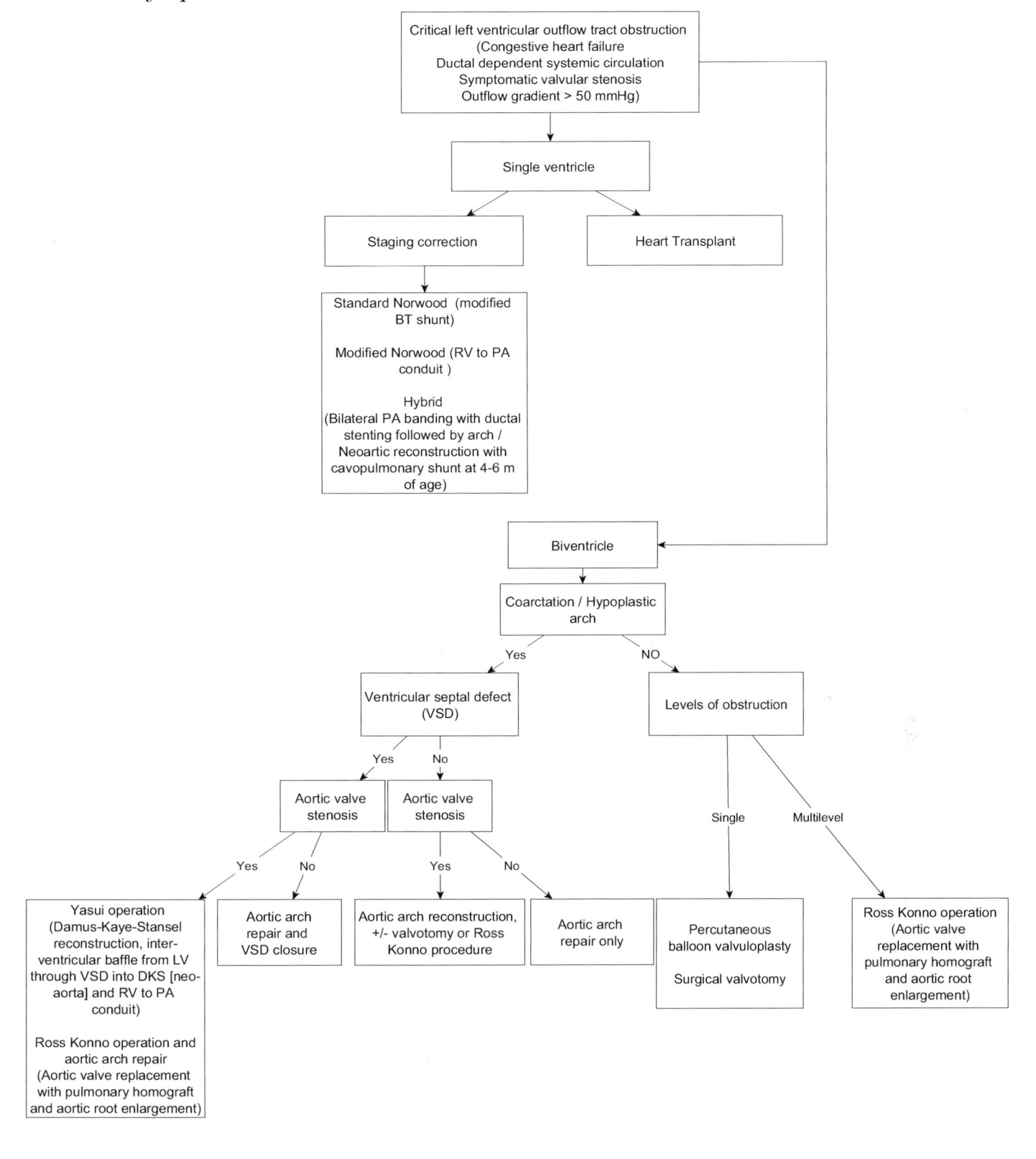

```
┌─────────────────────────────────────────┐
│ Critical left ventricular outflow tract │
│ obstruction                             │
│ (Congestive heart failure               │
│ Ductal dependent systemic circulation   │
│ Symptomatic valvular stenosis           │
│ Outflow gradient > 50 mmHg)             │
└─────────────────────────────────────────┘
                    │
              Single ventricle
               /          \
     Staging correction   Heart Transplant
              │
    ┌──────────────────────────────┐
    │ Standard Norwood (modified   │
    │ BT shunt)                    │
    │                              │
    │ Modified Norwood (RV to PA   │
    │ conduit)                     │
    │                              │
    │ Hybrid                       │
    │ (Bilateral PA banding with   │
    │ ductal stenting followed by  │
    │ arch / Neoartic reconstruct- │
    │ ion with cavopulmonary shunt │
    │ at 4-6 m of age)             │
    └──────────────────────────────┘
                    │
               Biventricle
                    │
         Coarctation / Hypoplastic arch
              Yes /        \ NO
                /            \
    Ventricular septal        Levels of obstruction
    defect (VSD)                    /        \
       Yes /  \ No              Single    Multilevel
         /      \
  Aortic valve  Aortic valve
  stenosis      stenosis
  Yes / \ No    Yes / \ No
```

- **Yasui operation** (Damus-Kaye-Stansel reconstruction, interventricular baffle from LV through VSD into DKS [neo-aorta] and RV to PA conduit)

  Ross Konno operation and aortic arch repair (Aortic valve replacement with pulmonary homograft and aortic root enlargement)

- **Aortic arch repair and VSD closure**

- **Aortic arch reconstruction, +/- valvotomy or Ross Konno procedure**

- **Aortic arch repair only**

- **Percutaneous balloon valvuloplasty**

  Surgical valvotomy

- **Ross Konno operation** (Aortic valve replacement with pulmonary homograft and aortic root enlargement)

Coronary Anomalies
Corinne Tan, Carlos M. Mery

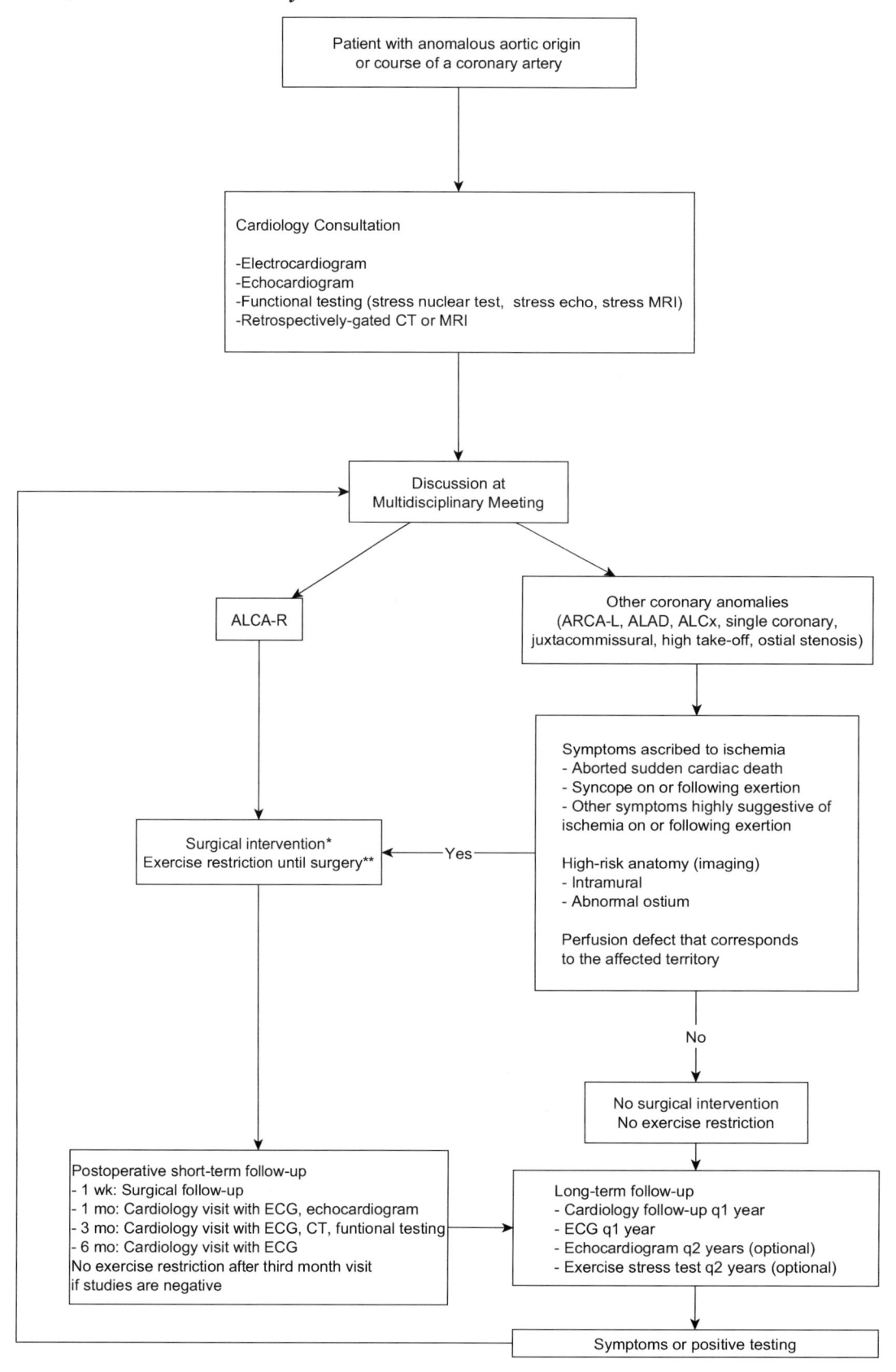

```
┌─────────────────────────────────────┐
│ Patient with anomalous aortic origin│
│  or course of a coronary artery     │
└─────────────────────────────────────┘
                 │
                 ▼
┌─────────────────────────────────────┐
│ Cardiology Consultation             │
│                                     │
│ -Electrocardiogram                  │
│ -Echocardiogram                     │
│ -Functional testing (stress nuclear │
│  test, stress echo, stress MRI)     │
│ -Retrospectively-gated CT or MRI    │
└─────────────────────────────────────┘
                 │
                 ▼
┌─────────────────────────────────────┐
│       Discussion at                 │
│   Multidisciplinary Meeting         │
└─────────────────────────────────────┘
          │                  │
          ▼                  ▼
      ┌───────┐   ┌──────────────────────────────┐
      │ALCA-R │   │ Other coronary anomalies     │
      └───────┘   │ (ARCA-L, ALAD, ALCx, single  │
          │       │ coronary, juxtacommissural,  │
          │       │ high take-off, ostial        │
          │       │ stenosis)                    │
          │       └──────────────────────────────┘
          │                  │
          │                  ▼
          │       ┌──────────────────────────────┐
          │       │ Symptoms ascribed to ischemia│
          │       │ - Aborted sudden cardiac     │
          │       │   death                      │
          │       │ - Syncope on or following    │
          │       │   exertion                   │
          │       │ - Other symptoms highly      │
          │       │   suggestive of ischemia on  │
          │       │   or following exertion      │
          │       │                              │
          │       │ High-risk anatomy (imaging)  │
          │       │ - Intramural                 │
          │       │ - Abnormal ostium            │
          │       │                              │
          │       │ Perfusion defect that        │
          │       │ corresponds to the affected  │
          │       │ territory                    │
          │       └──────────────────────────────┘
          ▼           Yes │              │ No
┌────────────────────────┐              │
│ Surgical intervention* │◄─────────────┘
│ Exercise restriction   │              ▼
│ until surgery**        │   ┌──────────────────────┐
└────────────────────────┘   │ No surgical          │
          │                  │ intervention         │
          │                  │ No exercise          │
          │                  │ restriction          │
          ▼                  └──────────────────────┘
┌──────────────────────────────────┐       │
│ Postoperative short-term         │       ▼
│ follow-up                        │   ┌──────────────────────────┐
│ - 1 wk: Surgical follow-up       │   │ Long-term follow-up      │
│ - 1 mo: Cardiology visit with    │──▶│ - Cardiology follow-up   │
│   ECG, echocardiogram            │   │   q1 year                │
│ - 3 mo: Cardiology visit with    │   │ - ECG q1 year            │
│   ECG, CT, funtional testing     │   │ - Echocardiogram q2      │
│ - 6 mo: Cardiology visit with ECG│   │   years (optional)       │
│ No exercise restriction after    │   │ - Exercise stress test   │
│ third month visit                │   │   q2 years (optional)    │
│ if studies are negative          │   └──────────────────────────┘
└──────────────────────────────────┘       │
          │                                ▼
          └────────────────►┌──────────────────────────────┐
                            │ Symptoms or positive testing │
                            └──────────────────────────────┘
```

Unroofing if significant intramural segment, neo-ostium creation or coronary translocation if intramural segment behind a commissure, coronary translocation or pulmonary artery translocation if short or no intramural segment.
** Restriction from participation in all competitive sports and in exercise with moderate or high dynamic component (>40% maximal oxygen uptake - e.g., soccer, tennis, swimming, basketball, American football).

ALAD, Anomalous left anterior descending artery; ALCA-R, Anomalous left coronary from the right sinus; ALCx, Anomalous left circumflex artery; ARCA-L, Anomalous right coronary from the left sinus

Hypoplastic Left Heart Syndrome
Peter Chen, John E. Mayer

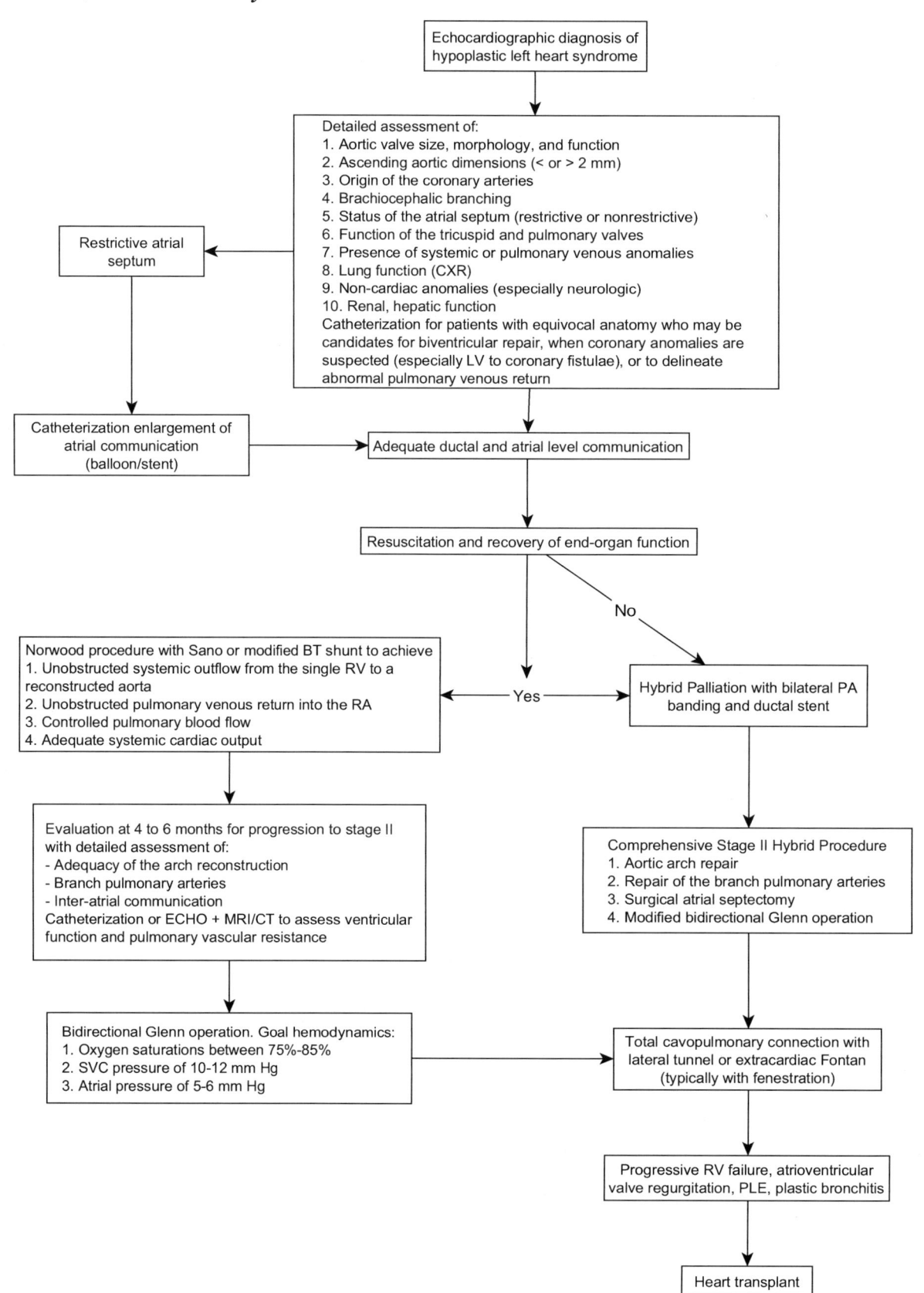

```
┌─────────────────────────────────────┐
│ Echocardiographic diagnosis of      │
│ hypoplastic left heart syndrome     │
└─────────────────────────────────────┘
                  │
                  ▼
┌──────────────────────────────────────────────────────────┐
│ Detailed assessment of:                                  │
│ 1. Aortic valve size, morphology, and function           │
│ 2. Ascending aortic dimensions (< or > 2 mm)             │
│ 3. Origin of the coronary arteries                       │
│ 4. Brachiocephalic branching                             │
│ 5. Status of the atrial septum (restrictive or           │
│    nonrestrictive)                                       │
│ 6. Function of the tricuspid and pulmonary valves        │
│ 7. Presence of systemic or pulmonary venous anomalies    │
│ 8. Lung function (CXR)                                   │
│ 9. Non-cardiac anomalies (especially neurologic)         │
│ 10. Renal, hepatic function                              │
│ Catheterization for patients with equivocal anatomy who  │
│ may be candidates for biventricular repair, when         │
│ coronary anomalies are suspected (especially LV to       │
│ coronary fistulae), or to delineate abnormal pulmonary   │
│ venous return                                            │
└──────────────────────────────────────────────────────────┘
```

- Restrictive atrial septum
- Catheterization enlargement of atrial communication (balloon/stent)
- Adequate ductal and atrial level communication
- Resuscitation and recovery of end-organ function

Yes: Norwood procedure with Sano or modified BT shunt to achieve
1. Unobstructed systemic outflow from the single RV to a reconstructed aorta
2. Unobstructed pulmonary venous return into the RA
3. Controlled pulmonary blood flow
4. Adequate systemic cardiac output

No: Hybrid Palliation with bilateral PA banding and ductal stent

Evaluation at 4 to 6 months for progression to stage II with detailed assessment of:
- Adequacy of the arch reconstruction
- Branch pulmonary arteries
- Inter-atrial communication

Catheterization or ECHO + MRI/CT to assess ventricular function and pulmonary vascular resistance

Comprehensive Stage II Hybrid Procedure
1. Aortic arch repair
2. Repair of the branch pulmonary arteries
3. Surgical atrial septectomy
4. Modified bidirectional Glenn operation

Bidirectional Glenn operation. Goal hemodynamics:
1. Oxygen saturations between 75%-85%
2. SVC pressure of 10-12 mm Hg
3. Atrial pressure of 5-6 mm Hg

Total cavopulmonary connection with lateral tunnel or extracardiac Fontan (typically with fenestration)

Progressive RV failure, atrioventricular valve regurgitation, PLE, plastic bronchitis

Heart transplant

CXR, chest x-ray; LV, left ventricular; PA, pulmonary artery; RV, right ventricle; PLE, protein losing enteropathy; BT, Blalock-Taussig; RA, right atrium

Vascular Rings and Pulmonary Artery Sling
Sudhan Nagarajan, Khanh Nguyen

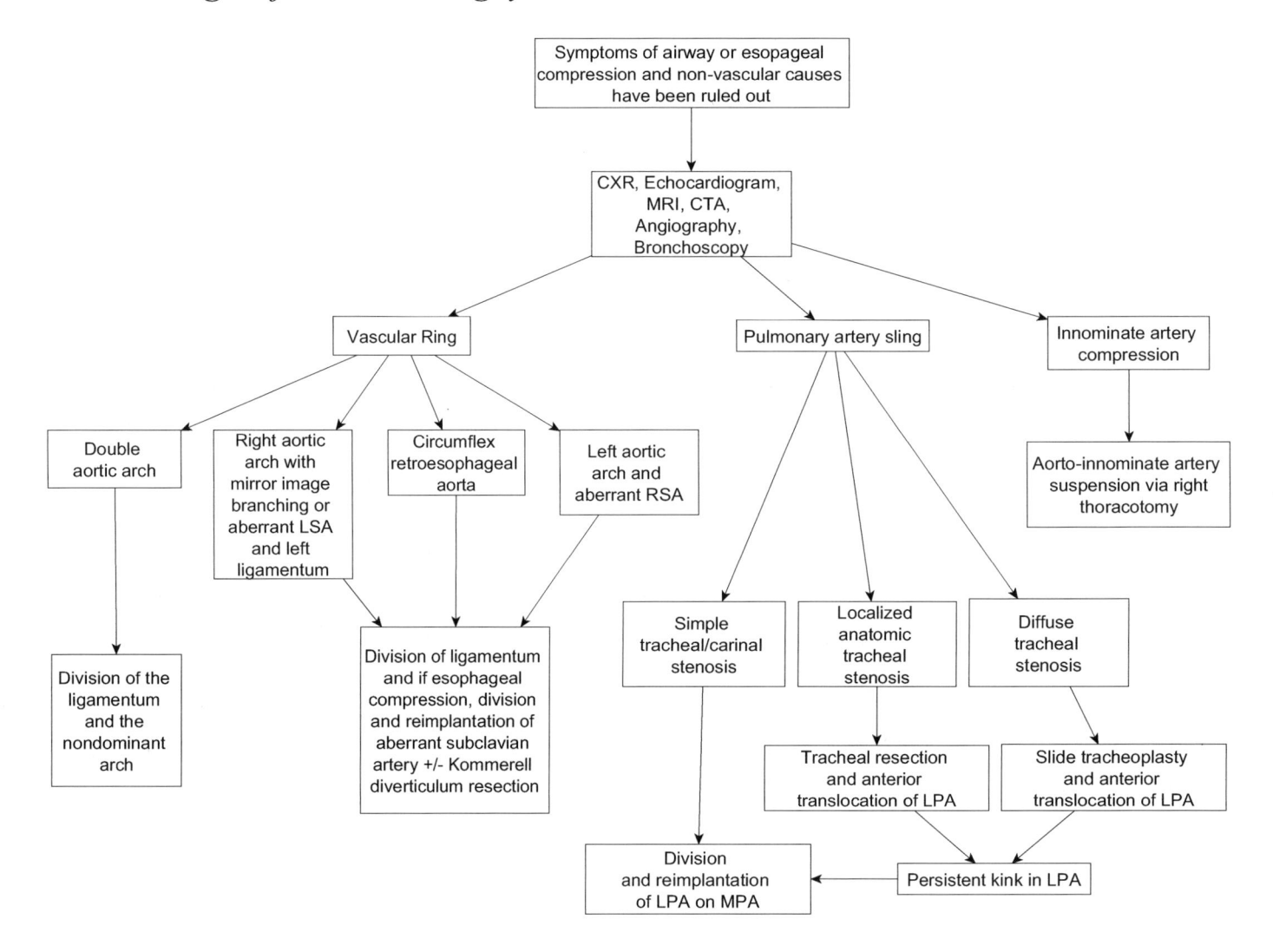

```
┌─────────────────────────────────┐
│ Symptoms of airway or esophageal│
│ compression and non-vascular    │
│ causes have been ruled out      │
└─────────────────────────────────┘
                │
                ▼
┌─────────────────────┐
│ CXR, Echocardiogram,│
│ MRI, CTA,           │
│ Angiography,        │
│ Bronchoscopy        │
└─────────────────────┘
        │
    ┌───┴────┬──────────────┐
    ▼        ▼              ▼
Vascular  Pulmonary    Innominate
 Ring    artery sling    artery
                       compression
                            │
                            ▼
                   Aorto-innominate artery
                   suspension via right
                   thoracotomy
```

Vascular Ring branches:
- **Double aortic arch** → Division of the ligamentum and the nondominant arch
- **Right aortic arch with mirror image branching or aberrant LSA and left ligamentum** → Division of ligamentum and if esophageal compression, division and reimplantation of aberrant subclavian artery +/- Kommerell diverticulum resection
- **Circumflex retroesophageal aorta** → (same box above)
- **Left aortic arch and aberrant RSA** → (same box above)

Pulmonary artery sling branches:
- **Simple tracheal/carinal stenosis** → Division and reimplantation of LPA on MPA
- **Localized anatomic tracheal stenosis** → Tracheal resection and anterior translocation of LPA → Persistent kink in LPA → Division and reimplantation of LPA on MPA
- **Diffuse tracheal stenosis** → Slide tracheoplasty and anterior translocation of LPA → Persistent kink in LPA → Division and reimplantation of LPA on MPA

Investigation of choice of all forms of vascular rings; Bronchoscopy - required for workup of pulmonary artery sling

Surgical approach - Thoracotomy same side of obstruction for all vascular rings; Sternotomy for pulmonary artery sling

CXR - Chest X ray; MRI - Magnetic resonance imaging; CTA - Computed tomographic angiogram; LSA - Left subclavian artery; RSA – Right subclavian artery; LPA - Left pulmonary artery; MPA - Main pulmonary artery; MRI

Pediatric heart Failure/Heart Transplant
Joshua Rosenblum, K Rose-Felker, Kirk Kanter

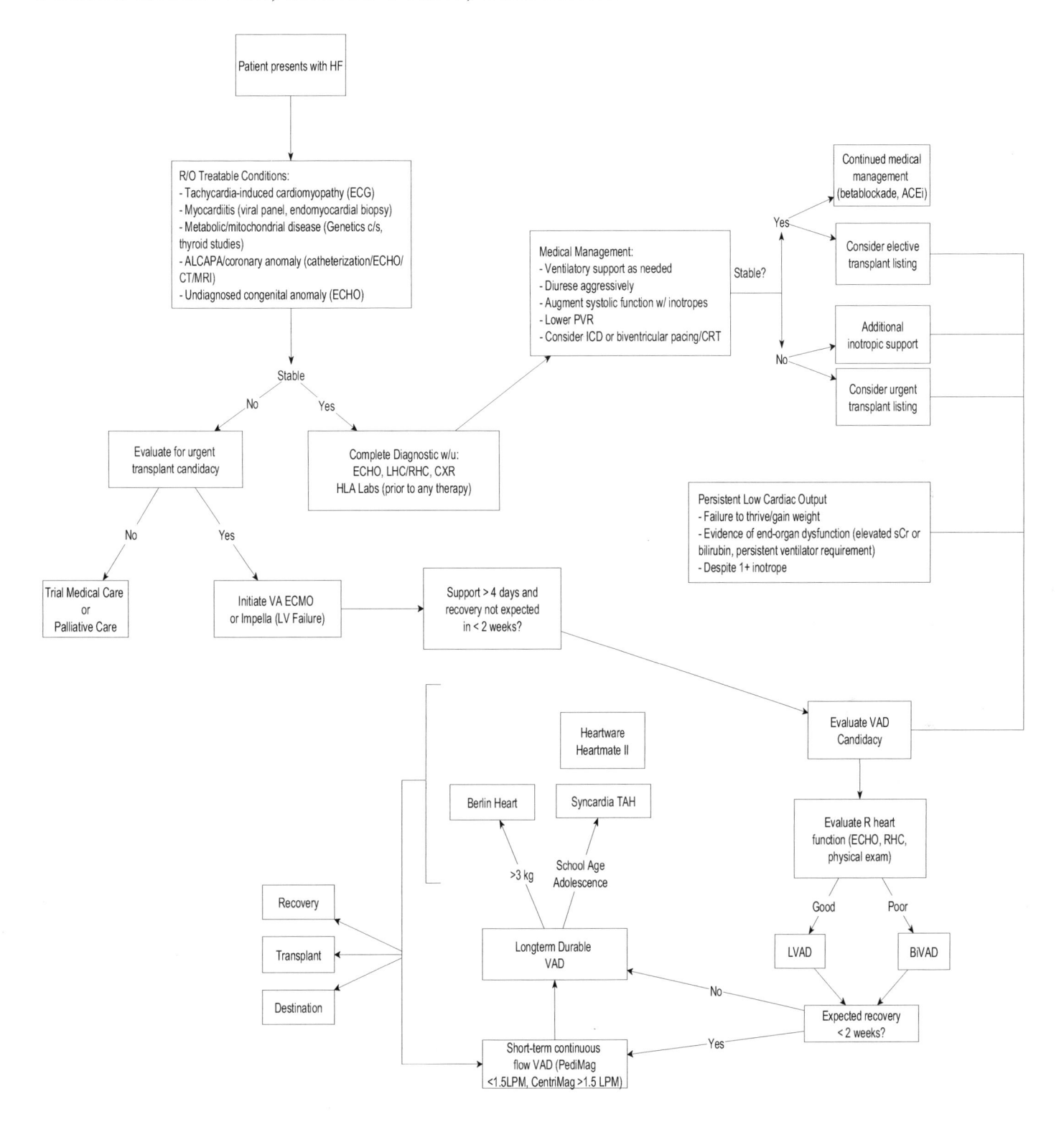

```
┌─────────────────────────┐
│ Patient presents with HF │
└───────────┬─────────────┘
            │
            ▼
┌──────────────────────────────────────────┐
│ R/O Treatable Conditions:                │
│  - Tachycardia-induced cardiomyopathy    │
│    (ECG)                                 │
│  - Myocarditis (viral panel,             │
│    endomyocardial biopsy)                │
│  - Metabolic/mitochondrial disease       │
│    (Genetics c/s, thyroid studies)       │
│  - ALCAPA/coronary anomaly               │
│    (catheterization/ECHO/CT/MRI)         │
│  - Undiagnosed congenital anomaly (ECHO) │
└──────────────────────────────────────────┘
          │ Stable
     No ──┴── Yes
     │         │
     ▼         ▼
 Evaluate   Complete Diagnostic w/u:
 for urgent ECHO, LHC/RHC, CXR
 transplant HLA Labs (prior to any therapy)
 candidacy
   │
 No│Yes
   │ │
   ▼ ▼
Trial    Initiate VA ECMO  ──► Support > 4 days and
Medical  or Impella              recovery not expected
Care or  (LV Failure)             in < 2 weeks?
Palliative
Care
```

Medical Management:
 - Ventilatory support as needed
 - Diurese aggressively
 - Augment systolic function w/ inotropes
 - Lower PVR
 - Consider ICD or biventricular pacing/CRT

Stable?
- Yes → Continued medical management (betablockade, ACEi)
- Yes → Consider elective transplant listing
- No → Additional inotropic support
- No → Consider urgent transplant listing

Persistent Low Cardiac Output
 - Failure to thrive/gain weight
 - Evidence of end-organ dysfunction (elevated sCr or bilirubin, persistent ventilator requirement)
 - Despite 1+ inotrope

Evaluate VAD Candidacy
 → Evaluate R heart function (ECHO, RHC, physical exam)
   - Good → LVAD
   - Poor → BiVAD
 → Expected recovery < 2 weeks?
   - Yes → Short-term continuous flow VAD (PediMag <1.5LPM, CentriMag >1.5 LPM)
   - No → Longterm Durable VAD

Longterm Durable VAD options:
 - Berlin Heart (>3 kg)
 - Heartware Heartmate II
 - Syncardia TAH (School Age, Adolescence)

Outcomes:
 - Recovery
 - Transplant
 - Destination

181

Contraindications to Tx:
Fixed, elevated PVR (irreversible PAH, high TPG)
Active sepsis
Mitochondrial disease
Severe neurological disease (CVA/IVH, refractory seizures)
Irreversible end-organ damage (heart/kidney and heart/liver tx per institution protocols)
BMI ≥ 35 kg/m2 (relative)
Diabetes with end-organ damage (relative)

ALCAPA, anomalous left coronary from the pulmonary artery; CF, continuous flow; CRT, cardiac resynchronization therapy; PAH, pulmonary arterial hypertension; PVR, pulmonary vascular resistance; TAH, total artificial heart; TPG, trans-pulmonary gradient

Interrupted Aortic Arch with VSD
Joshua Rosenblum, Kirk Kanter

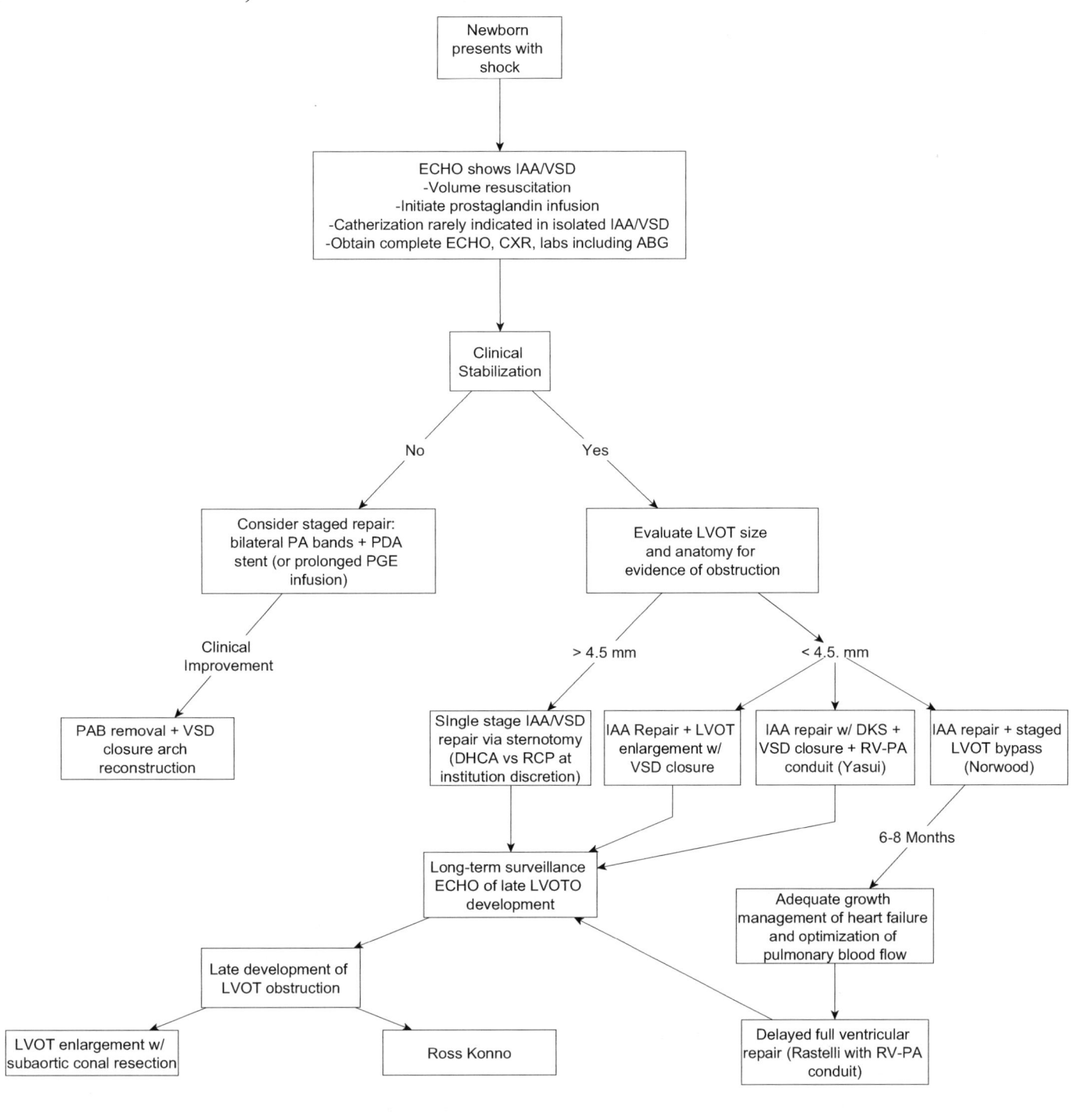

```
                    ┌─────────────────┐
                    │    Newborn      │
                    │  presents with  │
                    │     shock       │
                    └────────┬────────┘
                             │
                             ▼
         ┌──────────────────────────────────────────┐
         │          ECHO shows IAA/VSD              │
         │  -Volume resuscitation                   │
         │  -Initiate prostaglandin infusion        │
         │  -Catherization rarely indicated in      │
         │   isolated IAA/VSD                       │
         │  -Obtain complete ECHO, CXR, labs        │
         │   including ABG                          │
         └────────────────┬─────────────────────────┘
                          │
                          ▼
                  ┌───────────────┐
                  │   Clinical    │
                  │ Stabilization │
                  └───┬───────┬───┘
                 No  │       │  Yes
          ┌──────────┘       └──────────┐
          ▼                              ▼
┌──────────────────────┐      ┌────────────────────────┐
│ Consider staged      │      │  Evaluate LVOT size    │
│ repair: bilateral PA │      │  and anatomy for       │
│ bands + PDA stent    │      │  evidence of           │
│ (or prolonged PGE    │      │  obstruction           │
│ infusion)            │      └────────────────────────┘
└──────────────────────┘
```

Branches from "Evaluate LVOT size and anatomy for evidence of obstruction":
- **> 4.5 mm**: Single stage IAA/VSD repair via sternotomy (DHCA vs RCP at institution discretion)
- **< 4.5 mm**:
  - IAA Repair + LVOT enlargement w/ VSD closure
  - IAA repair w/ DKS + VSD closure + RV-PA conduit (Yasui)
  - IAA repair + staged LVOT bypass (Norwood)

From "Consider staged repair" → **Clinical Improvement** → PAB removal + VSD closure arch reconstruction

From Norwood → **6-8 Months** → Adequate growth management of heart failure and optimization of pulmonary blood flow → Delayed full ventricular repair (Rastelli with RV-PA conduit)

Single stage repair, IAA Repair + LVOT enlargement, and Yasui → Long-term surveillance ECHO of late LVOTO development

Long-term surveillance → Late development of LVOT obstruction:
- LVOT enlargement w/ subaortic conal resection
- Ross Konno

DHCA, Deep hypothermic circulatory arrest; DKS, Damus-Kaye-Stansel anastomosis; IAA, interrupted aortic arch; LVOT, left ventricular outflow tract; LVOTO, LVOT obstruction; PA, pulmonary artery; PAB, pulmonary artery band; RCP, regional/cerebral perfusion; VSD, ventricular septal defect

Functional Single Ventricle Palliation
Bartholomew V. Simon, Michael F. Swartz, George M. Alfieris

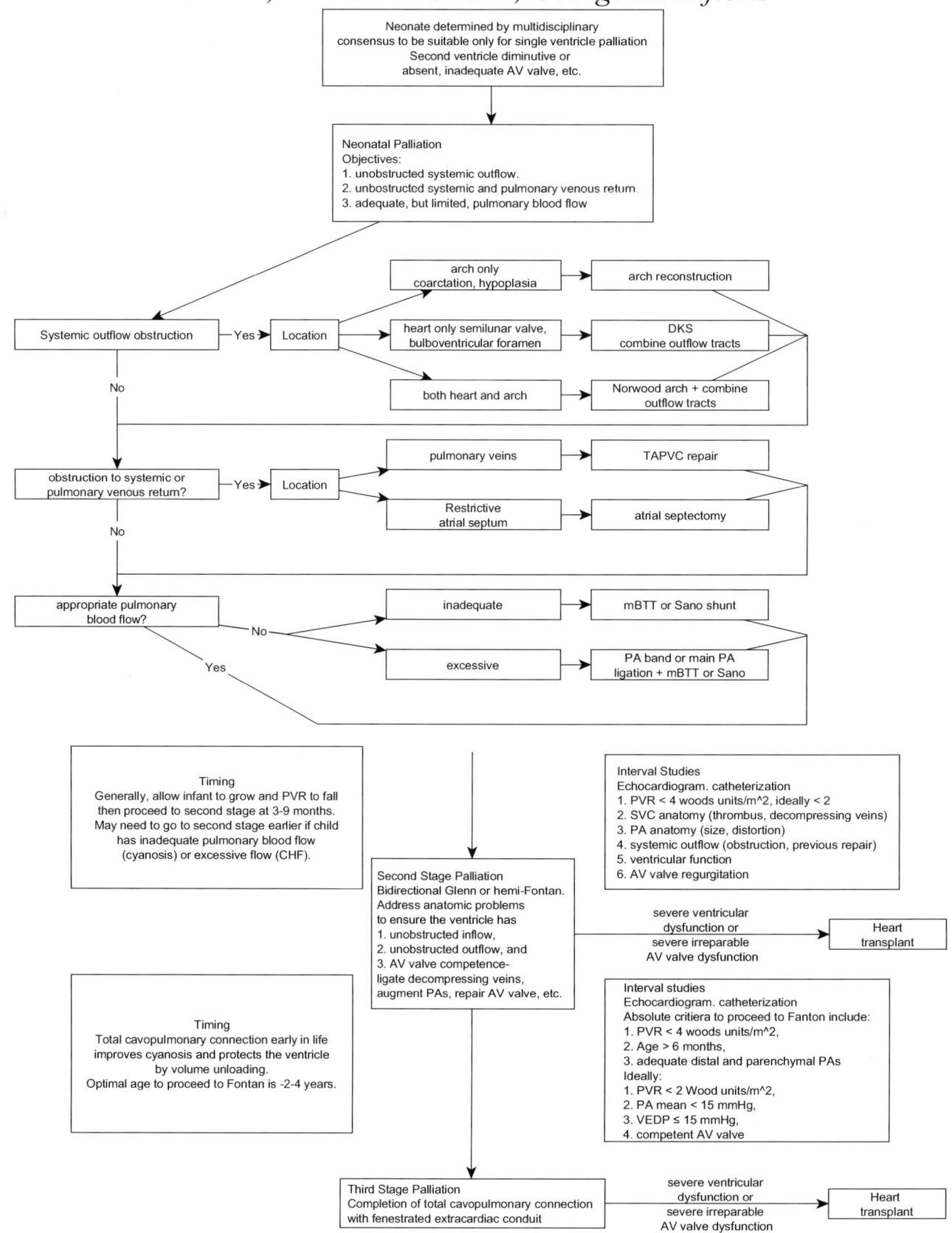

```
┌─────────────────────────────────────────┐
│ Neonate determined by multidisciplinary │
│ consensus to be suitable only for single│
│ ventricle palliation                    │
│ Second ventricle diminutive or          │
│ absent, inadequate AV valve, etc.       │
└─────────────────────────────────────────┘
                    │
                    ▼
┌─────────────────────────────────────────┐
│ Neonatal Palliation                     │
│ Objectives:                             │
│ 1. unobstructed systemic outflow.       │
│ 2. unobstructed systemic and pulmonary  │
│    venous return.                       │
│ 3. adequate, but limited, pulmonary     │
│    blood flow                           │
└─────────────────────────────────────────┘
```

Systemic outflow obstruction — Yes → Location →
- arch only coarctation, hypoplasia → arch reconstruction
- heart only semilunar valve, bulboventricular foramen → DKS combine outflow tracts
- both heart and arch → Norwood arch + combine outflow tracts

No ↓

obstruction to systemic or pulmonary venous return? — Yes → Location →
- pulmonary veins → TAPVC repair
- Restrictive atrial septum → atrial septectomy

No ↓

appropriate pulmonary blood flow? — No →
- inadequate → mBTT or Sano shunt
- excessive → PA band or main PA ligation + mBTT or Sano

Yes ↓

Timing
Generally, allow infant to grow and PVR to fall then proceed to second stage at 3-9 months. May need to go to second stage earlier if child has inadequate pulmonary blood flow (cyanosis) or excessive flow (CHF).

Second Stage Palliation
Bidirectional Glenn or hemi-Fontan.
Address anatomic problems to ensure the ventricle has
1. unobstructed inflow,
2. unobstructed outflow, and
3. AV valve competence-
ligate decompressing veins, augment PAs, repair AV valve, etc.

Interval Studies
Echocardiogram. catheterization
1. PVR < 4 woods units/m^2, ideally < 2
2. SVC anatomy (thrombus, decompressing veins)
3. PA anatomy (size, distortion)
4. systemic outflow (obstruction, previous repair)
5. ventricular function
6. AV valve regurgitation

→ severe ventricular dysfunction or severe irreparable AV valve dysfunction → Heart transplant

Timing
Total cavopulmonary connection early in life improves cyanosis and protects the ventricle by volume unloading.
Optimal age to proceed to Fontan is -2-4 years.

Interval studies
Echocardiogram. catheterization
Absolute critiera to proceed to Fanton include:
1. PVR < 4 woods units/m^2,
2. Age > 6 months,
3. adequate distal and parenchymal PAs
Ideally:
1. PVR < 2 Wood units/m^2,
2. PA mean < 15 mmHg,
3. VEDP ≤ 15 mmHg,
4. competent AV valve

Third Stage Palliation
Completion of total cavopulmonary connection with fenestrated extracardiac conduit

→ severe ventricular dysfunction or severe irreparable AV valve dysfunction → Heart transplant

```
┌─────────────────────────────────────────┐
│ Neonate determined by multidisciplinary │
│ consensus to be suitable only for single ventricle palliation │
│         Second ventricle diminutive or  │
│         absent, inadequate AV valve, etc.│
└─────────────────────────────────────────┘
                    │
                    ▼
┌─────────────────────────────────────────┐
│ Neonatal Palliation                     │
│ Objectives:                             │
│ 1. unobstructed systemic outflow.       │
│ 2. unobstructed systemic and pulmonary venous return. │
│ 3. adequate, but limited, pulmonary blood flow │
└─────────────────────────────────────────┘
```

Systemic outflow obstruction — Yes → Location →
- arch only coarctation, hypoplasia → arch reconstruction
- heart only semilunar valve, bulboventricular foramen → DKS combine outflow tracts
- both heart and arch → Norwood arch + combine outflow tracts

↓ No

obstruction to systemic or pulmonary venous return? — Yes → Location →
- pulmonary veins → TAPVC repair
- Restrictive atrial septum → atrial septectomy

↓ No

appropriate pulmonary blood flow? — No →
- inadequate → mBTT or Sano shunt
- excessive → PA band or main PA ligation + mBTT or Sano

↓ Yes

☆

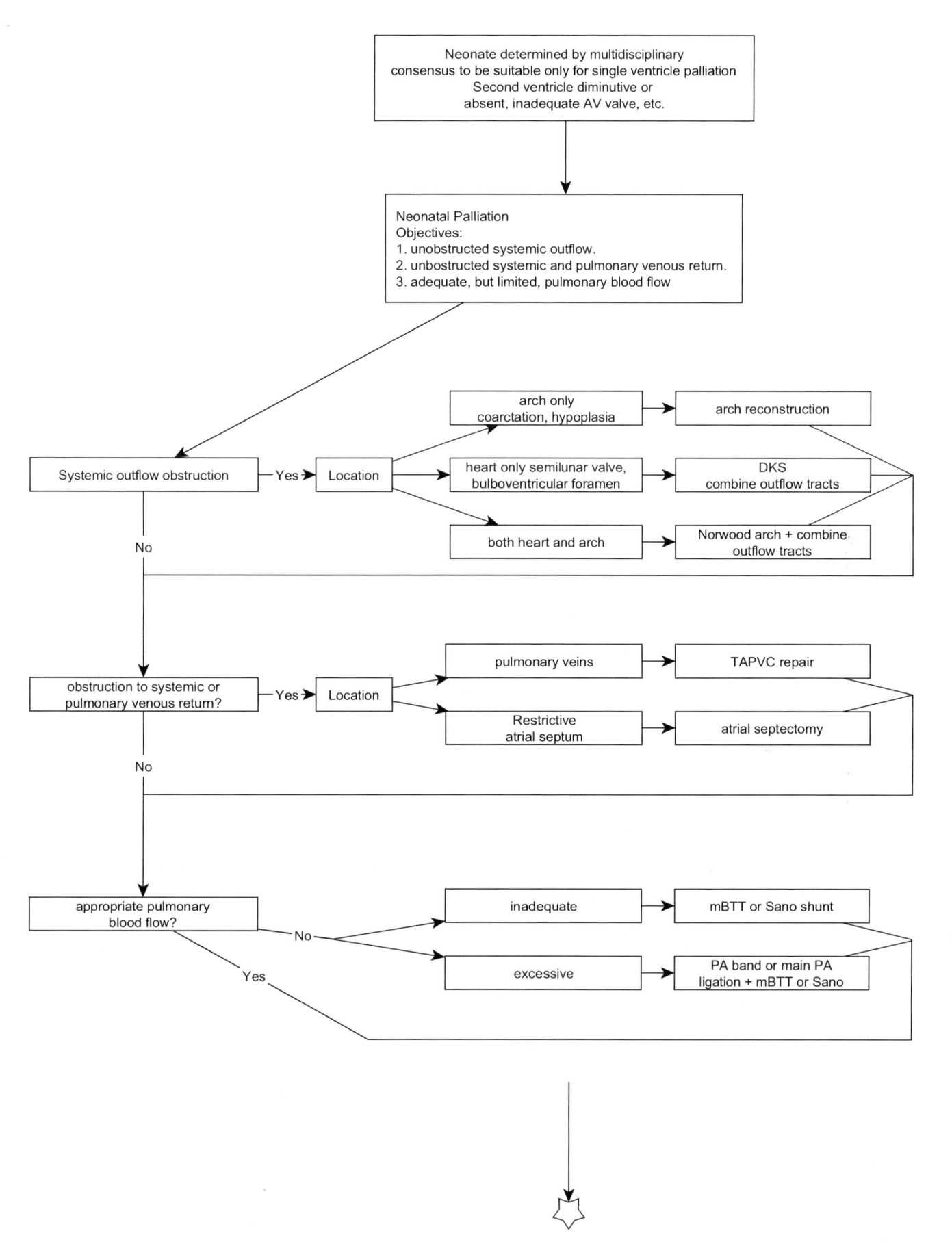

185

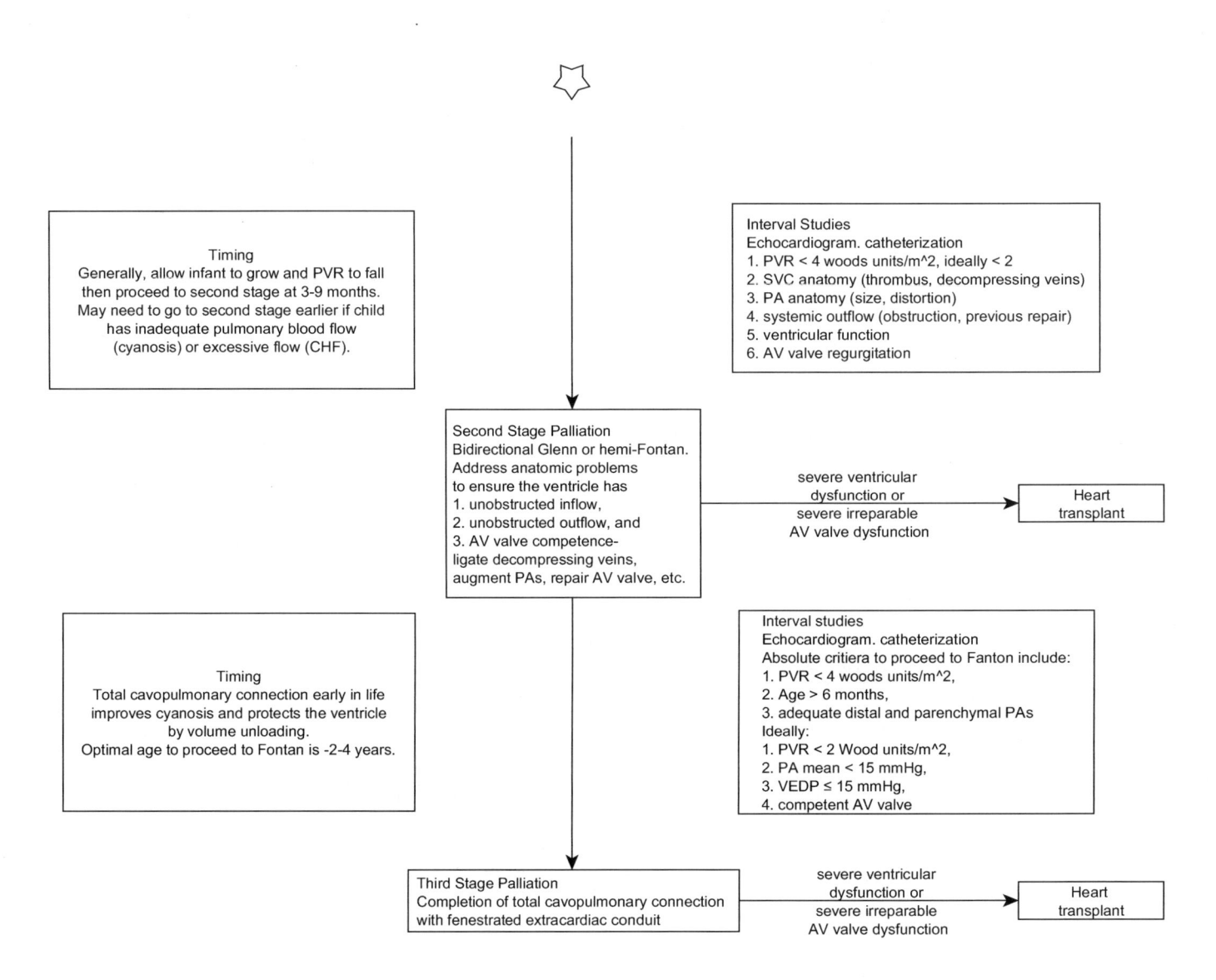

```
                                    ☆
                                    │
                                    │
┌─────────────────────────────┐     │     ┌──────────────────────────────────────┐
│         Timing              │     │     │ Interval Studies                     │
│ Generally, allow infant to  │     │     │ Echocardiogram. catheterization      │
│ grow and PVR to fall        │     │     │ 1. PVR < 4 woods units/m^2,          │
│ then proceed to second      │     │     │    ideally < 2                       │
│ stage at 3-9 months.        │     │     │ 2. SVC anatomy (thrombus,            │
│ May need to go to second    │     │     │    decompressing veins)              │
│ stage earlier if child      │     │     │ 3. PA anatomy (size, distortion)     │
│ has inadequate pulmonary    │     │     │ 4. systemic outflow (obstruction,    │
│ blood flow (cyanosis) or    │     │     │    previous repair)                  │
│ excessive flow (CHF).       │     │     │ 5. ventricular function              │
└─────────────────────────────┘     │     │ 6. AV valve regurgitation            │
                                    │     └──────────────────────────────────────┘
                                    ▼
                        ┌──────────────────────────┐
                        │ Second Stage Palliation  │
                        │ Bidirectional Glenn or   │      severe ventricular
                        │ hemi-Fontan.             │      dysfunction or              ┌───────────┐
                        │ Address anatomic problems├─────▶severe irreparable ─────────▶│   Heart   │
                        │ to ensure the ventricle  │      AV valve dysfunction        │ transplant│
                        │ has                      │                                  └───────────┘
                        │ 1. unobstructed inflow,  │
                        │ 2. unobstructed outflow, │
                        │ 3. AV valve competence-  │
                        │ ligate decompressing     │
                        │ veins, augment PAs,      │
                        │ repair AV valve, etc.    │
                        └──────────────────────────┘
                                    │
┌─────────────────────────────┐     │     ┌──────────────────────────────────────┐
│         Timing              │     │     │ Interval studies                     │
│ Total cavopulmonary         │     │     │ Echocardiogram. catheterization      │
│ connection early in life    │     │     │ Absolute critiera to proceed to      │
│ improves cyanosis and       │     │     │ Fanton include:                      │
│ protects the ventricle      │     │     │ 1. PVR < 4 woods units/m^2,          │
│ by volume unloading.        │     │     │ 2. Age > 6 months,                   │
│ Optimal age to proceed to   │     │     │ 3. adequate distal and parenchymal PAs│
│ Fontan is ~2-4 years.       │     │     │ Ideally:                             │
└─────────────────────────────┘     │     │ 1. PVR < 2 Wood units/m^2,           │
                                    │     │ 2. PA mean < 15 mmHg,                │
                                    │     │ 3. VEDP ≤ 15 mmHg,                   │
                                    │     │ 4. competent AV valve                │
                                    │     └──────────────────────────────────────┘
                                    ▼
                        ┌──────────────────────────┐      severe ventricular
                        │ Third Stage Palliation   │      dysfunction or              ┌───────────┐
                        │ Completion of total      ├─────▶severe irreparable ─────────▶│   Heart   │
                        │ cavopulmonary connection │      AV valve dysfunction        │ transplant│
                        │ with fenestrated         │                                  └───────────┘
                        │ extracardiac conduit     │
                        └──────────────────────────┘
```

AV, atrioventricular; DKS, Damus-Kaye-Stansel; TAPVC, total anomalous pulmonary venous connection; mBTT, modified Blalock-Thomas-Taussig; PA, pulmonary artery; CHF, congestive heart failure; PVR, pulmonary vascular resistance; SVC, superior vena cava; VEDP, Ventricular end diastolic pressure

Truncus Arteriosus
Christopher Greenleaf, Ali Dodge-Khatami

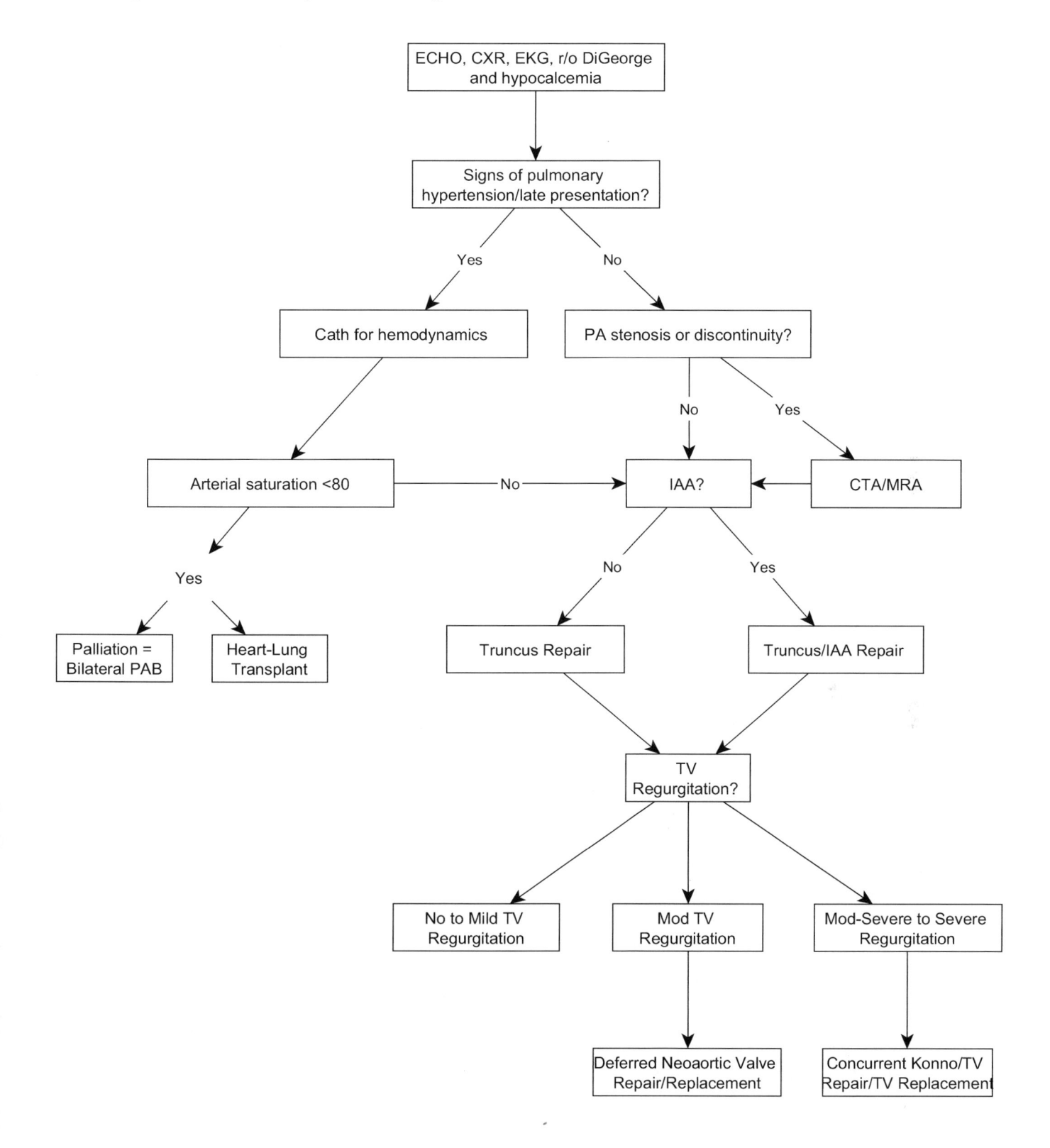

```
┌─────────────────────────────────┐
│ ECHO, CXR, EKG, r/o DiGeorge    │
│ and hypocalcemia                │
└─────────────────────────────────┘
                │
                ▼
┌─────────────────────────────────┐
│ Signs of pulmonary              │
│ hypertension/late presentation? │
└─────────────────────────────────┘
         │                │
        Yes               No
         │                │
         ▼                ▼
┌──────────────────┐  ┌──────────────────────────┐
│ Cath for         │  │ PA stenosis or           │
│ hemodynamics     │  │ discontinuity?           │
└──────────────────┘  └──────────────────────────┘
         │                │            │
         │               No           Yes
         ▼                │            │
┌──────────────────┐      │            ▼
│ Arterial         │──No──┼──►┌───────┐  ┌─────────┐
│ saturation <80   │      └──►│ IAA?  │◄─│ CTA/MRA │
└──────────────────┘          └───────┘  └─────────┘
         │                     │      │
        Yes                   No     Yes
         │                     │      │
         ▼                     ▼      ▼
┌──────────┐ ┌──────────┐  ┌────────────┐ ┌──────────────┐
│Palliation│ │Heart-Lung│  │Truncus     │ │Truncus/IAA   │
│= Bilat-  │ │Transplant│  │Repair      │ │Repair        │
│eral PAB  │ │          │  │            │ │              │
└──────────┘ └──────────┘  └────────────┘ └──────────────┘
                                 │             │
                                 ▼             ▼
                          ┌───────────────────────┐
                          │ TV Regurgitation?     │
                          └───────────────────────┘
                             │        │         │
                             ▼        ▼         ▼
                  ┌────────────┐ ┌──────────┐ ┌────────────────┐
                  │No to Mild  │ │Mod TV    │ │Mod-Severe to   │
                  │TV Regurgi- │ │Regurgi-  │ │Severe Regurgi- │
                  │tation      │ │tation    │ │tation          │
                  └────────────┘ └──────────┘ └────────────────┘
                                      │             │
                                      ▼             ▼
                            ┌──────────────────┐ ┌──────────────────┐
                            │Deferred Neoaortic│ │Concurrent Konno/ │
                            │Valve Repair/     │ │TV Repair/TV      │
                            │Replacement       │ │Replacement       │
                            └──────────────────┘ └──────────────────┘
```

PA, pulmonary artery; IAA - interrupted aortic arch; PAB, pulmonary artery band; TV, truncal valve; ECHO, echocardiography; CXR, chest x-ray; EKG, electrocardiogram; CTA, computed tomography angiogram; MRA, magnetic resonance angiogram; Mod, moderate

Complete Atrioventricular Canal Defect
Edo Bedzra, Lester Permut

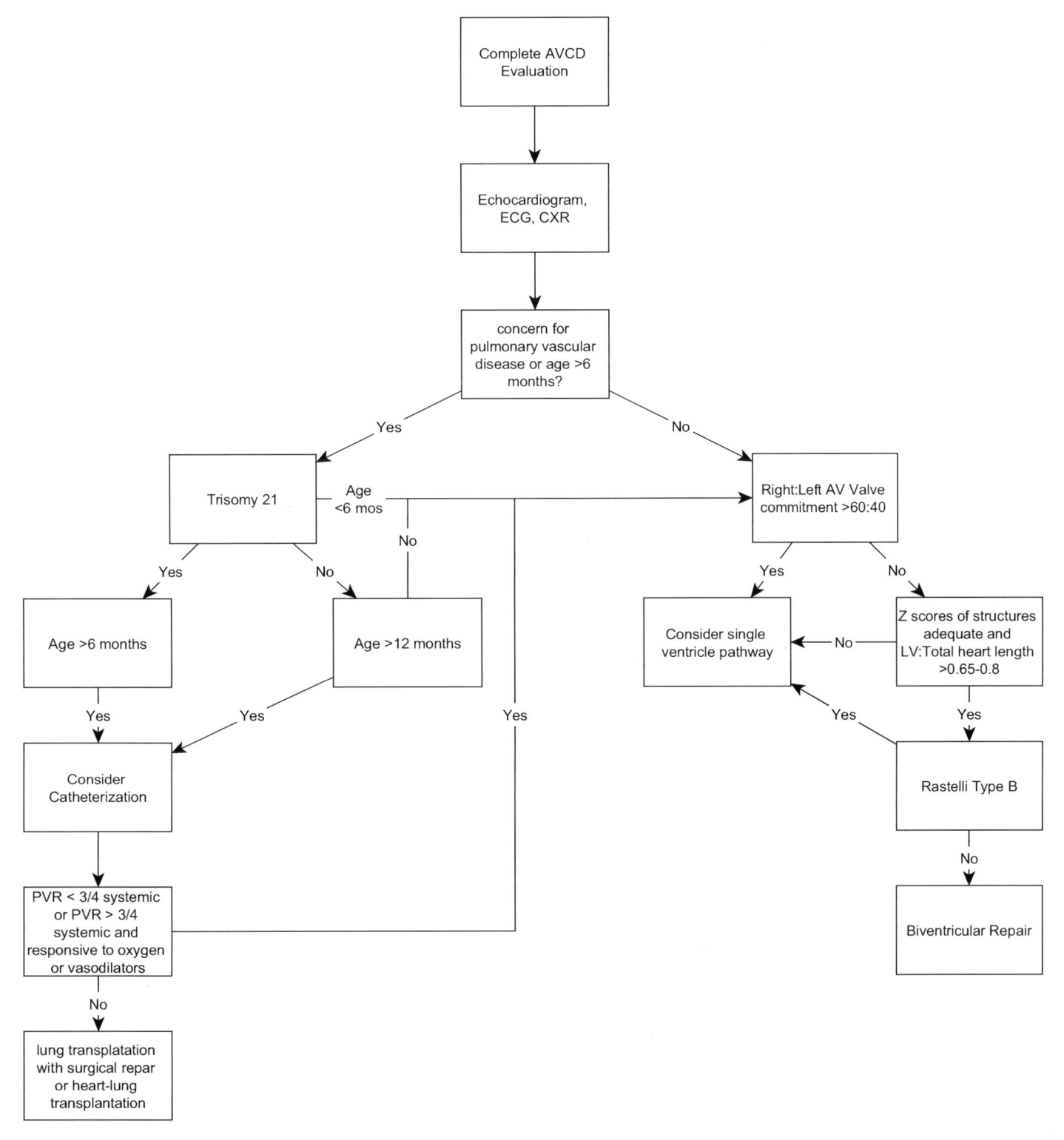

```
                    ┌─────────────────┐
                    │  Complete AVCD  │
                    │   Evaluation    │
                    └────────┬────────┘
                             ▼
                    ┌─────────────────┐
                    │  Echocardiogram,│
                    │     ECG, CXR    │
                    └────────┬────────┘
                             ▼
                    ┌─────────────────┐
                    │    concern for  │
                    │ pulmonary vascular│
                    │ disease or age >6│
                    │     months?     │
                    └────────┬────────┘
                   Yes              No
```

- concern for pulmonary vascular disease or age >6 months?
  - **Yes** → Trisomy 21?
    - **Yes** → Age >6 months → Consider Catheterization
    - **No** → Age <6 mos?
      - **No** → Age >12 months → Consider Catheterization
  - Consider Catheterization → PVR < 3/4 systemic or PVR > 3/4 systemic and responsive to oxygen or vasodilators
    - **Yes** → (proceed to Right:Left AV Valve commitment evaluation)
    - **No** → lung transplantation with surgical repair or heart-lung transplantation
  - **No** → Right:Left AV Valve commitment >60:40
    - **Yes** → Consider single ventricle pathway
    - **No** → Z scores of structures adequate and LV:Total heart length >0.65-0.8
      - **No** → Consider single ventricle pathway
      - **Yes** → Rastelli Type B
        - **Yes** → Consider single ventricle pathway
        - **No** → Biventricular Repair

AVCD, Atrioventricular canal defect; ECG, electrocardiogram; CXR, Chest X-ray; AV, Atrioventricular; PVR, Pulmonary vascular resistance; LV, Left ventricle

Double Outlet Right Ventricle (DORV)
Christopher Greenleaf, Ali Dodge-Khatami

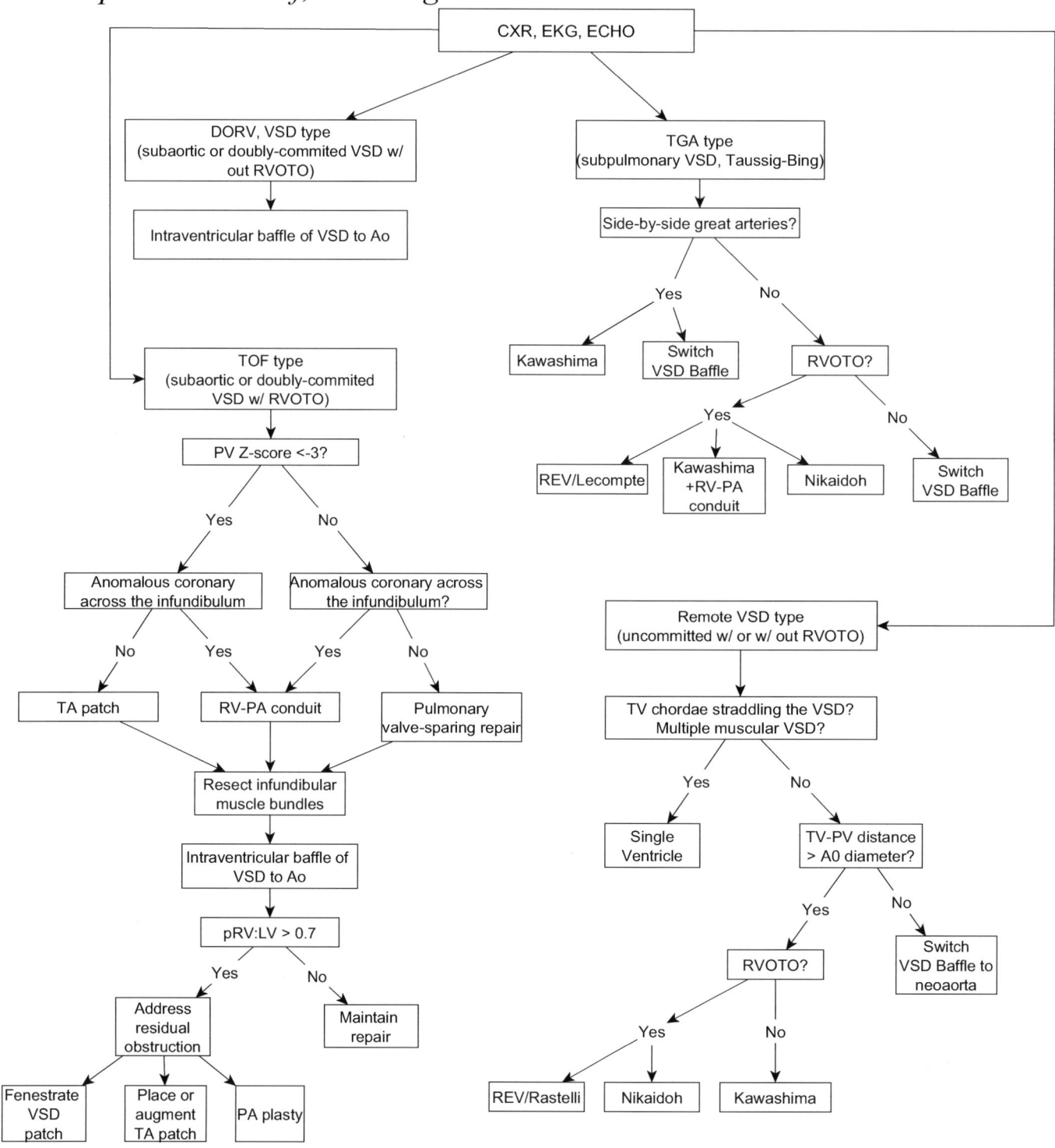

```
                          CXR, EKG, ECHO
          ┌───────────────────┼───────────────────┐
          ▼                                       ▼
 DORV, VSD type                           TGA type
 (subaortic or doubly-commited VSD w/     (subpulmonary VSD, Taussig-Bing)
  out RVOTO)                                      │
          │                                       ▼
          ▼                              Side-by-side great arteries?
 Intraventricular baffle of VSD to Ao      ┌──Yes──┬──No──┐
                                           ▼       ▼      ▼
                                       Kawashima  Switch  RVOTO?
                                                  VSD     ┌─Yes─┬──No──┐
                                                  Baffle  ▼           ▼
 TOF type                                                (REV/Lecompte,  Switch
 (subaortic or doubly-commited                            Kawashima      VSD Baffle
  VSD w/ RVOTO)                                           +RV-PA
          │                                               conduit,
          ▼                                               Nikaidoh)
 PV Z-score <-3?
   ┌──Yes──┬──No──┐
   ▼              ▼
 Anomalous      Anomalous coronary across
 coronary       the infundibulum?
 across the       ┌──Yes──┬──No──┐
 infundibulum    ▼              ▼
   ┌─No─┬─Yes─┐ RV-PA         Pulmonary
   ▼        ▼  conduit        valve-sparing repair
 TA patch  RV-PA conduit
                    │
                    ▼
          Resect infundibular
          muscle bundles
                    │
                    ▼
          Intraventricular baffle of VSD to Ao
                    │
                    ▼
               pRV:LV > 0.7
               ┌─Yes─┬─No─┐
               ▼          ▼
         Address       Maintain
         residual      repair
         obstruction
         ┌────┬────┬────┐
         ▼    ▼    ▼
 Fenestrate  Place or  PA plasty
 VSD patch   augment
             TA patch

 Remote VSD type
 (uncommitted w/ or w/ out RVOTO)
         │
         ▼
 TV chordae straddling the VSD?
 Multiple muscular VSD?
   ┌─Yes─┬──No──┐
   ▼            ▼
 Single      TV-PV distance > A0 diameter?
 Ventricle    ┌─Yes─┬──No──┐
              ▼           ▼
           RVOTO?      Switch VSD Baffle to neoaorta
           ┌─Yes─┬─No─┐
           ▼    ▼    ▼
      REV/   Nikaidoh  Kawashima
      Rastelli
```

☆

```
┌─────────────────────────────────┐
│         DORV, VSD type          │
│ (subaortic or doubly-commited VSD w/ │
│          out RVOTO)             │
└─────────────────────────────────┘
                │
                ▼
┌─────────────────────────────────┐
│ Intraventricular baffle of VSD to Ao │
└─────────────────────────────────┘
```

```
                    ☆  ☆

            ┌─────────────────────┐
            │       TOF type      │
            │ (subaortic or doubly-commited │
            │    VSD w/ RVOTO)    │
            └──────────┬──────────┘
                       ↓
            ┌─────────────────────┐
            │   PV Z-score <-3?   │
            └──────────┬──────────┘
                 Yes ↙   ↘ No
      ┌──────────────────┐  ┌──────────────────┐
      │ Anomalous coronary│  │Anomalous coronary across│
      │ across the infundibulum│ │  the infundibulum?  │
      └────┬─────────┬───┘  └────┬─────────┬───┘
        No ↙       ↘ Yes     Yes ↙       ↘ No
   ┌─────────┐   ┌──────────────┐     ┌──────────────┐
   │ TA patch│   │ RV-PA conduit│     │   Pulmonary  │
   │         │   │              │     │valve-sparing repair│
   └────┬────┘   └──────┬───────┘     └──────┬───────┘
        └───────────────┼────────────────────┘
                        ↓
            ┌─────────────────────┐
            │ Resect infundibular │
            │   muscle bundles    │
            └──────────┬──────────┘
                       ↓
            ┌─────────────────────┐
            │ Intraventricular baffle of│
            │      VSD to Ao      │
            └──────────┬──────────┘
                       ↓
            ┌─────────────────────┐
            │    pRV:LV > 0.7     │
            └────┬───────────┬────┘
             Yes ↙           ↘ No
      ┌──────────────┐      ┌──────────┐
      │   Address    │      │ Maintain │
      │   residual   │      │  repair  │
      │ obstruction  │      └──────────┘
      └──┬──────┬────┬──┘
         ↓      ↓    ↓
   ┌─────────┐┌────────┐┌─────────┐
   │Fenestrate││Place or││PA plasty│
   │  VSD    ││augment ││         │
   │ patch   ││TA patch││         │
   └─────────┘└────────┘└─────────┘
```

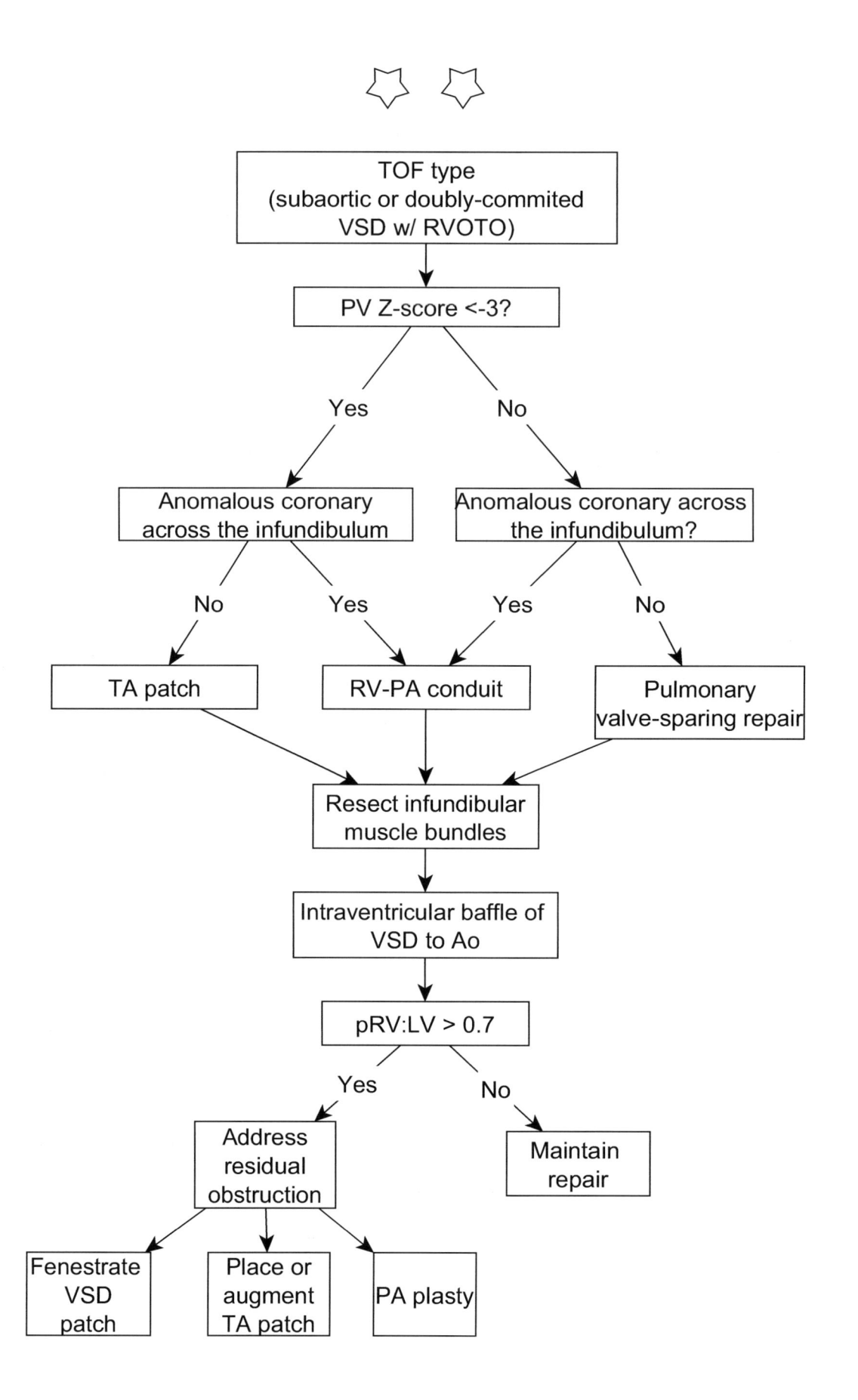

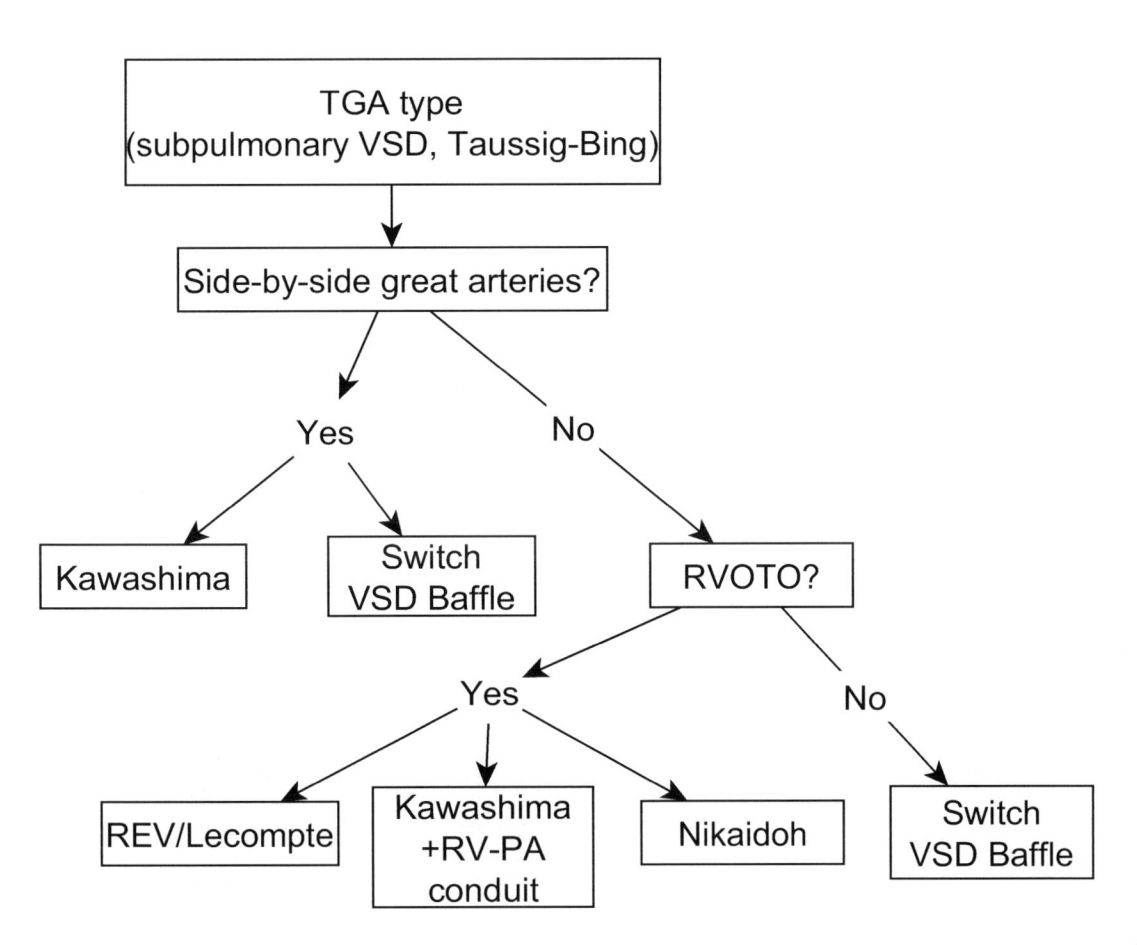

```
                    TGA type
            (subpulmonary VSD, Taussig-Bing)
                          |
                          v
              Side-by-side great arteries?
                   /              \
                Yes                No
                / \                 \
         Kawashima  Switch         RVOTO?
                    VSD Baffle     /     \
                                 Yes      No
                              /   |   \      \
                      REV/    Kawashima  Nikaidoh   Switch
                    Lecompte  +RV-PA                VSD Baffle
                              conduit
```

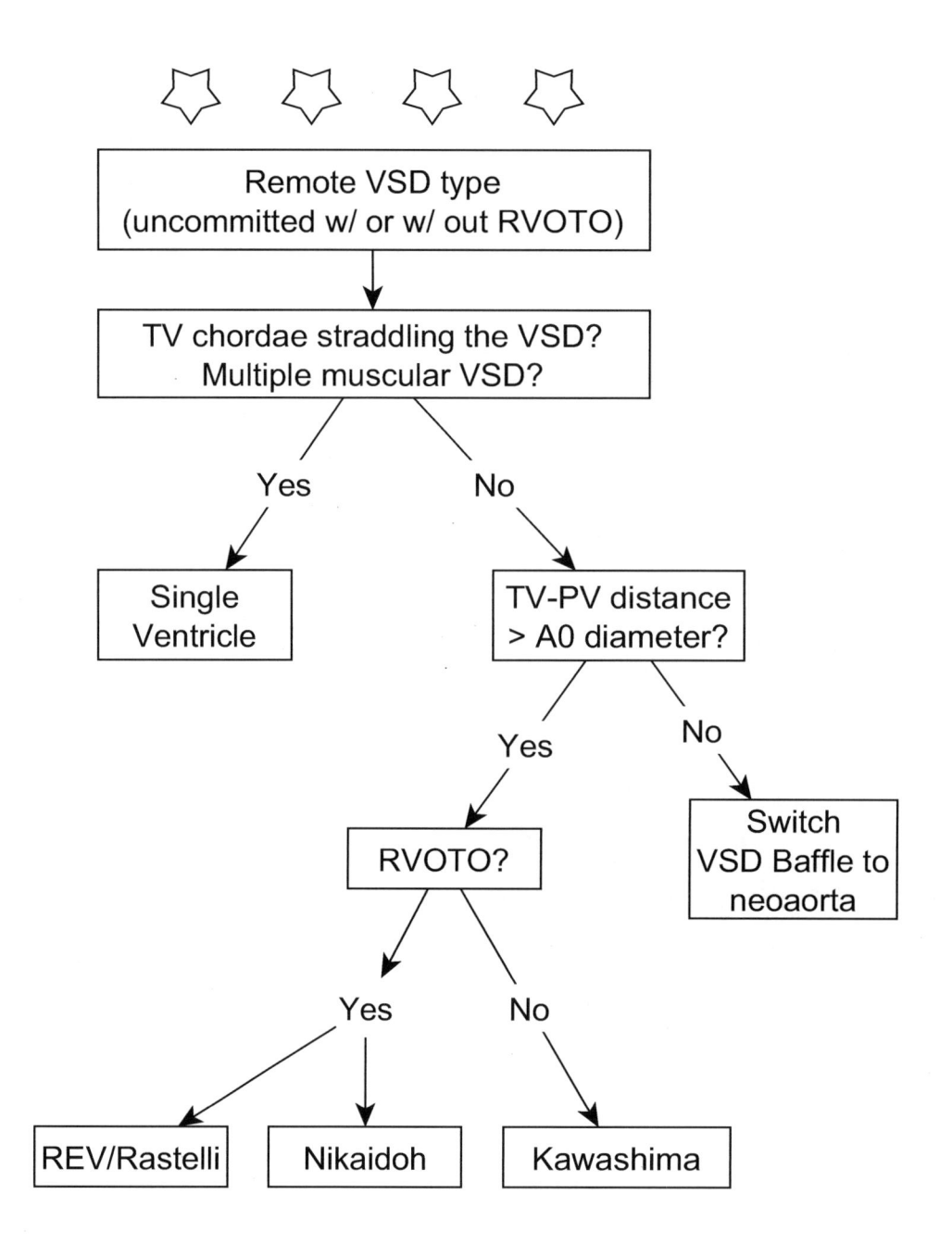

```
         ☆    ☆    ☆    ☆
    ┌─────────────────────────────┐
    │   Remote VSD type           │
    │ (uncommitted w/ or w/out RVOTO) │
    └─────────────────────────────┘
                 │
                 ▼
    ┌─────────────────────────────┐
    │ TV chordae straddling the VSD? │
    │     Multiple muscular VSD?   │
    └─────────────────────────────┘
         Yes            No
          │              │
          ▼              ▼
    ┌──────────┐   ┌──────────────┐
    │ Single   │   │ TV-PV distance│
    │Ventricle │   │  > A0 diameter?│
    └──────────┘   └──────────────┘
                    Yes        No
                     │          │
                     ▼          ▼
                 ┌───────┐  ┌──────────┐
                 │RVOTO? │  │ Switch   │
                 └───────┘  │VSD Baffle to│
                  Yes  No   │ neoaorta │
                   │   │    └──────────┘
          ┌────────┼───┴──────┐
          ▼        ▼          ▼
     ┌─────────┐┌────────┐┌──────────┐
     │REV/Rastelli││Nikaidoh││Kawashima │
     └─────────┘└────────┘└──────────┘
```

DORV, Double-outlet right ventricle; VSD, ventricular septal defect; RVOTO, right ventricular outflow tract obstruction; TOR, Tetralogy of Fallot; Ao, aorta; PV, pulmonary valve; TA, transannular; RV-PA, right ventricle-pulmonary artery; TGA, transposition of the great arteries; TV, tricuspid valve; REV, reparation a l'etage ventriculaire

Congenital Pulmonary Vein Anomalies
Bartholomew V. Simon, Michael F. Swartz, George M. Alfieris

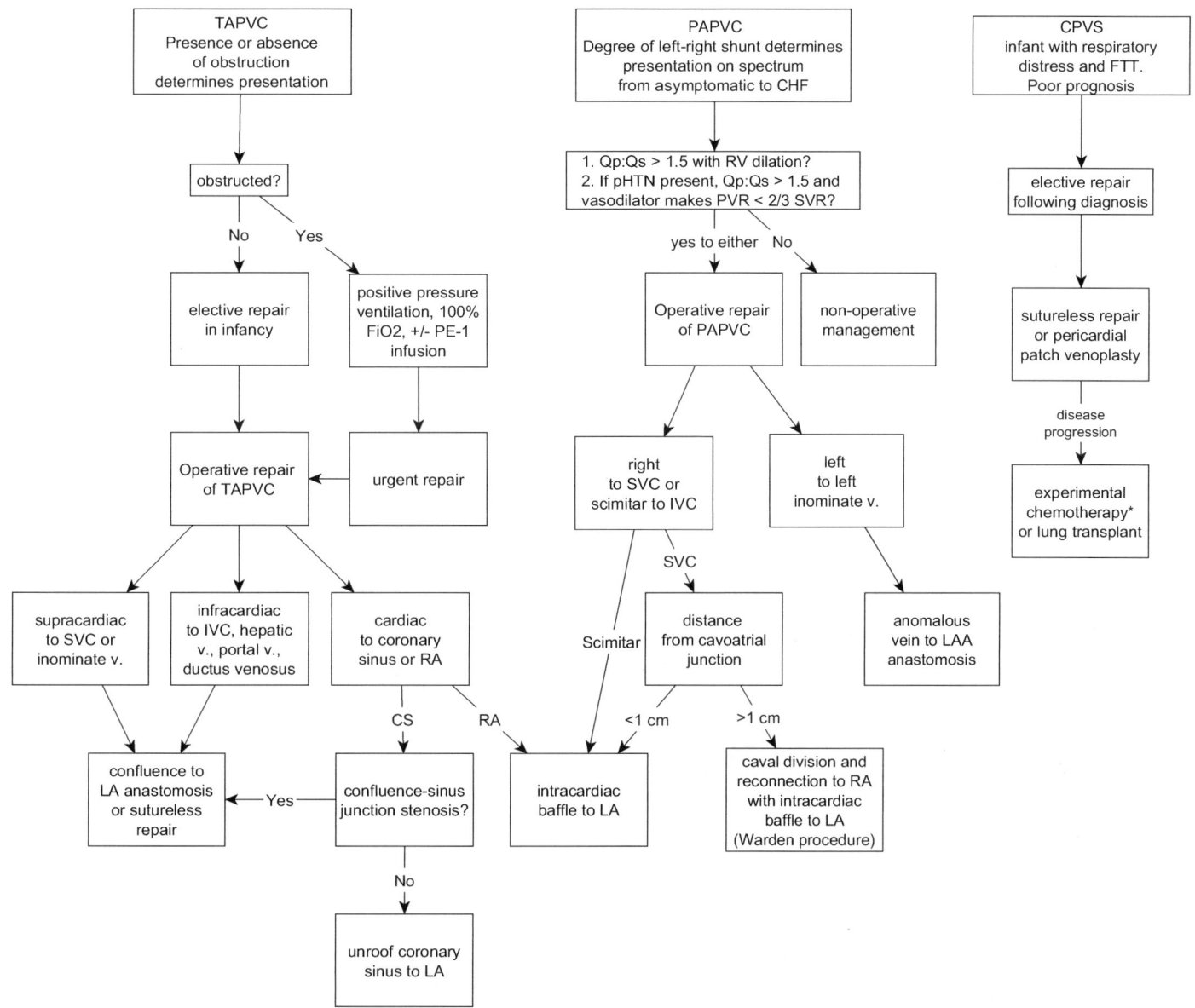

*Aimed at slowing myofibroblast proliferation and disease progression
CVPS, congenital pulmonary vein stenosis; TAPVC, total anomalous pulmonary venous connection; PAPVC, partial anomalous pulmonary venous connection; FTT, failure to thrive; RV, right ventricle; pHTN, pulmonary hypertension; PVR, pulmonary vascular resistance; SVR, systemic vascular resistance; SVC, superior vena cava; IVC, inferior vena cava; RA, right atrium; LAA, left atrial appendage

Congenital Mitral Stenosis
Kyle Riggs, David LS Morales

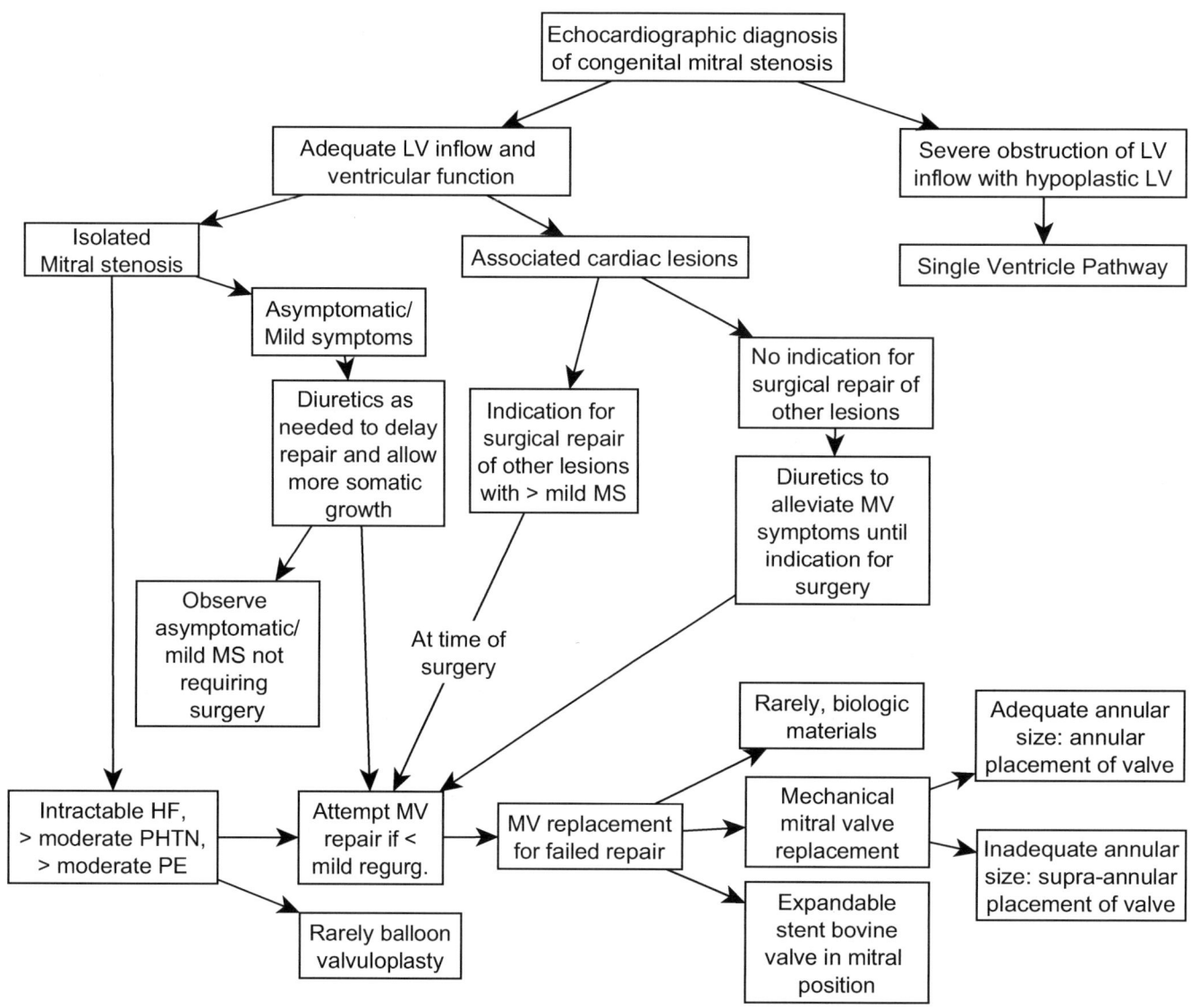

```
                    ┌─────────────────────────────┐
                    │ Echocardiographic diagnosis │
                    │ of congenital mitral stenosis│
                    └──────────────┬──────────────┘
                          ┌────────┴────────┐
          ┌───────────────▼──────┐   ┌──────▼──────────────────┐
          │ Adequate LV inflow and│   │ Severe obstruction of LV │
          │ ventricular function  │   │ inflow with hypoplastic LV│
          └──┬──────────────┬─────┘   └──────────┬──────────────┘
             │              │                    ▼
    ┌────────▼──┐   ┌───────▼──────────────┐  ┌──────────────────────┐
    │ Isolated  │   │ Associated cardiac   │  │ Single Ventricle     │
    │ Mitral    │   │ lesions              │  │ Pathway              │
    │ stenosis  │   └──┬────────────────┬──┘  └──────────────────────┘
    └────┬──────┘      │                │
         │       ┌─────▼──────┐   ┌─────▼──────────┐
         │       │Asymptomatic/│   │ No indication  │
         │       │Mild symptoms│   │ for surgical   │
         │       └─────┬──────┘   │ repair of      │
         │             │          │ other lesions  │
         │       ┌─────▼──────┐   └─────┬──────────┘
         │       │Diuretics as│   ┌─────▼──────────┐
         │       │needed to   │   │ Indication for │   │ Diuretics to   │
         │       │delay repair│   │ surgical repair│   │ alleviate MV   │
         │       │and allow   │   │ of other lesions│  │ symptoms until │
         │       │more somatic│   │ with > mild MS │   │ indication for │
         │       │growth      │   └─────┬──────────┘   │ surgery        │
         │       └─────┬──────┘         │              └────────────────┘
         │       ┌─────▼──────┐         │
         │       │ Observe    │         │
         │       │asymptomatic/│  At time of
         │       │mild MS not │   surgery
         │       │requiring   │         │
         │       │surgery     │         │
         │       └────────────┘         │
```

- Intractable HF, > moderate PHTN, > moderate PE → Attempt MV repair if < mild regurg. → MV replacement for failed repair
  - Rarely, biologic materials
  - Mechanical mitral valve replacement → Adequate annular size: annular placement of valve / Inadequate annular size: supra-annular placement of valve
  - Expandable stent bovine valve in mitral position
- Rarely balloon valvuloplasty

HF, heart failure; LV, left ventricle; MS, mitral stenosis; MV, mitral valve; PE, pulmonary edema; PHTN, pulmonary hypertension

References

CABG Guidelines

Hillis et al. JACC Vol. 58, No. 24, 2011
2011 ACCF/AHA CABG Guideline December 6, 2011:e123–210

Management of STEMI

Mehta SR, Bassand J-P, Chrolavicius S, et al. Dose comparisons of clopidogrel and aspirin in acute coronary syndromes. N Engl J Med. 2010; 363:930–42. Erratum in: N Engl J Med. 2010; 363:1585.

Levine, G. N., et al. (2016). "2016 ACC/AHA guideline focused update on duration of dual antiplatelet therapy in patients with coronary artery disease: A report of the American College of Cardiology/American Heart Association Task Force on Clinical Practice Guidelines." J Thorac Cardiovasc Surg 152(5): 1243-1275.

Indications for fibrinolytic therapy in suspected acute myocardial infarction: collaborative overview of early mortality and major morbidity results from all randomized trials of more than 1000 patients. Fibrinolytic Therapy Trialists' (FTT) Collaborative Group. Lancet. 1994; 343:311–22. Erratum in: Lancet. 1994; 343:742.

O'Gara, P. T., et al. (2013). "2013 ACCF/AHA guideline for the management of ST-elevation myocardial infarction: executive summary: a report of the American College of Cardiology Foundation/American Heart Association Task Force on Practice Guidelines." Circulation 127(4): 529-555.

Sjauw KD, Engström AE, Vis MM, et al. A systematic review and meta-analysis of intra-aortic balloon pump therapy in ST-elevation myocardial infarction: should we change the guidelines? Eur Heart J. 2009; 30:459–68.

Montalescot G, Barragan P, Wittenberg O, et al. Platelet glycoprotein IIb/IIIa inhibition with coronary stenting for acute myocardial infarction. N Engl J Med. 2001; 344:1895–903.

Nordmann AJ, Hengstler P, Harr T, et al. Clinical outcomes of primary stenting versus balloon angioplasty in patients with myocardial infarction: a meta-analysis of randomized controlled trials. Am J Med. 2004; 116:253–62.

Zhu MM, Feit A, Chadow H, et al. Primary stent implantation compared with primary balloon angioplasty for acute myocardial infarction: a meta-analysis of randomized clinical trials. Am J Cardiol. 2001; 88:297–301.

Hillis LD, Smith PK, Anderson JL, et al. 2011 ACCF/AHA guideline for coronary artery bypass graft surgery: a report of the American College of Cardiology Foundation/American Heart Association Task Force on Practice Guidelines. Circulation. 2011; 124:e652–735.

Hochman JS, Buller CE, Sleeper LA, et al. Cardiogenic shock complicating acute myocardial infarction: etiologies, management and outcome: a report from the SHOCK Trial Registry: Should we emergently revascularize Occluded Coronaries for cardiogenic shock? J Am CollCardiol. 2000; 36:1063–70.

Optimal Timing from Myocardial Infarction to Coronary Artery Bypass Grafting on Hospital Mortality Nichols, Elizabeth L. et al. The Annals of Thoracic Surgery, Volume 103, Issue 1 , 162 – 171

Aortic Stenosis

Nishimura RA, Otto CM, Bonow RO, Carabello BA, Erwin JP 3rd, Guyton RA, O'Gara PT, Ruiz CE,
Skubas NJ, Sorajja P, Sundt TM 3rd, Thomas JD; American College of Cardiology/American Heart
Association Task Force on Practice Guidelines. 2014 AHA/ACC guideline for the management of patients
with valvular heart disease: executive summary: a report of the American College of Cardiology/American Heart Association Task Force on Practice Guidelines. J Am Coll Cardiol. 2014 Jun
10;63(22):2438-88. doi: 10.1016/j.jacc.2014.02.537. Epub 2014 Mar 3.

Pump Thrombosis

Goldstein DJ, John R, Salerno C et al. Algorithm for the diagnosis and management of suspected pump thrombus. J Heart Lung Transplant 2013;32(7):667-670.

Endocarditis

2017 AHA/ACC Focused Update of the 2014 AHA/ACC Guidelines for the Management of Patients with Valvular Heart Disease

2014 ESC/ESA Guidelines on non-cardiac surgery: cardiovascular assessment and management: The Joint Task Force on non-cardiac surgery: cardiovascular assessment and management of the European Society of Cardiology (ESC) and the European Society of Anaesthesiology (ESA). European Heart Journal, Volume 35, Issue 35, 14 Sept 2014, Pages 2383–2431,

Indications for Surgical Intervention in the Treatment of Tricuspid Disease at the Time of Operation for Left-Sided Valvular Disease

Table: Stages of Tricuspid Regurgitation
Adapted from the 2014 AHA/ACC Guideline for the Management of Patients with Valvular Heart Disease: Executive Summary

Mitral Stenosis

Adapted from 2017 Update to the AHA/ACC Guideline for Management of Mitral Valve Disease

Pump Thrombosis

Goldstein DJ, John R, Salerno C et al. Algorithm for the diagnosis and management of suspected pump thrombus. J Heart Lung Transplant 2013;32(7):667-670.

Trachea Tumors

Berry MF, Friedberg JS. Overview. In: Sugarbaker DJ, Bueno R, Colson YL, Jaklitsch MT, Krasna MJ, Menter SJ, Williams M, Adams A. Eds. Adult Chest Surgery, Second Edition New York, NY: McGraw-Hill; 2014.

Freitag L, Darwiche K. Endoscopic Treatment of Tracheal Stenosis. Thorac Surg Clin. 2014; 24:27-40.

Grillo HC, Mathisen DJ. Primary Tracheal Tumors: Treatment and Results. Ann Thorac Surg 1990;49:69-77.

He J, Shen J, Huang J, et al. Prognosis of primary tracheal tumor: A population-based analysis. J Surg Oncol. 2017;9999:1-7.

Junker K. Pathology of Tracheal Tumors. Thorac Surg Clin 2014; 24:7-11.

Raz DJ, Weiser TS, Mathisen DJ. Tracheal Diseases. In: Yuh DD, Vricella LA, Yang SC, Doty JR. eds. Johns Hopkins Textbook of Cardiothoracic Surgery, Second Edition New York, NY: McGraw-Hill; 2014.

Wiedemann K, Mannle C. Anesthesia and Gas Exchange in Tracheal Surgery. Thorac Surg Clin. 2014; 24:13-25

Tracheal Stenosis

Karapantzos I, Karapantzou C, Zarogoulidis P, et al. Benign tracheal stenosis a case report and up to date management. Ann Transl Med. 2016; 4(22):451-456

Lorenz RR. Adult laryngotracheal stenosis: etiology and surgical management. Curr Opin Otolaryngol Head Neck Surg. 2003; 11:467-472

Puchalshki J, Musani A. Tracheal Stenosis: Causes and Advances in Management Clin Chest Med. 2013; 34:557-567.

Raz DJ, Weiser TS, Mathisen DJ. Tracheal Diseases. In: Yuh DD, Vricella LA, Yang SC, Doty JR. eds. Johns Hopkins Textbook of Cardiothoracic Surgery, Second Edition New York, NY: McGraw-Hill; 2014.

Rea F, Callegaro D, Loy M, et al. Benign tracheal and laryngotracheal stenosis: surgical treatment and results. Eur J Cardiothor Surg. (2002) 22:352-356.

Pulmonary Nodules

Naidich DP, Bankier AA, MacMahon H, et al. Recommendations for the management of subsolid pulmonary nodules detected at CT: a statement from the Fleischner Society. Radiology 2013;266 (1):304-317

Truong MT, Ko JP, Rossi SE, et al. Update in the evaluation of the solitary pulmonary nodule.

Radiographics 2014;34(6):1658-1679.

Herder GJ, Van Tinteren H, Golding RP, et al. Clinical predication model to characterize pulmonary nodules: validation and added value of 18F-fluorodeoxyglucose positron emission tomography. Chest 2005; 128(4):2490-2496

Jaklitsch MT, Jacobson FL, Austin JH, et al. The American Association for Thoracic Surgery guidelines for lung cancer screening using low-dose computed tomography scans for lung cancer survivors and other high-risk groups. J Thorac Cardiovasc Surg. 2012 144(1):33-38.

Callister ME, Baldwin DR, Akram AR, et al. British Thoracic Society guidelines for the investigation and management of pulmonary nodules. Thorax. 2015;70 Suppl 2 (Suppl 2): ii1-ii54.

Pleural Effusion

C Hooper, Y C G Lee, N Maskell, on behalf of the BTS Pleural Guideline Group. Investigation of a unilateral pleural effusion in adults: British Thoracic Society pleural disease guideline 2010. THORAX 2010; 65(Suppl 2): ii4-ii17. Doi:10.1136/thx.2010.136978

Shen et al. The American Association for Thoracic Surgery consensus guidelines for the management of empyema. J Thorac Cardiovasc Surg 2017; 153(6): e129 – e146

C Hooper, Y C G Lee, N Maskell, on behalf of the BTS Pleural Guideline Group. Management of a malignant pleural effusion: British Thoracic Society pleural disease guideline 2010. THORAX 2010; 65(Suppl 2): ii32-ii40.

Interstitial Lung Disease

Raghu G. Am J Respir Crit Care Med 1995; 151:909.

Sugarbaker, D. J., Bueno, R., Zellos, L., Krasna, M., & Mentzer, S. J. (2009). Adult chest surgery (1st ed., Vol. 1). New York: McGraw-Hill Medical.

Lung Volume Reduction Surgery

National Emphysema Treatment Trial Research Group. Rationale and designs of the National Emphysema Treatment Trial (NETT): a prospective, randomized trial of lung volume reduction surgery.

JThorac Cardiovasc Surg 1999; 118:518.

Shields, T. W. (2009). General Thoracic Surgery (7th ed., Vol. 2). Philadelphia, PA: Wolters Kluwer Health/Lippincott Williams & Wilkins.

Primary Esophageal Motility Disorders

Chicago Classification v3.0

Diaphragmatic Injury

Pachter HL, Frangos SG, and Simon R. Traumatic Injury to the Diaphragm. Fischer's Mastery of Surgery. 2012. 6th Edition. (1): 752-759.

Hanna WC, Ferri LE, Fata P, Razek T, Mulder DS. The Current Status of Traumatic Diaphragmatic Injury: Lessons Learned From 105 Patients Over 13 Years. Ann Thorac Surg. 2008;85(3):1044-1048.

Hanna WC, Ferri LE. Acute Traumatic Diaphragmatic Injury. Thorac Surg Clin. 2009;19(4):485-489.

Eren S, Esme H, Sehitogullari A, Durkan A. The risk factors and management of posttraumatic empyema in trauma patients. Injury. 2008;39(1):44-49.

Teicher, EJ., Madbak, FG., Dangleben, DA., Pasquale M. Human Acellular Dermal Matrix as a Prosthesis for Repair of a Traumatic Diaphragm Rupture. Am Surg. 2010;76(2):231-233.

Al-Nouri O, Hartman B, Freedman R, Thomas C, Esposito T. Diaphragmatic rupture: Is management with biological mesh feasible? Int J Surg Case Rep. 2012;3(8):349-353.

TSRA: A Resource for Thoracic Surgery Residents

Check out our latest resource

TSRA Online Question Bank

Tsranet.org

(Resources)

This website allows the user to test their knowledge base by answering multiple choice questions in the major disciplines associated with thoracic surgery: adult cardiac surgery, congenital cardiac surgery, general thoracic surgery, and trauma and critical care. Each of the four disciplines is based on subdivisions of important categories of each subject. The user selects the best answer and is notified if their choice was correct. The notification contains the correct answer and, usually, an explanation for the correct answer and the incorrect options.

There are a total of:

71 Trauma/Critical Care Questions

259 Thoracic Surgery Questions

177 Cardiac Surgery Questions

81 Congenital Heart Surgery Questions

Made in the USA
San Bernardino, CA
06 January 2020